Thoreau's Senior Living Options Planner

Decide How to Reside:
How to Evaluate Your Living Needs and Make the Best Living and Care Choices

By Philip Baker

Thoreau's Senior Living Options Planner

Title: Thoreau's Senior Living Options Planner
Subtitle: Decide How to Reside: How to Evaluate Your Living Needs and Make the Best Living and Care Choices
Author: Philip Baker
Published by Philip Baker

All rights reserved. No part of this book may be reproduced or transmitted in any form or by any means, electronic or mechanical, including photocopying, recording or by any information storage and retrieval system, without written permission from the author, except for the inclusion of brief quotations in a review.

ISBN: 9798509638640

Copyright © 2021 by Philip Baker
First Edition, 2021
Published in USA

Thoreau's Senior Living Options Planner

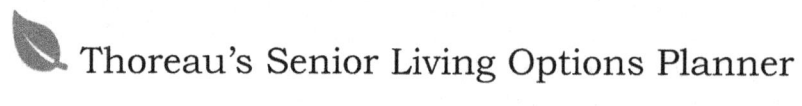

This Living Options Planner Belongs to:

"What lies behind us and what lies ahead of us are tiny matters compared to what lives within us."
– Henry David Thoreau

Thoreau's Senior Living Options Planner

Table of Contents

1. How to Use This Planner 10
    When to Start 12
    Where to Start 12
    Master TO DO List 14

2. How Can You Evaluate Your Living Needs? 16
    What are the Activities of Daily Living (ADLs)? 17
        Evaluating Activities of Daily Living (ADLs) Form 21
    What are the Instrumental Activities of Daily Living (IADLs)? . 22
        Instrumental Activities of Daily Living (IADLs) Form 26
        Living Wants and Needs Worksheet 28
    Special Section for Caregivers: 39
        What are The Ten Indicators That a Person Might Need Support or Supervision? 39
        Living Needs Evaluation Checklist for Caregivers 41

3. Is Staying in Your Home the Best Choice? 45
    How Can You Determine If Staying in Your Home is the Best Choice for You? 46
    Staying in Your Home: Personal Needs Checklist 48
    Staying in Your Home: Pets Checklist 50
    Staying in Your Home: Safety Checklist 51
    Staying in Your Home: Transportation Checklist 53
    Staying in Your Home: Social Interaction and Communication Checklist 54
    Staying in Your Home: Home Maintenance Needs 55
    Staying in Your Home: Disability or Mobility Needs 56
    Home Ownership Worksheet 60

Current Home Ownership Expenses Form 64

Other Home Ownership Options 66

4. Is Renting an Option for You? 70

What to Consider 71

Questions to Ask Landlords or Property Managers Form ... 73

Renting Financial Resources Worksheet 79

Selling Your Home and Renting or Moving to Care Facility: Cash Gain Worksheet 80

Current Monthly Expenses Worksheet A 81

Moving to a Rental Home, Apartment or in with Family: Estimate New Living Option Expenses Worksheet B 82

5. Are In-Home Care Options Right for You? 85

Why In-Home Care? 85

What is Home Care? 86

What to Consider 86

What is Home Health Care? 88

What to Consider 88

Choosing an Aid 90

Hiring Through an Agency Vs. Independent Caregiver 91

What to Ask 92

After the Hire 93

In-Home Care Costs Worksheet 95

Caregiver's List of Duties 96

Caregiver Interview Worksheet 102

6. What Should You Consider About Independent Living Communities? 108

Retirement Community 108

Naturally Occurring Retirement Communities (NORCs) or Villages 110

What to Ask Independent Living Communities Worksheet 112

Independent Living Community Cost Comparison Worksheet 119

7. What are Your Options for Group Living and Care Facilities? 121

What to Consider About a Facility 123

Assisted Living or Board and Care Homes 124

The Two Assisted Living Categories 124

Board and Care Homes 129

Adult Foster Care Homes 129

Residential Care Facility (RCF) 129

Assisted Living Facility (ALF) 129

Intermediate Care Facility (ICF) 130

Skilled Nursing Facility (SNF) 130

The Eden (or Greenhouse) Alternative 131

Continuing Care Retirement Communities (CCRCs) 131

Long-Term Care 131

Veteran's Communities 134

Visiting Facilities 134

What to Ask Assisted Living or Board and Care Homes 136

Assisted Living Cost Comparison Worksheet 141

Group Living Worksheet 142

Group Living Checklist 148

Disability or Mobility Needs Checklist 152

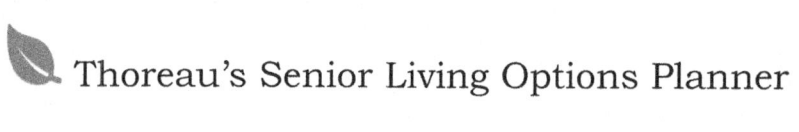

Community Requirements Checklist 155

Personal Needs Checklist 157

8. Living Options and Insurance **164**

Medicare 164

Medicaid 166

Other Insurance 168

For Family Caregivers: Family Medical Leave Act and
Family-Friendly Leave 169

9. What Do You Need to Know About Senior Mobile Home Parks and Communities? **171**

Senior Mobile Home Parks 171

Locations 171

What to Look For 172

What are All the Costs? 174

10. Is Moving in with Family the Right Option for You? **180**

Practical and Lifestyle Aspects of Moving in with Family 181

Practical and Lifestyle Aspects: What to Ask Yourself Before Moving in with Your Family Form 183

Practical and Lifestyle Questionnaire for Host Family Members Form 187

Living Space 191

Moving 191

Privacy 192

Home Prepping 192

Living with Family: Space Questionnaire 196

Safety, Disability and/or Mobility Considerations Questionnaire 198

Financial Considerations 201
    Financial Considerations for Your Family 201
    Home Preparation Costs Planning Form 203
    Living Expenses 206
    Living with Family Monthly Expenses Worksheet (for Families) 207
    Your Monthly Expenses When Living with Family 210

Relationships 213
    Living with Family Relationship Worksheet for You 215
    Living with Family Relationship Worksheet for Your Family 219
    Household Rules for Living with Family Form 224

Conclusion 232

Thoreau's Senior Living Options Planner

1. How to Use This Planner

"So thoroughly and sincerely are we compelled to live, reverencing our life, and denying the possibility of change. All change is a miracle to contemplate; a miracle which is taking place every instant."
— Henry David Thoreau

Was your idea of retirement anything like mine? My vision was spending afternoons in a rocking chair on the front porch overlooking my garden. I would sip my coffee while browsing through a travel guide contemplating my next trip to some tropical paradise. Color me Pollyanna!

While for many people retirement and senior years represent a dream of an easy paced lifestyle with steady consistency, the fact is that our 'golden years' are often fraught with frequent changes, sometimes unexpected. In addition to the slowing of lifestyle pace due to natural aging, we can experience instant upheavals that can be the most profound we experience in life. Changes can happen quickly and also occur for our friends, associates and loved ones.

Often the causes for life changes are health related when conditions arise; ailments and diseases progress, a loss of eyesight, hearing, or mobility occur, or due to injuries such as from a fall. There are other events that can cause the need to consider new living options such as a sudden loss of a loved one, support person, or caregiver, or a change in financial status, or any recent transformation in lifestyle needs.

Health conditions can result in an inability to maintain a lifestyle, loss of mobility, revocation of driving privileges, or the requirement of specific types of care. While many changes are sudden, some things happen over time such as deterioration from a progressive disease or disorder.

Thoreau's Senior Living Options Planner

Your living option choices might need to be made several times during your senior years as needs change. For example, a senior might move in with family or adult children after the loss of a spouse, mobility issues, or for certain care requirements. As health conditions progress this same person might need to move to a care facility to receive the support needed.

"Thoreau's Senior Living Options Planner" is designed to help seniors, empty nesters, adult children or relatives of seniors, and caregivers make the best living choices through valuable information, organization methods, and planning.

If you are a caregiver or adult child helping your parent or parents, this planner will also help you become informed, be supportive, assist with choices, and have an efficient plan.

There are lists, worksheets, and checklists designed for each step in this transition. *Since every situation is different, select the chapters, areas and forms that apply to you.*

While living and staying in your home is covered in this planner, many living options require moving. Moving is considered a high-stress life event. This relocation can be mixed with uncertainty, loneliness, possible illness, and a loss of independence. Due to the many additional decisions to be made, researching living options and moving can be complex. Whether you or loved ones are moving across town or across the country you will be:

- Tackling major living decisions.
- Comparing costs of living options and evaluating finances.
- Assessing living option arrangements and services.
- Possibly hiring caregivers and other help.
- Dealing with belongings; sorting through decades of family history, organizing, selling, giving way and discarding, and packing and unpacking.
- Organizing and cleaning.

- Reviewing leases, property contracts and other legal paperwork.
- Shutting off and turning on utilities.
- Stopping services and starting services.
- Changing addresses and notifying everyone.
- Gathering, organizing, and keeping important documents and records.

And with a myriad of other tasks all on a schedule, this is a formidable challenge for anyone and even paralyzing for many people.

When to Start

Every senior and family of a parent or elderly relative would benefit from learning about living options before a crisis makes choosing a new one an emergency. Yet we are not always afforded the luxury of time. This planner will provide you with what you need to know to make the best decisions and make your experience more organized, giving you a better outcome.

Where to Start

Please review the Table of Contents as this book covers a myriad of topics and options. Then begin with reviewing the following MASTER TO DO LIST. This list is designed to guide you through the major steps in the process. The steps are ordered; however, the dates in which you complete each item will depend on your situation.

While the process of aging and diminished capabilities might be natural, accepting new limitations can be a challenge. People that have been independent, proud, raised children, cared for loved ones, and self-sufficient can suddenly and sometimes for the first time in their adult lives need assistance from others.

Thoreau's Senior Living Options Planner

Denial of needing help can only temporarily insulate us from the inevitable. Only by facing your limitations and with candid answers can you accurately evaluate your needs and live safely and comfortably in the best situation for you.

Keep this planner with you, and whenever you think of something related to your options or move, write it down on the relevant form or worksheet.

The information and worksheets are integrated with quotes of wisdom from Henry David Thoreau.

Note:

Web pages, contact information and reference
phone numbers commonly change. If you find that a
phone number referred to herein is disconnected,
or a web address is no longer valid, please let me know.
My contact information is at the end of this book.

Thank you!

Hopefully, through this book, I can be of humble service to you.

Thoreau's Senior Living Options Planner

Master TO DO List

Date to Do	Completed	WHAT TO DO
		Let family, friends, caregivers, physicians, and advisers know you are considering a change.
		At the beginning of each chapter there is a list of the forms, worksheets, and questionnaires contained in that chapter.
		Evaluate your living needs and complete the forms in that chapter.
		Select from the remaining chapters that apply to your situation and read and complete the forms. As you complete the forms, check them off on the lists at the beginning of each chapter.
		If considering moving in with family, complete the forms in that chapter and have your family complete the applicable questionnaires also.
		Enlist the help of a friend, associate, or family member to accompany you on facility visits.
		Visit the home, facilities, etc. where you are considering moving. Gather information.
		Apply for any Financial Assistance Programs.
		Meet with any family, friends, caregivers, physicians, and advisers to present the information you have gathered and garner feedback.

Thoreau's Senior Living Options Planner

Date to Do	Completed	**WHAT TO DO: DECIDING WHERE TO MOVE**
		Decide if and where you will be moving.
		Set a tentative date on when you plan to move by. (Consider the time that will be needed to sell your home as well as time to sort and downsize possessions.)
		Coordinate your move with family members, caregivers, and facilitators.

2. How Can You Evaluate Your Living Needs?

"You must live in the present, launch yourself on every wave, find your eternity in each moment." – Henry David Thoreau

Evaluating Living Needs Forms

Completed ✓	This chapter contains the following checklists, forms, questionnaires, and/or worksheets:
	Evaluating Activities of Daily Living (ADLs) Form
	Instrumental Activities of Daily Living (IADLs) Form
	Living Wants and Needs Worksheet
	Living Needs Evaluation Checklist for Caregivers

This chapter describes the daily living needs and activities with which you might need or want assistance. You will also find questionnaires to help you and caregivers evaluate your situation. There is a separate checklist designed for caregivers. The 'Living Wants and Needs Worksheet' covers your needs and lifestyle desires.

The many options available for you depend on what support or care services might be needed now or are anticipated in the future, the cost, and your desires. There is staying in your home or apartment with ownership versus renting choices. Or you might consider moving in with family members or a roommate situation. There are numerous residential support and care communities for seniors.

Some are owned and managed by faith-based organizations with which you might be affiliated.

IMPORTANT: Review your answers to the forms in this chapter with your physician, caregivers, and family members; your answers will help them, and you, better evaluate any of the living options available to you throughout this book.

What are the Activities of Daily Living (ADLs)?

The Activities of Daily Living are the basic day-to-day actions necessary for independent living at home or in a community. They include bathing or showering, dressing, getting in and out of bed or a chair, walking, using the toilet, and eating.

If you have difficulty performing an activity by yourself without special equipment or cannot perform the activity at all due to health issues, you are deemed to have a limitation in that activity. Your limitations could be temporary or chronic. Strokes and falls make difficulty performing these basic tasks more likely.

Think of ADLs as the tasks you perform without having to think about them. One way to measure your independence in the Activities of Daily Living is to think of your regular morning routine. What actions that you would normally perform in the morning have become arduous or time-consuming?

Progressive Problems

Bathing independently is often the first challenge that seniors encounter. First, you use the assistance of a non-skid mat, handrails, and a shower chair. As strength and balance decline, human help is needed to step into and out of the bathtub.

The bathroom is the most dangerous room in the house for people of all ages. The wet floors and tight walls become even more difficult to navigate as you age.

Thoreau's Senior Living Options Planner

Has stepping in and out of the bathtub become too difficult? Even if you can get in and out by yourself right now, are you doing it safely? What would it mean for your health and your wallet if you took a fall? You would quickly find yourself in a position where you needed a lot more help and would maybe be in a worse position to afford the care you would need.

After you lose self-sufficiency in personal grooming, dressing yourself becomes more difficult, followed by toileting, moving and transferring, and eating.

There is a lot of specialty equipment available to you to help you stay independent in some or all the ADLs for as long as possible. A dressing stick and shoehorn can be purchased to allow you to dress yourself. You can have a raised toilet seat with arms installed to maintain self-sufficiency in using the bathroom while reducing the likelihood of injury. Adaptive feeding equipment can be used to decrease challenges at mealtime.

Not all seniors who move require help with ADLs. Receiving care *before* a problem arises is often a smart move. The need for assistance is cumulative.

Occupational Therapy

If you have had a recent medical event that has contributed to your ability to perform ADLs, consider teaming up with a health professional to regain or maintain your independence in addition to getting the help you need while retraining your brain and body. Chronic conditions can also be improved with hard work.

Working with an occupational therapist can help you to overcome hurdles to physical and mental barriers. In order to reap the benefits of OT, you must be honest with yourself, your practitioner, and your caretaker about your ability levels.

Plan of Care

Assessing your capabilities in carrying out ADLs and IADLs will help determine your Plan of Care. You may want help with dressing but not with toileting. You can discuss this with those you entrust your care to.

This information can be used to discover if you qualify for financial assistance from Medicaid or other state programs. Knowledge of where you are struggling can help your doctors diagnose problems and allow your caregivers to come up with a plan of management.

Social Security Disability Insurance and long-term care insurance also use an inability to complete ADLs as a trigger for qualification and payouts.

If you require help with more than three of your ADLs, you will be categorized as needing the highest level of care. This means you will be eligible for financial assistance for a nursing home or in-home care.

Whether you require help with ADLs is not just dependent on your ability to perform the task. The ability to recognize the need to perform a task is also essential to independent living. If you require prompting to eat, this needs to be recorded to accurately assess your need for care.

You will benefit from opening the discussion about your need for assistance with your adult children and other caregivers. When you initiate a discussion with family members in making your care plan, you avoid being left out. Ignoring the need for an honest talk about the issue at hand may leave you in a combative process with those who oversee your care.

Use the ADL assessment included in this chapter to get an overview of your needs. Once you have an overview of your needs, make an appointment to see a family doctor or occupational therapist. You can also inquire at your Local Area Agency on Aging (AAA). They will

Thoreau's Senior Living Options Planner

be able to give you information on the benefits you may qualify for and give you a referral.

There are five basic categories listed in the following form with questions to gauge living needs. Whether or not you can perform these activities by yourself or with assistance helps measure your level of independence. If you are considering living independently your answers will help you gauge your ability to do so. If you visit or apply to any assisted living facilities or communities, you might be asked many of these same questions.

While answering assessment questions, please answer "yes" if only *some* assistance is needed.

Thoreau's Senior Living Options Planner

Evaluating Activities of Daily Living (ADLs) Form

Yes or No	Questions
	Personal Hygiene: Do you need assistance bathing or showering?
	Do you need help with grooming such as brushing hair, shaving, trimming finger and toenails, etc.?
	Do you need help with oral care?
	Dressing: Can you choose the appropriate clothing for the weather and events?
	Can you physically dress and undress yourself?
	Can you replace clothing folded in storage and on hangers?
	Can you get accessories (watches, earrings, jewelry, ties) on and off?
	Mobility: Can you move yourself from a seated to standing position?
	Can you get in and out of bed without assistance?
	Can you walk (or move in a wheelchair) from one location to another within your home without assistance?
	Can you go outside your home and back in without help?
	Can you safely get up and down off the floor?
	Can you safely navigate all stairs and steps in your home?

Evaluating Activities of Daily Living (ADLs) Form (continued)	
Yes or No	Questions
	Eating: Can you feed yourself regularly?
	Can you handle drinks without spilling?
	Do you choose healthy foods and portions?
	Maintaining Continence: Do you always know when you need to use the restroom?
	Can you use the bathroom without assistance?
	Can you adequately clean yourself after using the restroom?

What are the Instrumental Activities of Daily Living (IADLs)?

Instrumental Activities of Daily Living (IADLs) are actions that are important to living independently, but not always required activities on a daily basis.

While loss of function with the IADLs is usually less noticeable than with the ADLs, they are usually the first activities to experience attrition. Trouble performing ADLs are usually connected to a decline in motor function, while IADLs are associated with cognitive impairments.

The IADLs include seven basic categories including basic communication skills, transportation, meal preparation, shopping, housework, medication management, and personal financial management.

Thoreau's Senior Living Options Planner

Transportation

Depending on what state you live in, you may find yourself worried about an upcoming visit to your local DMV and your ability to pass the eye examination. Perhaps you think the woman behind the counter will ask for a doctor's certificate that states you are physically and mentally capable of driving.

This is the situation a lot of seniors find themselves in. If you are concerned that you are going to be *found out* when you drive, then you should not be driving. You are putting your life and others on the line.

If you are considering living independently, you will be able to find help with transportation in your area through local and state programs or through a faith-based organization. Some in-home health care services also provide transportation for daily tasks.

Housekeeping

As driving proves to be more difficult, so does staying home. You might find that the cleanliness of your house is not quite up to your old standards. You used to be able to keep things neat and tidy with ease. Now, nooks-and-crannies of the homestead that used to be dusted go untouched. Changing sheets is difficult on your back. Doing the laundry proves more unforgiving as you bend down to load the washer. Clutter seems to be growing on its own.

If you live in a two or three-story house, things can be even more challenging. You might choose to downsize to a smaller home to make upkeep more manageable. Would you be able to maintain a smaller house?

Housekeeping services can be acquired separately from other in-house help, but the help may not fold the way you like. Take time to consider what you can reasonably do and what you can reasonably expect of others if you decide to look for a maid.

Meal Preparation

Many seniors find cooking for one or two demanding and discouraging. As your calorie needs have gone down, your meals are even smaller than before. You struggle to use up vegetables before they go bad.

Meal delivery services are popular. Companies provide pre-measured meals to your door which reduces waste. Some people choose to forgo them and buy freezer dinners, sacrificing their health when they need to be more careful than ever. How are you managing your diet?

Medication Management

Medication management is fraught with danger. You can take too many pills or too few. Without careful attention, you are liable to take expired medication.

Even your food or vitamins can cause adverse side effects when you are on certain medications. Pill organizers help simplify your daily regiment but there is a lot of information to remember about cross-reactions. Safety is extremely important. Are you confident you are not sacrificing?

Communication

Communication is an essential part of daily living. As vision and hearing decline, understanding others becomes more difficult. Cognitive impairments mean that conveying your meaning also becomes a struggle.

Even if you are hearing well and your speech is intelligible, communication must be practiced like every other skill. As family moves and friends pass away, you become a bit out of practice. Care in a facility and in-home care will both provide you with the connection you need to stay sharp.

Financial Management

You may have heard about scam artists targeting seniors on the news. While scary, this is not the only problem that seniors run into regarding their finances.

Debt, a lack of financial planning, and increasing health care costs can all be burdens. Recognizing fraudulent phone calls, staying within your allotted budget, and keeping accurate records are all skills that you need to keep yourself solvent. How do you feel you are managing your finances? Are you certain of where all your money is going?

Shopping

Shopping is intricately connected to financial management. Being on a fixed income is challenging as the price of basic goods like eggs and apples is always rising. You may have been able to splurge on an exotic fruit or decadent dessert before but that may be irresponsible now.

In addition to the financial considerations of shopping there is the physical aspect. Most anything can be delivered to your door these days. Depending on your location, grocery and necessity needs can be delivered to you or ordered and picked up from your local market.

Evaluation

As with your IADLs, be honest with yourself about the level at which you perform these tasks and if you need some help, answer "yes." IADLs can help determine with greater detail the level of assistance you might require. You should get yourself evaluated whenever you notice a deterioration or change in your abilities.

Thoreau's Senior Living Options Planner

Instrumental Activities of Daily Living (IADLs) Form

Yes or No	Questions
	Communication Skills: Can you use your phone or cell phone to answer and make calls?
	Can you navigate the internet?
	Can you use email?
	Can you use social media?
	Meals: Can you plan appropriate meals regularly?
	Can you safely use kitchen appliances and utensils?
	Can you cook and prepare your meals?
	Can you clean up after eating?
	Housework: Can you maintain a safe and clean home?
	Can you sweep, mop, and vacuum?
	Can you do laundry?
	Can you wash dishes?
	Do you recognize unsafe conditions or situations in your home and take proper action?

Thoreau's Senior Living Options Planner

Instrumental Activities of Daily Living (IADLs) Form (continued)	
Yes or No	Questions
	Managing Finances: Can you pay bills on time and keep accurate records?
	Can you manage necessary banking activities?
	Do you stay within your budget?
	Do you make bad financial decisions or borrow or lend money when you should not?
	Can you recognize and avoid over the phone, mail, email, and other scams?
	Managing Medications: Can you remember to take medications as prescribed?
	Can you always take the prescribed doses?
	Can you keep medications safely stored?
	Can you remember to have prescriptions refilled as needed?
	Transportation: Can you legally drive and maintain your car safely?
	Can you use public transportation safely alone?
	Can you arrange rides when needed?
	Shopping: Can you make appropriate buying decisions?
	Do you need to be accompanied when shopping?

Thoreau's Senior Living Options Planner

Living Wants and Needs Worksheet

What kind of lifestyle do you want? Do you want regular social interaction and events?

_____
_____
_____
_____

What living conditions will you be happy with?

_____
_____
_____
_____
_____
_____
_____

Thoreau's Senior Living Options Planner

Who else is involved in this decision? (Family members, Friends, Advisors) List each person and what role they will have in making these decisions:

Thoreau's Senior Living Options Planner

What factors are involved in location? How close would you like or need to be to family and friends, doctors, pharmacies, other medical facilities, shopping, senior centers, religious facilities, and other amenities?

Thoreau's Senior Living Options Planner

Does your current health status require certain features for mobility and if so, what are they?

_____

_____

_____

_____

_____

How much can you afford monthly for housing?

_____

_____

_____

Do you expect your expenses or income to change and by how much?

_____

_____

_____

Thoreau's Senior Living Options Planner

What health and medical services are required now?

___ Medication Management

___ Blood Pressure Monitoring

___ Blood Sugar Levels Monitoring

___ Diabetes Type I

___ Diabetes Type II

Other health and medical services needed:

_____

_____

_____

_____

_____

_____

_____

_____

Thoreau's Senior Living Options Planner

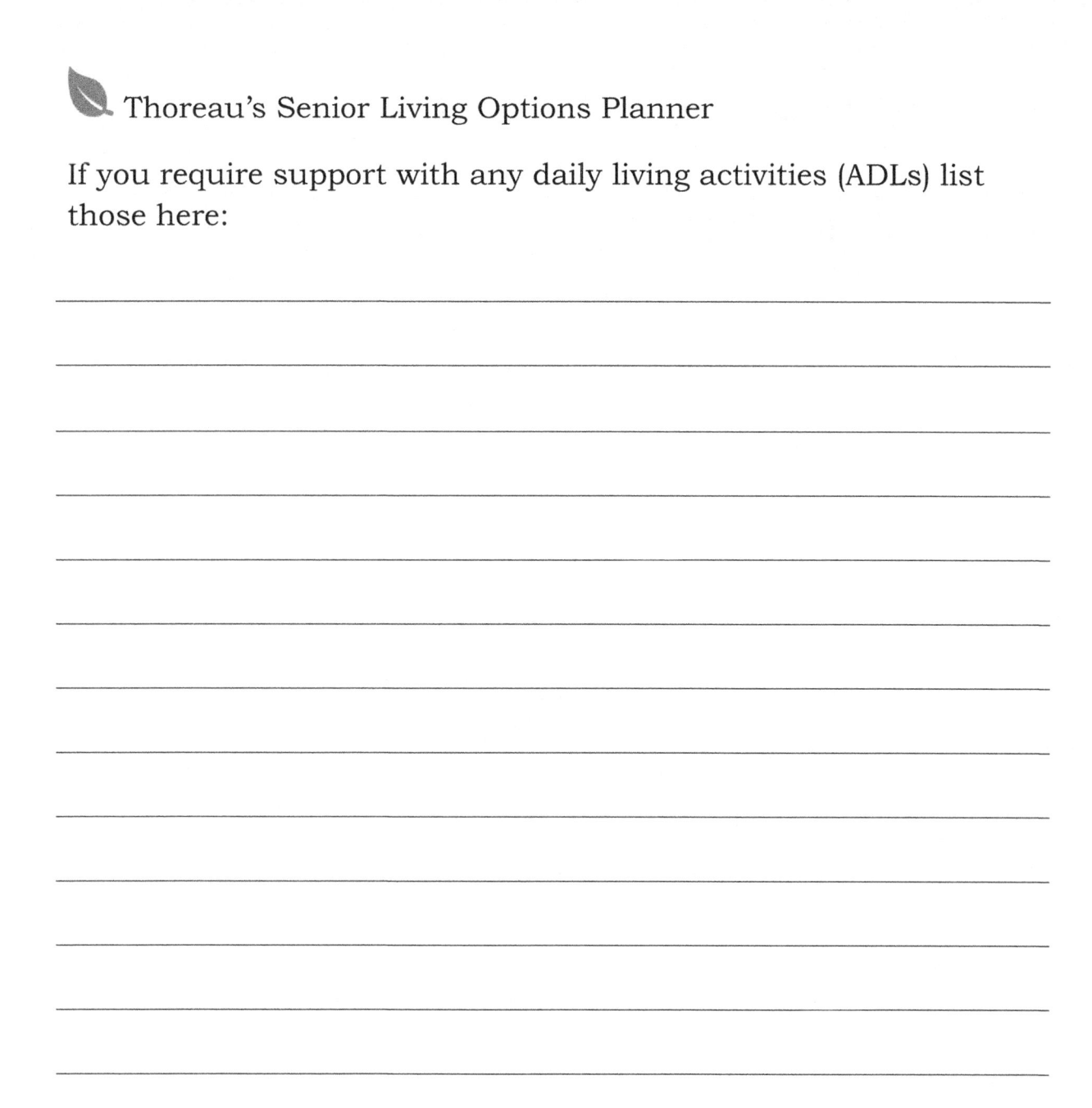

If you require support with any daily living activities (ADLs) list those here:

Thoreau's Senior Living Options Planner

List any additional health and medical services expected to be needed within the next 12 months:

Thoreau's Senior Living Options Planner

What other special support services are needed?

Thoreau's Senior Living Options Planner

Do you have an attorney that will explain your rights, any legal concerns, and review any leases, contracts or agreements?

_____
_____
_____
_____
_____
_____

List any publicly funded or subsidized services, such as Medicare or Medicaid you are eligible for:

_____
_____
_____
_____
_____
_____

Thoreau's Senior Living Options Planner

Notes About Living Wants and Needs

Notes About Living Wants and Needs

Thoreau's Senior Living Options Planner

Special Section for Caregivers:

What are The Ten Indicators That a Person Might Need Support or Supervision?

For caregivers and/or relatives: Before considering independent living as an option, there are a number of signs that can indicate the subject person needs a more supportive living situation.

When the time comes, moving your parent or relative into your home or a support facility are options, but how do you know when the time has come? If you are a family member or caregiver trying to decide if your client, loved one, or parent needs to move to a home with care and/or support, here are eight indicators:

1. Health
2. Mental Capacity
3. Safety and Mobility
4. Meals
5. Hygiene
6. Housekeeping
7. Finances
8. Social Life
9. Pets
10. Independence

Many senior citizens are in denial about their need for assistance. The loss of independence can feel like a loss of dignity. Unable to face their situation, they find themselves fighting against their loved ones.

Try to discuss your intentions in a cooperative manner with your parent, client, or loved one. Keep in perspective what becoming dependent means after years of independence.

Thoreau's Senior Living Options Planner

The following Living Evaluation Checklist for Family and Caregivers can help you with your decision. While a 'no' answer to any of the questions can raise a red flag, check with the person's physician, caregivers, relatives, and friends for additional input when needed.

Thoreau's Senior Living Options Planner

Living Needs Evaluation Checklist for Caregivers

Yes or No	Questions
	Health: Has a physician or other health care worker or caregiver recommend this person have live-in help or need extra care?
	Is he or she on medications and if so, able to take them as directed?
	Mental Capacity: Does this person forget things that could put his or her safety or home in jeopardy? (Such as leaving a stove burner on, forgetting to close or lock doors and windows, leaving objects in walking areas or on stairways, etc.)
	Are there any other mental health issues?
	Safety and Mobility: Does the subject person have trouble getting around the house?
	Has he or she fallen or been injured?
	Are there any vision or hearing problems severe enough to be a concern?
	Finances: Are bills being paid in a timely manner?
	Is spending responsible and recorded accurately?
	Is this person vulnerable to being scammed?

Thoreau's Senior Living Options Planner

Living Needs Evaluation Checklist for Caregivers (continued)	
Yes or No	**Questions**
	Meals: Is he or she currently eating a healthy diet?
	Is this person able to obtain food and prepare meals or capable of having them delivered?
	Housekeeping: Is the person able to maintain their home or do they have someone who does?
	Social Life: Has he or she kept their social life and events or are they becoming withdrawn?
	Are they unable to attend gatherings and events outside their home?
	Would they benefit from the social aspect of a group living environment?
	Hygiene: Is the person able to maintain his or her own hygiene?
	Pets: Are pets being properly taken care of? A lack of care for a pet is often a sign that a person is struggling to take care of him or herself.
	Independence: Is this person able to go out of the house alone and get back without becoming disoriented?

Thoreau's Senior Living Options Planner

Notes About Living Evaluation Needs

Thoreau's Senior Living Options Planner

Notes About Living Evaluation Needs

Thoreau's Senior Living Options Planner

3. Is Staying in Your Home the Best Choice?

"Only that traveling is good which reveals to me the value of home and enables me to enjoy it better." – Henry David Thoreau

Staying in Your Home Forms

Completed ✓	This chapter contains the following checklists, forms, questionnaires, and/or worksheets:
	Staying in Your Home: Personal Needs Checklist
	Staying in Your Home: Pets Checklist
	Staying in Your Home: Safety Checklist
	Staying in Your Home: Transportation Checklist
	Staying in Your Home: Social Interaction and Communication Checklist
	Staying in Your Home: Home Maintenance Needs
	Staying in Your Home: Disability or Mobility Needs
	Home Ownership Worksheet
	Current Home Ownership Expenses Form

Thoreau's Senior Living Options Planner

How Can You Determine If Staying in Your Home is the Best Choice for You?

This chapter will help you determine if staying in your home is the best living option for you now considering your health, safety, social interaction, abilities, near future expectations and finances.

Review this chapter and the checklists and worksheets with a relative, physician, caregiver, or other friend or associate that can provide an impartial and informed point of view.

Most seniors would rather live in their own homes if feasible. There are communities that offer services such as transportation, meal delivery, and more for seniors. Sometimes due to physical or mental capabilities 'in-home care' is needed. In-home caregivers and other services are available for fees from support businesses and by hiring individual caregivers.

When a person is not capable of taking care of a home, there are a host of options that can help him or her stay in the home, or moving from a single-family home to a small apartment or condo might be choices to consider. Sharing an apartment or house with a roommate, friend or relative can be a possibility. In some areas there are agencies that will help seniors find these arrangements.

Couples often want to stay together; however, their health requirements commonly differ. At some point one spouse might require different living arrangements than the other and separation becomes unavoidable.

Thoreau's Senior Living Options Planner

Some of the considerations in determining whether staying in your home is an option include:

- Assistance or care needed
- Degree of mobility
- Affordability
- Safety
- Access to social contact
- Home upkeep and maintenance required
- Transportation available
- Other occupants in home
- Local services available
- Location

IMPORTANT: Review your answers with your physician, caregivers, and family members to these two forms from the previous chapter:

Evaluating Activities of Daily Living (ADLs) Form
Instrumental Activities of Daily Living (IADLs) Form

Your answers will help you and your physician, caregivers, and family members gauge whether staying in your home is the best decision at this time and if so, what you might need to live safely and comfortably.

The following forms will further help you evaluate whether staying in your home is best for you, your health, your family, and your finances.

Thoreau's Senior Living Options Planner

Staying in Your Home: Personal Needs Checklist

Yes/No	What to Consider About Your (or the Subject Person's) Personal Needs (For Staying in Your Home)
	Do you live alone?
	If you live with another person or other people, can they provide any assistance?
Do you need assistance with:	
	Medications
	Health Procedures
	Hygiene
	Meal Preparation
	Eating
	Mobility
	Transportation
	Basic Decisions
	Basic Communication
	Emergency Communication
	Bathroom
	Paying Bills or for Services and Handling Money
	Safety Concerns
	Using the Phone

Thoreau's Senior Living Options Planner

Yes/No	What to Consider (For Staying in Your Home)
	Personal Needs
	Are any progressive diseases present that will soon affect decision making skills (such as dementia or Alzheimer's)?
	If you live with another person or other people, can they provide any assistance (with as listed below)?
	Do you currently have any deteriorating conditions that will affect your independence in the next year?
	Do you require prescriptions or medications?
	Are you capable of remembering to take prescriptions and medications and keeping records?
	Do you need assistance with personal hygiene?
	Are you capable of preparing your own meals?
	Do you need help cleaning up after meals?
	Do you need general home cleaning assistance?
	Are you able to do your own laundry?
	Do you need any assistance dressing and undressing?
	Do you need daily support with contact lenses, hearing aids, or any medical devices?
	Are you able to determine if food is unsafe to eat? (Expired or spoiled)

Thoreau's Senior Living Options Planner

Staying in Your Home: Pets Checklist

Yes/No	What to Consider (For Staying in Your Home)
	Pets
	Do you have any pets and if so, are you able to provide proper care for them?
	Do you remember to feed and give water to your pets as needed?
	Are you able to take pets outdoors safely if needed?
	Are you able to get pets to a veterinarian for checkups, shots, and in an emergency?
	Are you able to clean up after your pets?
	Do your pets present any issues for visitors or caregivers?
	Are you able to walk your pets if needed?
	Do you have a plan in place for your pets should anything happen to you?
	Do you have a plan for help with your pets if needed?

Thoreau's Senior Living Options Planner

Staying in Your Home: Safety Checklist

Yes/No	What to Consider (For Staying in Your Home)
	Safety
	Do you feel safe in your home?
	Are emergency services (Police, Fire, Ambulance) close by (within 10 minutes)?
	Is your home secure and are you able to maintain that security (locking doors and windows at night, seeing who is at the door before answering, etc.)?
	Can you easily escape your home from any room in the case of fire or other emergency?
	Are you near relatives that can help if needed?
	Do you need a personal emergency alert system?
	Do you have neighbors that can assist you in an emergency and are aware of your possible needs?
	Do you have the contact information of neighbors, relatives, and emergency numbers and able to use a phone and communicate with them?
	Do you keep a phone with you at all times?
	Do you have an emergency alert system?
	Are you capable and in the habit of keeping your home decluttered?

Thoreau's Senior Living Options Planner

Yes/No	What to Consider (For Staying in Your Home)
	Safety (continued)
	Is your home equipped with working smoke detectors and carbon monoxide detectors and will they wake you in an emergency?
	Are you able to inspect all areas of your home (such as a basement for possible leaks, pests, etc.)?
	Are you able to spot safety concerns and address them (such as a door in disrepair, items in walkways, broken glass, spilled chemicals in the garage, etc.)?
	Are you able to safely use kitchen appliances and utensils?
	Can you safely plug and unplug all electrical appliances, lights, electronics, and other electrical items in and about your home?
	Fire Extinguisher Checklist ___ Kitchen (Near stove) ___ Garage ___ Each floor of home ___ Bedroom ___ Other _____
	Will you need motion-sensor lights for lighting when entering or exiting your home and for security? Doorbell: A flashing light initiated by the doorbell can alert you if your hearing is diminished.

Staying in Your Home: Transportation Checklist

	Staying in Your Home Living Needs Checklist **Transportation**
	Transportation (Your Own Vehicle)
	Do you have a current driver's license and drive safely?
	Do you own a motor vehicle?
	If you still drive, are you able to easily access and operate your vehicle in a safe manner?
	Are you able to spot simple vehicle maintenance needs?
	Can you drive at night?
	Have you had an eye exam in the last 12 months?
	Are you able to put fuel in your vehicle without assistance?
	Are you able to change a flat tire or have emergency road service available?
	Do you carry a cell phone when you leave home?
	Transportation (Other)
	If you do not drive do you have access to easy transportation when needed?
	Do you have any special needs for transportation and if so, is such transportation available when you need it?

Thoreau's Senior Living Options Planner

Staying in Your Home: Social Interaction and Communication Checklist

	Staying in Your Home Living Needs Checklist **Social Interaction and Communication**
	Do you have a phone handy and are you completely capable of making and receiving calls?
	Will someone be checking in with you on a daily basis either in person or by phone?
	Do you attend events or gatherings outside your home at least once per week?
	Do you live alone?
	Are you active on social media such as Facebook?
	Do you communicate with relatives and friends by email?
	Are you near relatives that can help if needed?

Staying in Your Home: Home Maintenance Needs

Yes/No	What to Consider About Staying in Your Home
	Maintenance
	Can you make good home maintenance decisions?
	Are you able to see when home repairs are needed and when maintenance is required such as lawn mowing and take appropriate action?
	Are you able to inspect all areas of your home (such as a basement for possible leaks, pests, etc. or see your roof for any foreign objects or damage)?
	Can you recognize unsafe situations and take appropriate action?
	Do you have a reliable handyman with references?
	Are you able to safely use basic tools?
	Can you haul your trash containers to the curb if needed?
	Can you change light bulbs?

Thoreau's Senior Living Options Planner

Staying in Your Home: Disability or Mobility Needs

Yes or No	Safety, Disability and/or Mobility Need Considerations (For Staying in Your Home)
	Do you need to and are you capable of navigating steps or stairs safely?
	Do you feel comfortable using all the steps and stairs in your home?
	Do all steps and stairways have safe railings, bannisters, lifts, and safe stair treads?
	Can you easily and safely 'lock and unlock' and 'open and close' all doors in your home?
	Do you remember to keep your doors and windows locked?
	Can you easily navigate and exit your home in an emergency from any location?
	Can you easily reach all interior and exterior light switches, door handles, locks, and faucets in your home? If not, list the location of any that you cannot reach: _____ _____ _____ _____ _____

Thoreau's Senior Living Options Planner

Yes or No	Safety, Disability and/or Mobility Need Considerations (For Staying in Your Home)
	Can you smell natural gas?
	Can you easily smell smoke?
	Can you feel when water is too hot?
	Can you hear all alarms, alerts, doorbells, and phones in your home?
	If you need a walker or wheelchair is your home completely accessible?
	Can you read, reach, and adjust all thermostats and/or temperature controls?
	Do you need a wheelchair-accessible bathroom and/or shower?
	Do you need a taller toilet or raised seat?

Thoreau's Senior Living Options Planner

Yes or No	Safety, Disability and/or Mobility Need Considerations (For Staying in Your Home)
	Is your home 'walker safe'? (No throw rugs or dangerous thresholds.)
	If a wheelchair is needed do all rooms, hallways, and doorways have adequate clearance?
	Do you need different door handles anywhere in your home?
	Do you need handrails or grab bars for assistance in any areas of your home such as the bathroom?
	Are laundry facilities easily accessible?
	Are gates needed at the top of any stairways?
	Do you need special locks, door chimes and/or other alert and prevention devices?
	Have you done a hazard review: Dangling Cords, Poisons, Slippery Surfaces, Unsteady Chairs, Throw Rugs, Electrical Cords, etc.
	Do you have auto shut offs for stove tops, coffee makers, etc.
	Do you have adequate interior and exterior lighting?
	Are temperature controls easily accessible?

Thoreau's Senior Living Options Planner

	Disability or Mobility Needs

Thoreau's Senior Living Options Planner

Home Ownership Worksheet

Is remaining at home a short-term (less than two years) or a long-term plan (two years or more)?

If you remain at home, how will your social, health and financial needs be met?

Is sharing your home (roommate) an option to consider?

Do you have equity in your home? If so, what are ways to obtain a loan and use that money?

Thoreau's Senior Living Options Planner

Are you eligible for any home repair programs that are completed by volunteers?

_____
_____
_____
_____

Are there programs available to help you pay for the costs of home repairs, home modifications, heating expenses, weatherization, utility bills and other expenses of maintaining a home?

_____
_____
_____

Would modifying your home permit you to continue living there? If so, how do you find a qualified remodeler? Is the remodeler you are considering a Certified 'Aging-in-Place' Specialist? Are there volunteers from any local 'Area Agency on Aging' who can help you?

_____
_____
_____
_____

Thoreau's Senior Living Options Planner

What products and features from the previous 'Staying in Your Home: Safety Checklist' and 'Staying in Your Home: Disability or Mobility Needs Checklist' should you consider, that will make your home safer and more comfortable?

_____
_____
_____
_____
_____
_____
_____
_____
_____

Am I eligible for any property tax relief programs in my state?

_____
_____

Thoreau's Senior Living Options Planner

Am I eligible for any 'in-home' support services through federal, state or local programs, such as Medicare or Medicaid?

_____
_____
_____
_____

Can I use my long-term care insurance policy to pay for in-home support services?

_____
_____
_____

Thoreau's Senior Living Options Planner

Current Home Ownership Expenses Form

Monthly Amount	Current Home Ownership Expenses Description

Thoreau's Senior Living Options Planner

Monthly Amount	Current Home Ownership Expenses Description

Other Home Ownership Options

As people age the upkeep and maintenance of a home can be an increasing expense as they become less able and must pay for some services such as lawn care, painting, cleaning, etc.

In addition, some people require some form of in-home care. While controversial in some areas or according to certain experts, a reverse mortgage loan can be used for living expenses, medical and long-term care needs, and home repairs and modifications. Note: A reverse mortgage loan or the income from house sharing (roommates) might affect eligibility for public benefits.

There are other considerations such as the effect of receiving Medicaid services on the transfer of the title of the home after the homeowner dies or; the use of a life estate to allow the homeowner to remain in the home if the sale or transfer of the property is being considered.

Because of the unique situations and complexities of the effects of a reverse mortgage, consult with your accountant or tax advisor and a lawyer before making this decision.

Notes About Staying in Home

Thoreau's Senior Living Options Planner

Notes About Staying in Home

Thoreau's Senior Living Options Planner

Notes About Staying in Home

Thoreau's Senior Living Options Planner

4. Is Renting an Option for You?

"All change is a miracle to contemplate; but it is a miracle which is taking place every instant." – Henry David Thoreau

Renting Options Forms

Completed ✓	This chapter contains the following checklists, forms, questionnaires, and/or worksheets:
	Questions to Ask Landlords or Property Managers Form
	Renting Financial Resources Worksheet
	Selling Your Home and Renting or Moving to Care Facility: Cash Gain Worksheet
	Current Monthly Expenses Worksheet A
	Moving to a Rental Home, Apartment or in with Family: Estimate New Living Option Expenses Worksheet B

Maybe you have a home you want to sell so that you can cash in your equity or perhaps you want to relocate closer to services or relatives. Renting can also reduce your responsibilities and chores. Renting a single-family home, apartment, mobile home in a park, condominium, or a unit in a retirement community can relieve you of maintenance, repairs, snow shoveling and yard work.

Thoreau's Senior Living Options Planner

What to Consider

Renting Pros:

Little or no maintenance: If you do not want to deal with home maintenance issues, renting eliminates responsibility for most upkeep and repairs.

Flexibility: When you rent you can commonly move more quickly and easily than when you need to sell your property first. Many leases allow a one- or two-months' notice to move especially if you are renting on a month-to-month basis.

Protection from house price declines: When home values decline you do not lose equity or get upside down (owing more on your mortgage than your home value) with your property.

Sense of community: Renters often have a sense of community especially in a senior rental area or building.

Discounted rent: Some communities offer discounts for seniors and some communities are specifically designed for adults over 55 years of age. These communities often offer a quieter environment, lower rental rates, and amenities and services aimed at seniors. Amenities and services can include transportation services, workout areas, Internet connections, swimming pools, community centers, special groups and events.

You could be eligible for public housing or subsidized housing such as Section 8. You can get more information here including about your state and the area that you would like to live:

https://www.hud.gov/topics/rental_assistance

Renting Cons:

Limited or no home improvements and preferences: While you will have little maintenance, you will also have few options for making improvements or changing paint colors.

Thoreau's Senior Living Options Planner

Less stability: Depending on your lease and any rent control, your rent can be increased periodically. This can make living on a fixed income difficult and at the least make budgeting unpredictable. In addition, when your lease expires, your landlord might not renew causing you to need to find a new home.

No opportunity for equity: You miss out on the advantage you get when you own of building equity.

No tax benefits: You miss out on any tax deductions for mortgage interest.

Limited options for pets: Many rental properties do not allow pets and those that do often charge more for deposits and/or rent.

Questions to Ask Landlords or Property Managers Form

How soon is the unit or home available?

_____

What is your application process and screening practices?

_____

_____

_____

What payment methods will you accept rent?

_____

_____

What is the shortest lease term you accept?

_____

Is the lease renewable or go to a month-to-month at the end?

_____

What is your policy on subletting?

_____

_____

_____

Is early lease termination permitted and if so, what are the fees?

_____

_____

Thoreau's Senior Living Options Planner

Is there a break clause in the lease?

What's your late fee policy?

What is the monthly rent?

What all is included in the rent?

What deposit is required?

What is your policy for refunding deposits and is that in writing?

Thoreau's Senior Living Options Planner

What utilities am I responsible for and what do they average per month?

_____

_____

_____

What's your pet policy, and do you require a pet deposit?

_____

_____

_____

Is there assigned parking or where is parking?

_____

_____

Is there guest parking?

_____

_____

Is there a guest policy?

_____

_____

What am I allowed to decorate?

_____

_____

_____

Thoreau's Senior Living Options Planner

What are the rules for the balcony or patio?

_____

_____

Is a BBQ or outdoor cooking allowed?

_____

_____

Which furnishings or appliances are included?

_____

_____

_____

_____

How's the crime in the neighborhood, and has this property experienced any break-ins, theft, or assaults? (You can also check local public police records for the area.)

_____

_____

_____

What's the procedure for submitting a maintenance request, and who typically makes repairs?

_____

_____

_____

Thoreau's Senior Living Options Planner

What repairs am I responsible for?

_____
_____
_____

How much notice do you usually give before you or your representative shows up at the property?

_____
_____
_____

What are the common areas and what services, or amenities are included?

_____
_____
_____

What security measures are in place such as security guards or CCTV cameras?

_____
_____
_____

Thoreau's Senior Living Options Planner

What local transportation is available?

_____

_____

_____

How close are grocery stores and other services?

_____

_____

_____

Is there a safe jogging or walking area?

_____

Are in-home support services allowed in the lease? Is there additional parking for caregivers?

_____

_____

_____

If I need to make physical changes to the unit to make it more accessible, who is responsible for the cost of the modifications?

_____

_____

_____

Thoreau's Senior Living Options Planner

Renting Financial Resources Worksheet

Are there any federal, state, or local programs that I am eligible for regarding in-home support services?

_____
_____
_____
_____

Will my long-term care insurance pay for any in-home support services?

_____
_____
_____

Am I eligible for any state or federal rent subsidy programs?

_____
_____
_____

The following worksheets will help you estimate if you will gain any cash on hand from selling your home, belongings and other assets when moving to a rental or care facility or other option and any difference in monthly expenses. You can complete these whenever you have the information needed.

Thoreau's Senior Living Options Planner

Selling Your Home and Renting or Moving to Care Facility: Cash Gain Worksheet

Additional Cash After Selling Your Home Will selling property and belongings put money in your pocket?	
Sale of Home Net Equity (After paying any mortgages and taxes)	$
Selling Belongings Estimate	$
Deposits Refunded	$
Other (List Below)	
	$
	$
	$
	$
	$
	$
	$
	$
Total of All Amounts Above (Total Cash)	$
Subtract Estimated Cost of Moving	- $
Total Net Cash Gain	$

Thoreau's Senior Living Options Planner

Current Monthly Expenses Worksheet A

Current Monthly Expenses	
Description	**Monthly Amount**
Utilities Average Cost	$
Housing Cost (Mortgage, Rent, etc.)	$
Home Maintenance Expenses	$
Monthly Insurance Expense (Property, Renter's)	$
Property Taxes	$
Average Monthly Home Repairs	$
Lawn Maintenance	$
All Other Home Monthly Expenses:	$
Current Vehicle Ownership Expenses (Only if you will be selling your vehicle or will be downsizing to one vehicle or a smaller vehicle)	
Average Monthly Maintenance	$
Monthly Fuel	$
Monthly Payment	$
Monthly Auto Insurance	$
Auto Taxes, License, Registration (Monthly Cost)	$
Add All Above for Total Current Monthly Expenses Before Any Move	$

Moving to a Rental Home, Apartment or in with Family: Estimate New Living Option Expenses Worksheet B

Monthly Expenses After Moving	
Description	**Monthly Amount**
Utilities Average Cost	$
Housing Cost (Mortgage, Rent, Care, etc.) Fees	$
Home Maintenance Expenses	$
Monthly Insurance Expense (Property, Renter's)	$
Property Taxes	$
Home Repairs	$
Lawn Maintenance	$
Other:	$
Other:	$
Other:	$
Other:	$
	$
	$
	$
	$
	$
	$
	$

Thoreau's Senior Living Options Planner

Vehicle Ownership Expenses (Enter Zero for these expenses if you will be selling your vehicle or the estimated amounts if you downsize to one vehicle or a smaller vehicle)	
Monthly Maintenance	$
Monthly Fuel	$
Monthly Payment	$
Monthly Insurance	$
Monthly Vehicle Registration	$
Monthly Vehicle Taxes	$
Total All Monthly Expenses After Moving (Add all monthly amounts on this Worksheet B)	$

Now subtract the total on Worksheet B from the total on Worksheet A.

The result will be an estimate of how much you will be saving or how much your move will cost you monthly.

Total Worksheet A	$
Subtract Total Worksheet B	- $
Estimated Monthly Savings or Cost of Your Move	$

Thoreau's Senior Living Options Planner

Notes About Renting

Thoreau's Senior Living Options Planner

5. Are In-Home Care Options Right for You?

"You must live in the present, launch yourself on every wave, find your eternity in each moment." – Henry David Thoreau

In-Home Care Forms

Completed ✓	This chapter contains the following checklists, forms, questionnaires, and/or worksheets:
	In-Home Care Costs Worksheet
	Caregiver's List of Duties
	Caregiver Interview Worksheet

Why In-Home Care?

Getting assistance at home can help you maintain some of the independence you currently enjoy. Due to the one-on-one nature of the arrangement, your care is often more personalized. While in a larger community you might have to accept the standards of the institution, while you are in your own home, there is more flexibility in setting guidelines for your care.

Another reason that you might enjoy individualized care is that you will have the full attention of your caregiver. The staff at senior residential facilities often find themselves pulled in more than one direction at a time, making it harder to do a job thoroughly or have a conversation.

Home care can help meet your assistance needs so that you do not become a burden on your family, friends, and neighbors. Our loved ones want to help and saying "No" can be difficult for them. This can put undue care on them, their families, and your relationship with them.

What is Home Care?

There are non-medical support staff, personal attendants, nurse assistants and caregivers available. These are assistance or companion roles. They can help with hygiene, mobility, and simple chores. These types of caregivers are not allowed to dispense medications. They can advise you when it is time to take medications. Hire licensed personnel that are authorized to distribute medication and perform any medical assistance if you need them.

Home care business requirements are regulated at the state level and vary between states.

You can dictate the times, days and hours care is needed. Some companies have minimum visit requirements such as four hours per visit.

What to Consider

Keep in mind that 'Home Care' is generally companionship with some responsibilities. These caregivers are non-medical personnel. While some caregivers are independent, others work for a service. You will need to hire, manage and if needed, terminate the employee or caregiver.

Thoreau's Senior Living Options Planner

If you hire an individual (that is not working for a service) you will become an employer with legal requirements. If you are unfamiliar with being an employer, meet with your accountant, tax advisor, and lawyer so that you understand your legal, record keeping, and tax liabilities and obligations before going down this road.

Home care can be a benefit after a hospital stay during your recovery.

Home care is a good option for you if you are still able to perform some or all your Activities of Daily Living and have limited medical issues, but you are at risk of becoming socially isolated.

This arrangement is also beneficial for couples where one partner needs help, but the other does not. Getting home care can help relieve some of the responsibilities of your partner. This will allow you to stay at home together while you get the care you need.

In other situations, the quantity of care needed is a financial consideration. Around-the-clock care can cost $15,000–$18,000 a month and can drain your savings. 24-hour care is frequently far more expensive than moving into assisted living or a skilled nursing facility. Employing live-in caregivers can save you some money, but you will lose privacy.

Also, if you are suffering from dementia, you will need a trusted relative or friend to manage home care services for you.

What to Ask

Complete the Caregiver's List of Duties in this chapter and the Caregiver Interview Worksheet.

Thoreau's Senior Living Options Planner

What is Home Health Care?

There was a time when doctors came to you… and those visits were known as 'house calls.' That is similar to home health care. You stay in your home and nurses, therapists, and other health care professionals come to you. Home health care is one level better than home care and of course costs more.

What to Consider

Most seniors get home health care professionals for short-term periods. Long-term home health care that involves certified professionals is costly.

Medicare Part A (Hospital Insurance) and Medicare Part B (Medical Insurance) covers eligible home health services such as part-time or intermittent skilled nursing care and physical therapy, occupational therapy, speech-language pathology services, and medical social services.

A home health care agency can direct services prescribed or ordered for you by your doctor. Medicare will not pay for 24-hour care at home or for personal non-medical care.

Medicare doesn't pay for:

- 24-hour-a-day care at home
- Meals delivered to your home
- Homemaker services
- Personal care

You can find additional information regarding Medicare coverage and costs here:

https://www.medicare.gov/coverage/home-health-services.html

Thoreau's Senior Living Options Planner

There are additional resources that might help pay for home caregivers including:

- Commercial insurance
- Long-term care insurance
- Medicaid waivers
- A Medicaid state plan
- Older American's Act (OAA)
- Title B Supportive Services; Title III E Family Caregiver funds
- Veterans benefits (contact your local VA Hospital)

A key factor for many families in deciding to pay for in-home care is the state of your immune system. Over a quarter of a million seniors pass away from infections caught in nursing homes each year. While pneumonia, staph, and flu are common among the elderly, rates of infection are much higher in nursing homes.

If you do suffer from a weakened immune system, find out whether you qualify for the Program for All-Inclusive Care for the Elderly (PACE). You can join PACE with Medicaid or Medicare. Check to see if the program is available in your area.

If you decide that your care should stay a family matter, Medicaid can help. You can hire a family member as your personal care provider, and they can submit timesheets to Medicaid to be paid for services rendered. Keep in mind that while your adult children may fulfill this role, your spouse or legal guardian may not.

Home health care would benefit you if you are able to regain skills affected by motor or cognitive decline. Enrolling in occupational therapy qualifies you for home health care eligibility under Medicare.

Thoreau's Senior Living Options Planner

What to Ask

Complete the Caregiver's List of Duties in this chapter and the Caregiver Interview Worksheet.

You may decide that both Home Health Care and Home Care would suit your needs best. Since payment for these services may come from different sources, such an arrangement could be economically feasible.

Choosing an Aid

What to Look For

Here are a few characteristics you need to look for in medical or non-medical staff:

Patience: A lot of activities take you more time than they used to and may take even longer as you age. This can be frustrating for *you*. You need someone who remains patient as you recover or maintain your independence.

Cleanliness: Whether you need assistance administering insulin or washing the dishes, you need someone who is sanitary and has a similar standard of tidiness as you. Someone's attire, hair, and handbag can all be signs of their cleanliness.

Punctuality: As you come to depend on an assistant, their punctuality becomes important. You may count on them for transportation to and from appointments or to administer medicine. If someone shows up to your first meeting late, that is a bad sign. If you are working with an agency, let them know immediately if your caregiver makes a habit of tardiness.

A good listener: You may have to hire non-medical staff primarily to be socially engaged. Inside your own home and regarding your own body, you will need someone to understand specific directions.

Look for someone who actively listens and asks detailed questions on the first interview.

Ability to handle difficult situations: You may fall. You may require emergency help. You may wander off or forget where you are. All of these are stressful situations for you and your caregiver. You need someone with a cool head. Make sure to ask questions about how a candidate would respond to trying situations that they may find themselves in.

Hiring Through an Agency Vs. Independent Caregiver

You will have to decide whether you want to hire through an agency or independently. Each approach has pros and cons.

When you hire through an agency, the upfront cost is 20–30% higher than hiring independently. But this number does not include the hidden cost to being an employer, which includes paying taxes on your personal aid earnings as well as applying for, managing, and maintaining whatever documentation is necessary for your state.

If you are looking for medical personnel, you might find working with an agency easier. Independent caregivers are less likely to be certified, though web-based services may be able to match you up with someone who suits your needs.

There is no definite difference in the quality of care you should expect to receive from a caregiver hired independently or through an agency. Each person is unique. Your ability to connect with and communicate with them is unrelated to their employment status.

If you require a lot of flexibility, you may find that an independent caregiver is right for you. As they work for themselves, there is no restriction on the non-medical services they are able to provide.

Agencies may have strict requirements on what their employees can and cannot help with. For instance, many agencies will not allow caregivers to help with transportation as the liability cost is too high.

On the other hand, there are serious limitations to household employees that you need to consider. What happens when they call in for a sick day? In the case of a frail senior, coming in to work with a cough would be irresponsible. An agency would be able to send in backup.

Some people will say that agencies providing background checks for you is a benefit to working with agencies. While this is true, particularly in regard to certification and driving and criminal records, keep in mind that you should perform your own background checks regardless of the decision that you make. You will want to ask for referrals. Take care to talk to both the seniors who have received care from a particular caregiver and their adult children who typically oversee their care to get a balanced view of the situation.

What to Ask

You want to be certain you are hiring a reputable firm or individual. Here are some questions that you should ask when interviewing for either:

- How will emergencies be handled?
- What mechanism is in place to address and resolve conflict?
- How often are you willing to update a written plan of care?
- Will you provide us with a Patient's Bill of Rights to provide? (This is a document that lists the rights and responsibilities of all parties involved.)

Agency:

Is the agency licensed through the state?

How does the agency train caregivers? What are the ways they monitor the level of care?

Are there any resources to help pay for care? Is a payment plan available?

Individual:

Are you licensed and certified? (Check with the licensing body.)

Can you provide references to previous employers?

What are your expectations involving holidays and sick days?

After the Hire

After you have hired a caregiver, come up with a plan to evaluate them. Periodically measure the caregiver's skill in areas of communication, administration, safety, dependability, and responsiveness. Enroll the help of a family member to perform these evaluations if you are unsure of your ability to do so.

Make sure that you have a contract with the agency or your independent caregiver that includes all important information such as start dates, compensation, and schedules and responsibilities. If there is a standard contract with the agency, ask to include specifics like the restrictions on social media and phone usage. Caregivers spending too much time on their devices is one of the top complaints elderly patients have about home care.

A complaint about home care from both the clients and the caregivers is a lack of communication. Try to find a way to facilitate clear guidelines about what help is required. Some days your regular caregiver may call in and you'll have to bring a new person up to speed. Consider keeping a copy of the contract, a schedule, or a checklist around to help facilitate any conversation about responsibilities.

As your relationship with your caregiver gets more personal, the aide may come to think of themselves as part of the family and may come to occupy a place of trust for you. This is great for all parties involved. You want them to be personally invested in your care. However, this can result in a lack of professionalism. Remember that as an employer you are allowed to make demands on them. If you have trouble asserting yourself, you need to let a family member know.

These people have access to your home, your bedroom, all your belongings. Come up with a plan of action to fire your caregiver.

The following 'In-Home Care Costs Worksheet' will help you determine how long you can afford services. On a long-term basis, or if your needs should increase, another senior living option such as moving to a senior community or care facility might be more economical.

Thoreau's Senior Living Options Planner

In-Home Care Costs Worksheet

Weekly Cost	
1. Total Hours Needed per Week (Note: Certain caregivers require a minimum time per visit such as four hours.)	Hours: _____
2. Hourly Wage	$
3. Multiply Line 1 Times Line 2.	$

Financial Resource	Amount Weekly
4. Insurance	$
5. Long-Term Care Insurance	$
6. Medicaid	$
7. Older Americans Act OAA	$
8. Title B Supportive Services; Title III E Family Caregiver Funds	$
9. Veterans Benefits	$
10. Other Insurance or Benefits	$
11. Add Lines 4 through 10.	$
12. Enter Line 3 Total from Above: Weekly Cost	- $
Subtract Line 12 from Line 11 = Total Weekly Out of Pocket Cost	$

Thoreau's Senior Living Options Planner

Caregiver's List of Duties

Yes/No	Caregiver List of Duties
	General Supervision and Health Monitoring

Describe Supervision and Health Monitoring Needed:

Thoreau's Senior Living Options Planner

Yes/No	Caregiver List of Duties
	Medication Reminders
Current Medication: (Note: Unlicensed Caregivers Can Not Administer Medications)	

Thoreau's Senior Living Options Planner

Yes/No	Caregiver List of Duties
	Food Preparation

Describe Food Preparation:

Thoreau's Senior Living Options Planner

Yes/No	Caregiver List of Duties
	Mobility Assistance
Describe Special Mobility Needs:	
	Exercise
	Personal Preferences

Thoreau's Senior Living Options Planner

Yes/No	Caregiver List of Duties
	Hygiene and Bathroom Assistance

Describe Hygiene and Bathroom Needs:

Thoreau's Senior Living Options Planner

Yes/No	Caregiver List of Duties

Thoreau's Senior Living Options Planner

Caregiver Interview Worksheet

Are you a smoker? Yes _____ No _____

Do you have a driver's license from this state and a clean driving record? Yes _____ No _____

If you do not have a clean driving record, do you have any DUIs (Driving Under the Influence) or DWIs (Driving While Intoxicated)? Yes _____ No _____

Do you have reliable transportation and insurance? Yes _____ No _____

Ask for a copy of proof of insurance.

How far from here do you live?
_____
_____

Will you be comfortable using your own car to run errands if needed? Do you have proof of insurance?
_____
_____

Are you able to work the hours needed?
_____
_____

Thoreau's Senior Living Options Planner

Are you flexible with the days and work schedule?

_____

_____

What are your other work responsibilities and outside of work requirements?

_____

_____

Are you available for respite care, or extended stays?

_____

_____

When are you available to start working?

_____

_____

Do you need any specific days off?

_____

_____

Do you expect any vacation time?

_____

_____

Thoreau's Senior Living Options Planner

Are you comfortable signing our contract that you will not bring any guests or other people to the home without my prior written approval?

_____

_____

Will you sign a contract that allows you to only accept payment for services as agreed and no other gifts or monies?

_____

_____

Do you have experience caring for a person with (conditions similar to your loved one's care: elderly, mobility issues, etc.)? If so, please describe.

_____

_____

Please review this list of expected care tasks and duties and tell me if you have any concerns or questions?

_____

_____

Are you comfortable with pets (if applicable)?

_____

_____

🍃 Thoreau's Senior Living Options Planner

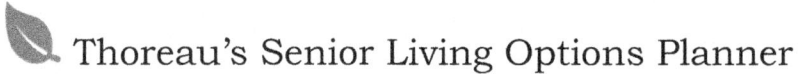

What certification, education and training do you have? Do you have CPR or first-aid training?

_____

_____

Request references and contact them. Perform a background check on the person and companies' reputations. At Care.com you can locate candidates and request free, unlimited standard background checks.

Note: If you need intermittent in-home nursing care at home, contact a home health agency or service that can deliver a certified professional.

Notes About Caregivers

Thoreau's Senior Living Options Planner

Notes About Caregivers

Thoreau's Senior Living Options Planner

6. What Should You Consider About Independent Living Communities?

"The future is worth expecting." – Henry David Thoreau

Independent Living Communities Forms

Completed ✓	This chapter contains the following checklists, forms, questionnaires, and/or worksheets:
	What to Ask Independent Living Communities Worksheet
	Independent Living Community Cost Comparison Worksheet

Retirement Community

Independent retirement communities are often like apartments. Services such as group meals, transportation, housekeeping and social activities are commonly available. Residents are free to come and go as they please with amenities and prices that vary. Some retirement communities offer access to a nurse or nurse practitioner. Additional services are often available. Some subsidized housing programs may be available for low-income individuals.

Thoreau's Senior Living Options Planner

Some are available on a month-to-month contract. The sizes can vary from studios to two-bedroom apartments. Some communities have stand-alone homes.

Independent living retirement communities usually provide:

- One or more meals each day
- Social areas, events, and activities
- Outings on a community van or bus
- Some form of transportation to health appointments
- Maintenance
- Utilities

Some independent living communities provide:

- Routine care
- Exercise programs
- Music therapy
- Housekeeping
- Personal laundry
- Emergency call systems

If additional services are needed, you can hire your own caregiver. Some of these communities do contract with a local agency and this cost is additional. You will still need to manage the caregivers.

Costs for independent retirement communities vary widely depending on unit sizes, amenities, services offered and the area.

Naturally Occurring Retirement Communities (NORCs) or Villages

NORCs are commonly a group of seniors with homes in the same neighborhood or other proximity. Services such as home repair, transportation and social educational activities are scrutinized and shared. There organizations require a fee for membership. This can be a great benefit for maintaining independent living.

NORCs include apartment buildings, condominiums, or cooperatives not designed as retirement communities but where at least 50 percent of the residents are 62 years old or older (which often include amenities such as grocery stores, pharmacies, limousine service, or shopping services on the premises) and/or recent technological advances (such as Velcro fasteners, lightweight wheelchairs, walk-in bathtubs, devices to control appliances, and dial telephone numbers) are available to help the elderly person stay in his/her home often make aging in place easier.

Home care services are available in many communities, providing appropriate, supervised personnel to help older persons with either health care (giving medications, changing dressings, catheter care, etc.) or personal care (bathing, dressing, and grooming).

Meals and transportation are available to older people to help them retain some independence. Group or home-delivered meal programs help ensure an adequate diet. Meals-On-Wheels programs are available in most parts of the United States. Several communities offer door-to-door transportation services to help older people get to and from medical facilities, community facilities, and other services.

Adult day care is comparable to child day care. The elderly person goes to a community facility daily or as needed. Activities consist of exercise programs, singing, guest lectures, and current events

Thoreau's Senior Living Options Planner

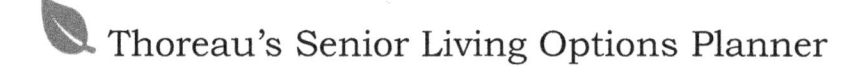

discussions. Cost varies and there are frequently long waiting lists to get in.

Respite care brings a trained person into your home, so the full-time caregiver can have time off. Respite care is commonly offered through area Departments of Social Services on a sliding fee scale.

Thoreau's Senior Living Options Planner

What to Ask Independent Living Communities Worksheet

	What to Ask Independent Living Communities
	Facilities
	What is the approximate square footage of living space?
	Are stairs a consideration?
	Does the unit provide comfortable privacy?
	What kind of parking is available if needed? _____ _____
	Is there adequate parking for visitors?
	Are there any visitor restrictions? (Number of visitors or times)
	Do I have a private outdoor area?
	Is this a detached home or multi-unit?
	Are laundry facilities easily accessible?
	Does the space accommodate all my needs?
	Is the bathroom safe for me?
	Is there adequate storage space?
	Can I access and use all of the kitchen space and appliances?
	Are the kitchen appliances what I need?

Thoreau's Senior Living Options Planner

	What to Ask Independent Living Communities
	Facilities
	Is interior and exterior lighting adequate?
	Is there an emergency call system that is staffed 24/7?
	Who will have keys to my unit? _____ _____ _____
	Is there a secure space for valuables?
	What maintenance am I responsible for? _____ _____ _____ _____
	Are common areas available and if so, what times and days?
	Are common areas well lit, safe, and clean?
	Is there a social or community center?
	Are there community events, therapy or classes offered and do they cost extra? _____ _____ _____

Thoreau's Senior Living Options Planner

	What to Ask Independent Living Communities
	Services
	What utilities are not included and what are the estimated monthly costs? _____ _____ _____
	What Internet services are available? _____ _____
	Are pets allowed and if so, are there any limitations? _____
	Is a pet deposit required?
	What is the policy for service animals?
	Is trash removal included and how often is this performed?
	What transportation services are included and/or available? _____ _____ _____
	What additional costs are involved for transportation? _____ _____

Thoreau's Senior Living Options Planner

	What to Ask Independent Living Communities
	Staff Services
	Are caregiver services available? If so, how much are the services? _____ _____ _____ _____
	Is there a licensed nurse available on staff? If so, what are the days and hours of availability and what services are available? Contact the nurse for more information. _____ _____ _____ _____
	Is medication management available?
	What if any other medical staff is available, what are their licenses, and what are their hours? _____ _____ _____
	Who is the director of the facility or community? _____ _____

Thoreau's Senior Living Options Planner

	What to Ask Independent Living Communities
	Meals
	What meals are provided, how often, and at what times? _____ _____ _____ _____ _____ _____
	Are meals served in a common dining area?
	Are meals delivered to me if needed?
	If meals are delivered, will dishes, trays etc. be picked up and how soon and how does that work?
	Are special diets accommodated?
	If food is included or you plan on partaking often, schedule a time when you can eat and sample the food. _____
	Is there a dietician on staff?
	Is food delivery available from local establishments?

Thoreau's Senior Living Options Planner

	What to Ask Independent Living Communities
	Costs
	What is the base monthly rental and deposit if any? _____ _____ How long is the monthly rate guaranteed not to increase? _____
	What is the monthly rental amount including all services and fees (including any daily care)? _____ _____ _____ _____ Is the contract month to month and if not, what is the term? _____ _____ _____ _____
	What forms of payment do you accept?
	When are payments due?
	What are late fees?

Thoreau's Senior Living Options Planner

	What to Ask Independent Living Communities
	General
	How soon is a unit available and is there a waiting list? _____ _____ _____
	Request a copy of rules and policies.
	Are there any questions I have not asked? _____ _____ _____ _____ _____ _____ _____
	Notes _____ _____ _____ _____ _____ _____ _____

Thoreau's Senior Living Options Planner

Independent Living Community Cost Comparison Worksheet

Cost (Before Insurance) Comparison Worksheet Compare Up to 4 Communities				
Name of Choice 1				
Name of Choice 2				
Name of Choice 3				
Name of Choice 4				
Amounts				
	Choice 1	**Choice 2**	**Choice 3**	**Choice 4**
Monthly Rent	$	$	$	$
Utilities Not Included (Estimate)	$	$	$	$
Care Not Included	$	$	$	$
Transportation Not Included	$	$	$	$
Amenities Not Included	$	$	$	$
Therapy Not Included	$	$	$	$
Other _____	$	$	$	$
Other _____	$	$	$	$
Other _____	$	$	$	$
Totals (Add the columns)	**$**	**$**	**$**	**$**

Notes and Conclusions About Independent Living Communities

Thoreau's Senior Living Options Planner

7. What are Your Options for Group Living and Care Facilities?

"But the place which you have selected for your camp, though never so rough and grim, begins at once to have its attractions, and becomes a very center of civilization to you: 'Home is home, be it never so homely.'" – Henry David Thoreau

Group Living and Care Facilities Forms

Completed ✓	This chapter contains the following checklists, forms, questionnaires, and/or worksheets:
	What to Consider About a Facility
	What to Ask Assisted Living Communities or Board and Care Homes
	Assisted Living Cost Comparison Worksheet
	Group Living Worksheet
	Group Living Checklist
	Disability or Mobility Needs Checklist
	Community Requirements Checklist
	Personal Needs Checklist

There are several types of senior housing and care facilities that cover the spectrum of needs and preferences. Group living arrangements provide housing, a range of support services, care, and some social activities. There are more than two dozen terms or names that states use for these types of group settings and each state describes and licenses group housing for older adults differently.

Group housing options present an assortment of support services and housing types. They also provide residents occasions for socializing. Group settings can often limit privacy and not all will be affordable for everyone.

Thoreau's Senior Living Options Planner

What to Consider About a Facility

	What to Consider About a Facility
	Facility Needs
	Approximate Square Footage
	Level of Privacy
	Single Level
	Garage or Parking
	Kitchen
	Exterior and Lawn Maintenance
	Multi-Unit
	Detached Home
	Secure Space for Valuables
	Near Any Relatives
	Internet Services
	Pets
	Transportation
	Medical Staff

Thoreau's Senior Living Options Planner

The following general descriptions of the various group care settings demonstrate some of the basic differences between each one. You will need to assess each one based on the services provided, your needs, location, and cost. Do not depend on advertisements and/or brochures to find out about these housing options. Narrow down your choices by completing the lists and forms in this chapter and then obtaining objective information.

Assisted Living or Board and Care Homes

Assisted living communities (or board and care) offer independent living with assistance based on your specific needs. They typically assist with medication management, hygiene, dressing, and meals or the "Activities of Daily Living" or ADLS. Rooms are typically private, and bathrooms might be private or shared.

Generally, these homes are state regulated. States evaluate these homes periodically. The staff records all resident medications, any changes in the residents' health or conditions, and all physician's orders.

See the State Guide to Assisted Living Records & Reports:

http://www.aplaceformom.com/assisted-living-state-licensing

The Two Assisted Living Categories

The first decision for choosing an assisted living facility is the level of need for medical assistance. Commonly, assisted living residents require some help with medication management. Determine if staff will supervise and dispense the proper medications. Communities and states vary in requirements for who may do this. Ask questions about who does this and if the person is on-site a minimum of 40 hours a week.

Thoreau's Senior Living Options Planner

1. Medical Model Assisted Living: The medical model provides medical care and support. These are usually facility type buildings where residents are assigned private or shared rooms that are similar to a nursing home. You might see medication dispensaries or carts and a nursing station.

2. Social Model Assisted Living Communities: These communities are typically apartment type buildings. Active lifestyle recreational programs are provided, and some have community dining. Health care staff such as a nurse is often available during weekdays.

Other Assisted Living Types or Models

Independent Living: As the description defines, people in these communities do not need any or little assistance with daily living (eating, bathing, dressing, bathroom, or continence). These facilities commonly offer one hour of basic daily assistance.

The facilities are often similar to apartments with kitchens and bathrooms. Staff usually provides only minimal supervision.

Recreational and social activities and group transportation to events are sometimes included. A community meal center is also available at some independent living facilities.

Traditional Assisted Living Facilities:

These are popular in the Unites States and are basically small studio, one-bedroom or two-bedroom apartments. Some apartments may be shared by roommates or couples. Meals, activities, and transportation are often available or provided.

Some residents have daily activity needs. A medical evaluation is often part of the application process. Specific support services are billed in addition to any monthly rent.

Memory Assisted Living: For individuals with memory issues, Alzheimer's and dementia, people reside in private or shared rooms with 24-hour supervision. This can be in a separate and secure area within a community or a dedicated facility. Activities for memory afflictions such as music, art, and song therapy are frequently available. Costs are more for memory impaired care.

Services and Costs

Assisted living retirement communities typically provide:

- Three meals per day and sometimes snacks.
- On and off-site social activities.
- Transportation for medical and dental appointments.

Assisted living or board and care homes commonly provide:

- Unit and community space maintenance.
- Utilities, except the phone and sometimes Wi-Fi.
- Cognitive impairment care.
- Housekeeping one time per week; linen service as needed.
- 24-7 staff.
- On-site nurse usually at least during business hours.
- Incontinence care.
- Emergency call system.

Some of these services may or may not be included in the monthly fee. Costs and services greatly vary between communities. The majority have a base monthly rate and specific care services are added.

Most base rates include room and meals for a fairly independent senior. Additional support and care will be charged for based on the specific care, a package price, or sometimes a point system.

The base rate usually does not include:

- Shower assistance
- Dressing and grooming assistance
- Medication management
- Other personal services

Get Full Disclosure of Costs

Assisted living communities are required by law to provide you with a written disclosure of the care service they offer. Admitting anyone they cannot care for is illegal.

At each facility you visit, request all full costs. Compare costs between 'all-inclusive rate' communities and 'base rates plus services' communities. Frequently an all-inclusive rate community can be more economical when additional services are needed.

Veterans

If you or your spouse is a veteran, you might qualify for VA benefits under the Aid and Attendance Program/VA. There are specific financial and health requirements.

If you need help with your daily activities, or you're housebound, you may qualify for Aid and Attendance or Housebound allowances in addition to your pension benefits. Find out if you can get these monthly payments added to the amount of your monthly pension.

Finding out if you qualify is a free service. You may qualify for Aid and Attendance if you get a VA pension, and you meet at least one of the requirements listed below.

At least one of these must be true:

- You need another person to help you perform daily activities, like bathing, feeding, and dressing, or

- You have to stay in bed—or spend a large portion of the day in bed—because of illness, or
- You are a patient in a nursing home due to the loss of mental or physical abilities related to a disability, or
- Your eyesight is limited (even with glasses or contact lenses you have only 5/200 or less in both eyes; or concentric contraction of the visual field to 5 degrees or less)

You may qualify for Housebound benefits if you get a VA pension and you spend most of your time in your home because of a permanent disability (a disability that doesn't go away).

Note: You cannot get Aid and Attendance benefits and Housebound benefits at the same time.

Who is covered:

- Qualified veterans
- Qualified surviving spouses

There are 2 ways you can get this benefit:

1. Write to your Pension Management Center (PMC). You can write to the PMC for your state.

Include this information:

Evidence, like a doctor's report, that shows you need Aid and Attendance or Housebound care, or VA Form 21-2680 (Examination for Housebound Status or Permanent Need for Regular Aid and Attendance), which your doctor can fill out.

Download VA Form 21-2680.

Details about what you normally do during the day and how you get places. Details that help show what kind of illness, injury, or mental or physical disability affects your ability to do things, like take a bath, on your own.

2. Apply in person; you can bring your information to a VA regional benefit office near you.

Board and Care Homes

Board and care homes are private and in residential settings. A board and care home can be a converted single-family home, duplex or apartment. These homes generally provide a room, meals, and living assistance. There is often a manager in place that helps with arranging for transportation, medications, and daily checks for well-being.

Adult Foster Care Homes

An adult foster care home offers a room and support services usually in a family setting. Foster care is for adults that need occasional or routine assistance with daily living. There is commonly more support in foster care than in a board and care home. There are adult foster care homes that have more complex care available with staff or visiting nurses.

Residential Care Facility (RCF)

A residential care facility is a group residence sometimes referred to as a board and care home or adult foster home. Rooms can be private or shared. The support is for meals, medication, bathing, dressing, eating, bathroom and care for people who cannot be left alone but do not necessitate skilled nursing care. Residential care facilities commonly also provide socialization and recreational activities.

Assisted Living Facility (ALF)

Assisted living facilities are designed for individuals that are somewhat self-sufficient but need some supervision and assistance. In certain states, the term 'assisted living' or 'assisted living facility' includes all types of group settings that provide support services. In other states, assisted living facilities are specially licensed and regulated by state law. In these states, assisted living facilities must provide the services and features the state requires. These facilities generally cater to people that do not need the same level of continuous nursing care that is found in a nursing home. People with Alzheimer's disease, or that need 'dementia care' are often housed in dedicated areas.

Medication management, personal care, bathing, grooming, eating or using the toilet, and is given as needed. Medical staff may be on-site or on call. People live in rooms or apartment-style accommodations. They provide group meals and often, social activities. The monthly charge for assisted living is determined by how much care a person requires and varies widely.

Assisted living facilities are generally private apartments with a bedroom, bathroom, small kitchen and living area. Others might have semiprivate sleeping areas and shared bathrooms.

Intermediate Care Facility (ICF)

This ICF provides 24-hour care for people that need help with bathing, grooming, toilet, and mobility. This is a choice for those seniors that cannot live independently. While skilled nursing is generally available, an ICF is not typically staffed 24 hours a day with a nurse. That would be the next step up in care or a 'Skilled Nursing Facility.'

Skilled Nursing Facility (SNF)

A skilled nursing facility or SNF is also referred to as a nursing home. There are nursing services available 24 hours a day for personal and medical care including administration of injections, blood pressure monitoring, managing ventilators and intravenous feedings. Medicaid or Medi-Cal in California might help with costs if you qualify.

The Eden (or Greenhouse) Alternative

The Eden Alternative is a program implemented by certain nursing facilities with the goal of a less institutional environment and more homelike. They encourage independence and interaction for residents and contact with plants, animals and children.

Continuing Care Retirement Communities (CCRCs)

CCRCs provide higher levels of care. A continuing care retirement community offers wide-ranging services including housing and nursing care. CCRCs require contracts that specify the services that will be provided and at what costs. These housing communities are often campus-like settings. Residents are assigned housing based on their needs and desires. Care can graduate as per a resident's needs. So, while you might move in living independently if daily care becomes compulsory, you can move to an assisted living section.

Some CCRCs require a sizeable upfront payment before moving in.

Long-Term Care

Long-term care is a description of a range of services and supports you might need to meet your personal care needs. Most long-term care is not medical care, but rather assistance with the basic personal tasks of everyday life, or the Activities of Daily Living (ADLs), such as:

- Bathing
- Dressing
- Using the toilet
- Transferring (to or from bed or chair)

- Caring for incontinence
- Eating

Other common long-term care services and supports are assistance with everyday tasks, sometimes called Instrumental Activities of Daily Living (IADLs) including:

- Housework
- Managing money
- Taking medication
- Preparing and cleaning up after meals
- Shopping for groceries or clothes
- Using the telephone or other communication devices
- Caring for pets
- Responding to emergency alerts such as fire alarms

According to LongTermCare.gov the national average costs for long-term care in the United States as of 2017 are:

- $225 a day or $6,844 per month for a semi-private room in a nursing home
- $253 a day or $7,698 per month for a private room in a nursing home
- $119 a day or $3,628 per month for care in an assisted living facility (for a one-bedroom unit)
- $20.50 an hour for a health aide
- $20 an hour for homemaker services
- $68 per day for services in an adult day health care center

The cost of long-term care depends on the type and duration of care you need, the provider you use, and where you live. Costs can be affected by certain factors, such as:

- Time of day. Home health and home care services, provided in two-to-four-hour blocks of time referred to as

"visits," are generally more expensive in the evening, on weekends, and on holidays
- Extra charges for services provided beyond the basic room, food and housekeeping charges at facilities, although some may have "all inclusive" fees
- Variable rates in some community programs, such as adult day service, are provided at a per-day rate, but can be more based on extra events and activities

Most long-term care is provided at home. Other kinds of long-term care services and supports are provided by community service organizations and in long-term care facilities. Examples of home care services include:

- An unpaid caregiver who may be a family member or friend
- A nurse, home health or home care aide, and/or therapist who comes to the home

Community support services include:

- Adult day care service centers
- Transportation services
- Home care agencies that provide services on a daily basis or as needed

Often these services supplement the care you receive at home or provide time off for your family caregivers.

Outside the home, a variety of facility-based programs offer more options:

- Nursing homes provide the most comprehensive range of services, including nursing care and 24-hour supervision
- Other facility-based choices include assisted living, board and care homes, and continuing care retirement communities. With these providers, the level of choice over who delivers your care varies by the type of facility. You may not get to choose

who will deliver services, and you may have limited say in when they arrive.

Participant Directed Services are a way to provide services that lets you control what services you receive, who provides them, and how and when those services are delivered. They provide you with information and assistance to choose and plan for the services and supports that work best for you including:

- Who you want to provide your services (can include family and friends)
- Whether you want to use a home care service agency

In facility-based services you generally do not have the option to hire someone independently, but you should have choices about:

- Which staff members provide your care
- The schedule you keep
- The meals you eat

In home and community-based settings, you should have the ability to participate or direct the development of a service plan, provide feedback on services and activities, and request changes as needed.

Veteran's Communities

There are veteran's communities in some states. These offer different levels of care starting with independent living with supportive health and social services, to complete skilled nursing facilities.

Visiting Facilities

When you have narrowed your choices, visit each facility and ask questions. Talk to residents and their family members whenever possible. The community should be clean and smell nice. Staff should be engaging with residents in a friendly and professional manner.

Additional information and assistance: Eldercare Locator at 800.677.1116 or www.eldercare.gov. The Eldercare Locator will direct you to the proper Area Agency on Aging in your location. They have information about state licensing and regulatory requirements and which facilities accept Medicaid.

Thoreau's Senior Living Options Planner

What to Ask Assisted Living or Board and Care Homes

	What to Ask Assisted Living or Board and Care Homes
	Is this community a social model or medical model?
	What type of licensed nurses are on staff? Examples: Registered nurse (RN) Licensed Practical or Vocational nurse (LPN/LVN) _____ _____ _____ _____ _____ _____ What days and hours are medical staff available? _____ _____ _____ _____ _____ _____
	What is the monthly rental amount including all services and fees (including any daily care)? _____ _____
	Is the contract month to month and if not, what is the term? _____

Thoreau's Senior Living Options Planner

What to Ask
Assisted Living or Board and Care Homes

Are meals and/or snacks included? How many meals per day?

_____

If so, what is the food? Ask for a menu or past weekly meal list.

_____
_____
_____
_____

Are special diet needs addressed?

_____
_____
_____
_____

Is there a dietician on staff?

_____
_____
_____

Are meals delivered to the room and/or is there a community dining area?

_____
_____
_____

Thoreau's Senior Living Options Planner

What to Ask
Assisted Living or Board and Care Homes

What transportation is included or available?

_____
_____
_____
_____

Within what radius is transportation included for medical and dental appointments?

_____
_____
_____

What is the emergency call system?

_____
_____
_____

Is the emergency call system staffed 24 hours a day?

What to Ask
Assisted Living or Board and Care Homes

What housekeeping, if any, is included and how often?

_____
_____
_____
_____
_____

What unit maintenance is included and what, if any, is not?

_____
_____
_____
_____
_____
_____
_____

Are any utilities not included?

_____
_____
_____

What social activities outside the facility are included? What acuity challenges and physical abilities are supported for these outings?

_____
_____
_____
_____
_____
_____
_____

Thoreau's Senior Living Options Planner

	What to Ask Assisted Living or Board and Care Homes
	What is the monthly base rate for this unit?
	What is the total monthly cost of my daily care including the base rate and all extras?
	What is the maximum monthly cost of all care you provide?
	At what point with what conditions and/or circumstances would I need to leave?
	Notes:

Thoreau's Senior Living Options Planner

Assisted Living Cost Comparison Worksheet

Cost (Before Insurance) Comparison Worksheet Compare Up to 4 Assisted Living Facilities or Communities				
Name of Choice 1				
Name of Choice 2				
Name of Choice 3				
Name of Choice 4				
	Amounts			
	Choice 1	**Choice 2**	**Choice 3**	**Choice 4**
Monthly Rent	$	$	$	$
Utilities Not Included (Estimate)	$	$	$	$
Extra Care Not Included	$	$	$	$
Transportation Not Included	$	$	$	$
Amenities Not Included	$	$	$	$
Therapy Not Included	$	$	$	$
Medication Management	$	$	$	$
Other _____	$	$	$	$
Other _____	$	$	$	$
Other _____	$	$	$	$
Totals (Add the columns)	**$**	**$**	**$**	**$**

Thoreau's Senior Living Options Planner

Group Living Worksheet

What is the basic monthly rate and what support services and amenities are included in that rate?

How many hours of service are included?

Can I save hours that I do not use during a day or week for a later time when I do need them?

Is there an entrance fee? Is it refundable?

Is there a waiting list?

Am I eligible for any support services through federal, state or local programs?

Thoreau's Senior Living Options Planner

Can I use my long-term care insurance policy to pay for support services? If so, what types of services and how many hours a day or week are they available? What would those additional costs be and how would I be billed?

_____
_____
_____
_____
_____

What happens if my needs change or increase?

_____
_____
_____

Will I be asked to sign an admissions agreement or a contract before I move in? Are there resources available to help me understand the contract?

_____
_____

Are my utilities included?

_____

Thoreau's Senior Living Options Planner

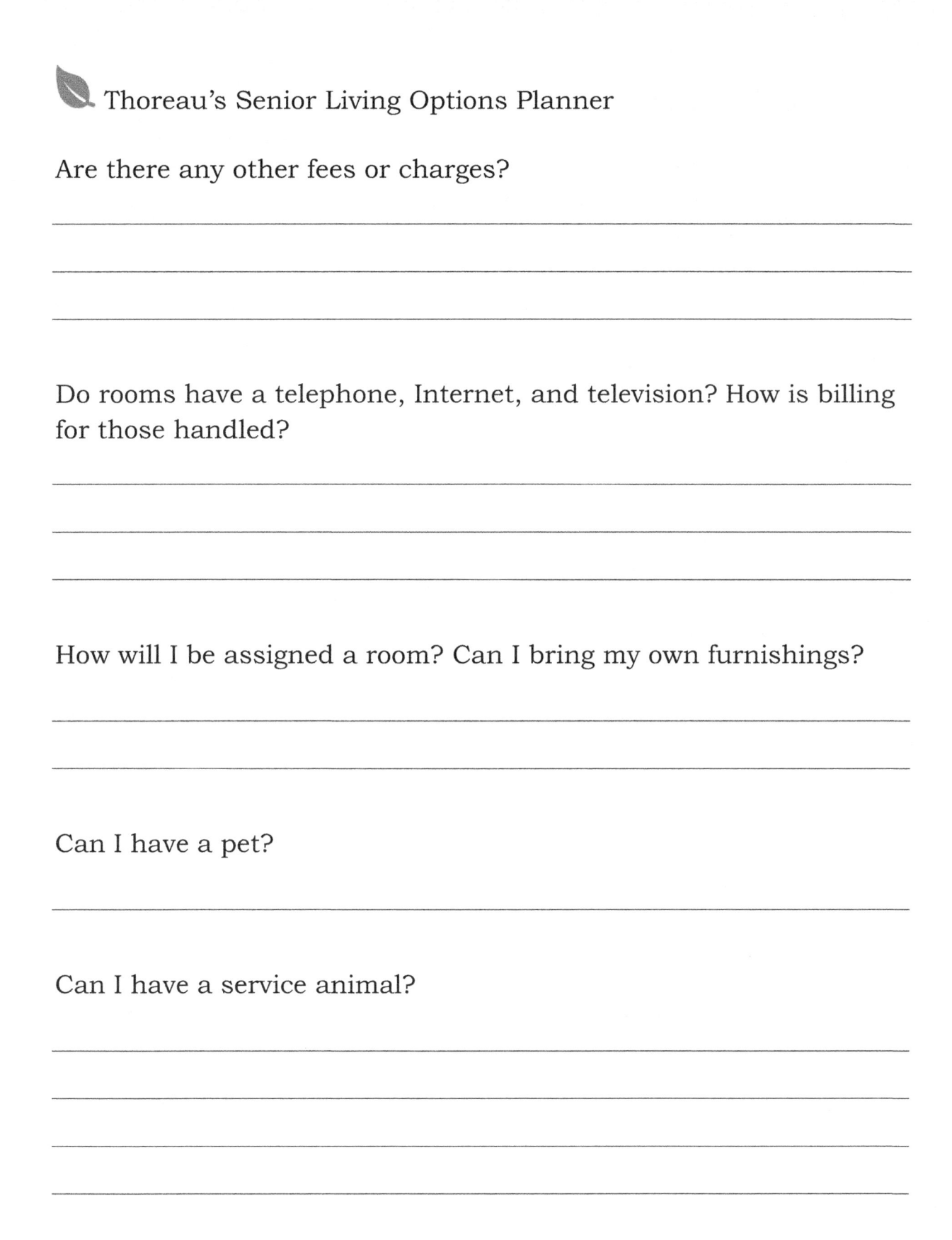

Are there any other fees or charges?

_____
_____
_____

Do rooms have a telephone, Internet, and television? How is billing for those handled?

_____
_____
_____

How will I be assigned a room? Can I bring my own furnishings?

_____
_____

Can I have a pet?

_____

Can I have a service animal?

_____
_____
_____
_____

Thoreau's Senior Living Options Planner

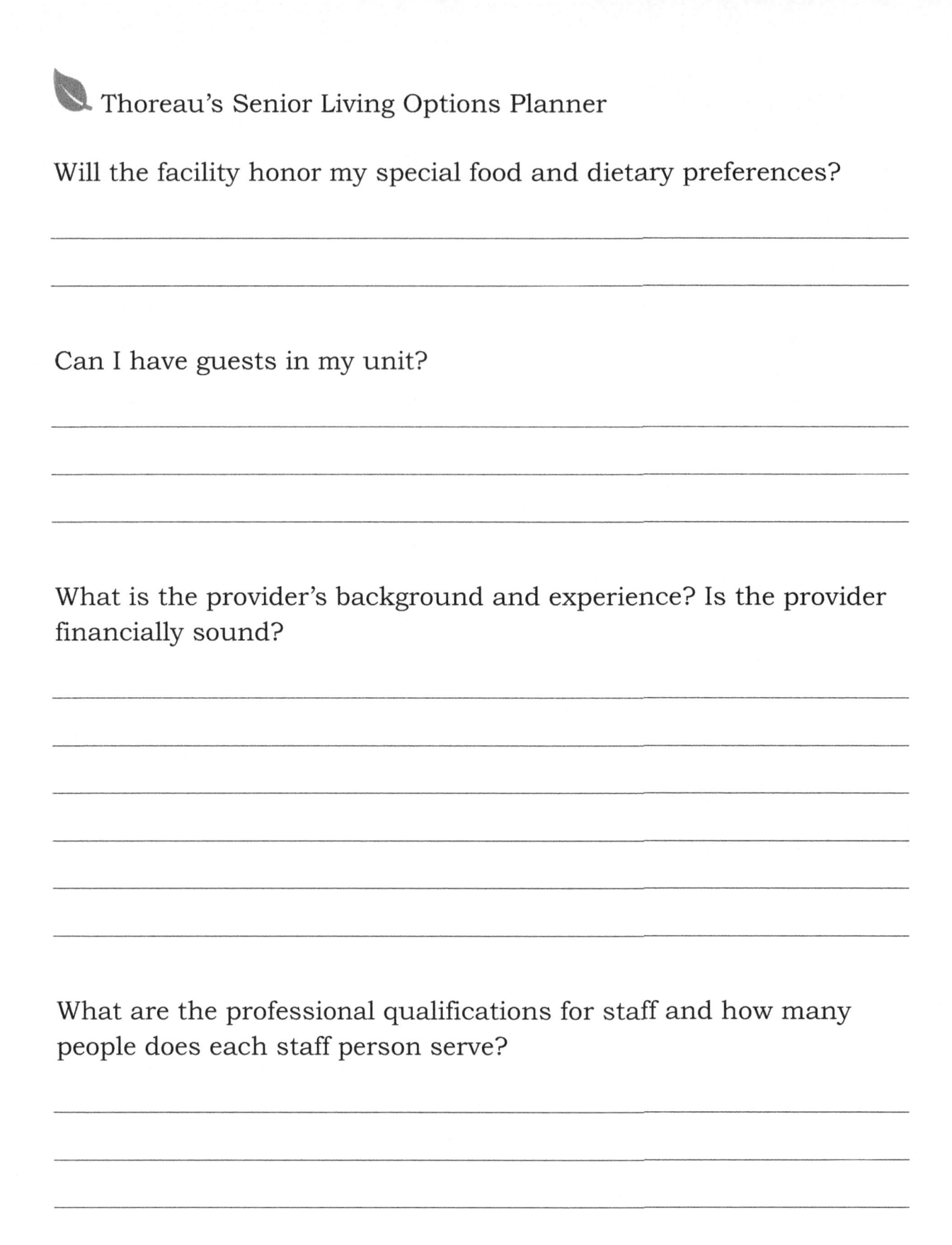

Will the facility honor my special food and dietary preferences?

Can I have guests in my unit?

What is the provider's background and experience? Is the provider financially sound?

What are the professional qualifications for staff and how many people does each staff person serve?

Thoreau's Senior Living Options Planner

What are the training requirements for the facility administrator and for the staff?

___

Does the facility have safety features? Does it have a disaster relief plan?

___

Is the facility close to shopping, senior centers, religious facilities, medical facilities, and other amenities that are important to me?

___

What happens if the facility asks me to leave?

___

Thoreau's Senior Living Options Planner

Have I received a copy of the facility's statement of resident rights?

___
___
___

Is there a resident council? Can I participate in facility management and decision making?

___
___
___

Thoreau's Senior Living Options Planner

Group Living Checklist

	Group Living Checklist
	Approximate Square Footage
	Level of Privacy
	Single Level
	Garage or Parking
	Kitchen
	Exterior and Lawn Maintenance
	Multi-Unit
	Detached Home
	Secure Space for Valuables
	Near Relatives
	Internet Services
	Pets
	Visitor Rules

Thoreau's Senior Living Options Planner

Group Living Checklist

Thoreau's Senior Living Options Planner

Notes About Group Living

Thoreau's Senior Living Options Planner

Notes About Group Living

Thoreau's Senior Living Options Planner

Disability or Mobility Needs Checklist

	Disability or Mobility Needs
	Accessory Dwelling Unit/Wheelchair Accessible
	Wheelchair-Accessible Bathroom and Shower
	Different Door Handles
	Lower Light Switches
	Bathroom Grab Bars
	Handrails
	Raised Toilet Seats
	Hall and Doorway Wheelchair Clearance
	Special Locks, Door Chimes and/or other Alert and Prevention Devices
	Hazard Review: Dangling Cords, Poisons, Slippery Surfaces, Unsteady Chairs, Throw Rugs, Electrical Cords, etc.
	Auto Shut Offs for Stove Tops, Coffee Makers, etc.
	Interior and Exterior Lighting
	Temperature Control
	Personal Emergency Notification System
	Facility Emergency Notification System

Thoreau's Senior Living Options Planner

	Disability or Mobility Needs

Thoreau's Senior Living Options Planner

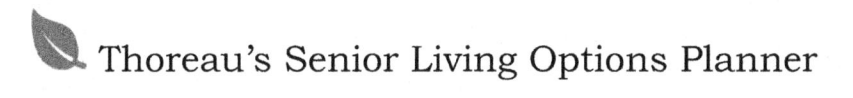

Thoreau's Senior Living Options Planner

Notes About Disability or Mobility

Thoreau's Senior Living Options Planner

Community Requirements Checklist

	Community Requirements
	Accessible Transportation
	Skilled Nursing Available
	Meals
	Socialization and Recreation
	Physician Location
	Place of Worship
	Family
	Grocery Shopping
	Other Shopping
	Prescription Availability and/or Delivery
	Health Specialists

Thoreau's Senior Living Options Planner

	Other Community Requirements

Thoreau's Senior Living Options Planner

Personal Needs Checklist

Yes or No	Personal Needs
	Mobility Assistance
	Grooming Assistance
	Eating Assistance
	Bathroom Assistance
	Meal Preparation
	Laundry Assistance
	Shopping Assistance
	Internet Access
	Phone
	Housekeeping
	Getting In and Out of Bed
	Dressing
	Managing Money

Thoreau's Senior Living Options Planner

Yes or No	Health and Medical Needs
	Medication Assistance
	Injection Assistance
	Equipment Monitoring
	Blood Pressure Monitoring
	Intravenous Feeding

Thoreau's Senior Living Options Planner

Notes About Personal, Health and Medical Needs

Notes About Personal, Health and Medical Needs

Thoreau's Senior Living Options Planner

Notes About Group Housing

Thoreau's Senior Living Options Planner

Notes About Group Housing

Thoreau's Senior Living Options Planner

Notes About Group Housing

8. Living Options and Insurance

"To know that we know what we know, and that we do not know what we do not know, that is true knowledge."
– Henry David Thoreau

Note: As insurance offerings and rules and regulations are ever changing, and can get complex, this is only an introduction and brief description of insurance options.

Medicare

Medicare is a Federal health insurance program, which helps defray many of the medical expenses of most Americans over the age of 65. Medicare has two parts:

(Part A) Hospital Insurance helps pay the cost of inpatient hospital care. The number of days in the hospital paid for by Medicare is governed by a system based upon patient diagnosis and medical necessity for hospital care. Once it is no longer medically necessary for the person to remain in the hospital, the physician will begin the discharge process. If the person or the family disagrees with this decision, they may appeal to the state's Peer Review Organization.

Medicare does not pay for custodial care or nursing home care. It will, however, help cover the expenses of a stay in a skilled nursing facility after a qualifying hospital stay (inpatient care in a hospital for three or more days).

There are strict requirements for getting your stay covered. You must check into the skilled nursing facility within 30 days of being discharged from the hospital. The first 20 days of your stay will be covered completely by Medicare. Around 80% of the cost of your stay will be covered for up to 80 days. After that, you will be responsible for full payment.

Thoreau's Senior Living Options Planner

The condition that the facility helps to care for must be the same that you were admitted to the hospital in order to address. Care must be administered every day in order to continue qualifying for coverage and must be administered by a "skilled" worker such as a physician, physical therapist, licensed practical nurse, or registered nurse.

(Part B) Medical Insurance pays for many medically necessary doctors' services, outpatient services, and some other medical services. Enrollees pay a monthly premium.

Medicare will cover the cost of part-time home health care for homebound seniors. Homebound or housebound refers to anyone who is unable to leave their home without assistance and are thus "confined." Your doctor must certify that you are homebound. You must have a physician who regularly updates and reviews your plan of care and certifies that you need skilled nursing, physical therapy, speech pathology, or continuing occupational therapy in order to qualify.

For your therapy treatments to be covered, they need to be considered safe, effective, and reliable ways to treat your condition with a clear and "reasonable" timeline established for your improvement or recovery. You will need to work with a home health care agency that has been certified by Medicare.

Medicare may cover 100% of the cost of home health care if you meet all qualifications and up to 20% of the cost of durable medical equipment such as commode chairs, oxygen equipment, and walkers.

Before signing up with an agency, have a discussion with them about any services they provide that are not covered by Medicare. Make sure to get documentation regarding any charges you may be responsible for. All providers should issue you an Advance Beneficiary Notice (ABN) before you receive any goods and services that may not be covered by Medicare.

Adult day health care centers are also covered under Medicare if the care there is prescribed and medically necessary as determined by your physician and state guidelines. These centers provide medical as well as non-medical services such as crafts, social services, and help with Activities of Daily Living.

Medicaid

Medicaid is a joint federal-state health care program for people with a low income. The program is administered by each state and the type of services covered differs. There are strict income requirements, so it may be necessary for the person to "spend down" all income and assets to poverty levels before becoming eligible. Medicaid is the major payer of nursing home care.

While Medicaid coverage varies state-by-state, there are certain federal requirements that force all states to pay for nursing home care or home health care services for all who medically and financially qualify. Those who do not qualify for a nursing home care may be eligible for financial aid to minimize the costs of assisted living facilities or housekeeping services.

In every state, Medicaid is required to cover the cost of adult day cares. These are institutions that provide structure and care to seniors and give respite to family caretakers. Every state has Home and Community Based Services Waiver Programs that help individuals continue to live in their homes. Nursing Home Diversion Programs may also exist in your state that will help pay for the cost of adult day care.

Rules defining nursing home care as "medically necessary" for an individual varies across states. Talk to your care provider to find out if you qualify. All states require that your physician certifies your need.

Income guidelines to qualify for Medicaid vary by the kind of long-term care that you need and by state. Most states have more flexibility on income limits regarding long-term care reimbursement than they do with Medicaid eligibility. Contact your local Medicaid office to discuss the specifics of your situation.

Seniors often pay privately when they enter a nursing facility and then "spend down" until they have reached the Medicaid guidelines for financial assistance. Be aware that you can spend your money on anything to reach requirements, not just your care. You cannot, however, give away assets or sell them at below market value in order to qualify. Medicaid will look at the sale of assets for the past five years to determine whether you have sold them at "fair market price."

If Medicaid finds that you have sold assets below market value, you will be penalized. The value of any assets you transferred will be divided by the monthly cost of nursing care in your state. Using this calculation, Medicaid will arrive at a penalty period for which you will be unable to receive benefits.

There are several categories of assets that are not counted when calculating your eligibility for Medicaid. Your house, one car, personal assets, properly structured 401Ks, and IRAs, assets that cannot be sold, and rental properties are all non-countable. A Medicaid lawyer can help you to legally convert countable assets into non-countable.

The Medicaid requirement to "spend down" all income and assets created great hardship for the spouse of a person needing nursing home care. Changes in the Medicaid rules now allow the spouse to keep a monthly income and some assets, including the primary residence. The amounts allowed change, so you must check for current levels.

In addition to spousal impoverishment protection rules regarding assets, all states have rules in place to protect the income of a healthy spouse. Your state will determine the amount of income a healthy spouse can earn by calculating their "Minimum Monthly Maintenance Needs Allowance (MMMNA)." That income will be exempt, and Medicaid will disregard that money when they calculate the Medicaid eligibility of the needy spouse.

Another option to avoid spending down is to establish a Qualified Income Trust (QIT) or Miller Trust. This is a restricted funds account. Each month, any money that you earn in excess of the allowable limits to qualify for Medicaid will be deposited into this account and may only be used for medical bills and care costs. QITs are irreversible. Make sure to talk to your family members and a lawyer before establishing such a trust.

Other Insurance

Why buy other insurance? The purchase of additional insurance gives the policyholder access to a greater choice of facilities without dipping into additional financial resources.

Medigap is privately purchased supplemental health insurance designed to help cover some of the gaps in Medicare coverage but does not cover long-term care. Study Medigap policies carefully to be sure they provide the protection needed and do not duplicate other health insurance.

Medigap plans usually help to cover expenses that would otherwise be out-of-pocket such as co-payments, coinsurances, and deductibles. Those who enroll in the program within 6 months of turning 65, or within 6 months of enrolling in Medicare Part B will get the best rates. Medigap plans are guaranteed to be renewable, which means that health problems will not get you removed from coverage.

Long-Term Care Insurance is private insurance that is usually either an indemnity policy or part of an individual life insurance policy. An indemnity policy pays a set amount per day for nursing home or home health care. Under the life insurance policy, a certain percentage of the death benefit is paid for each month the policyholder requires long-term care. Policies are priced differently depending on the age of the policyholder, the deductible periods are chosen, and indemnity value or duration of benefits.

Long-Term Care Insurance will allow you more flexibility in choosing the terms of your care and your care providers. Most policies will not cover those with certain pre-existing conditions such as Alzheimer's, dementia, MS, or Parkinson's. Before purchasing a Long-Term Care Insurance policy, be sure that there is a guarantee that the policy cannot be terminated based on deteriorating mental or physical health.

Purchasing a life insurance policy with long-term care benefits is expensive but has benefits. You will pay a large upfront fee to establish the account (on average, $75,000), but you will avoid the pain of rate hikes later.

This is an attractive option if you have an established life insurance plan. You can "roll over" the cash value of your old plan to purchase a hybrid policy tax-free. In this case, your beneficiary will not receive any money that you used on long-term care. If you are currently healthy, you may be able to get a discount on a plan if you submit yourself to a medical exam and present your medical records to the insurance company.

Long-Term Care Partnership Programs: Many states have Long-Term Care Partnership Programs. This is an initiative that allows you to protect yourself from having to spend down some of your assets should you need to apply for Medicaid after using up your Maximum Lifetime Benefits. The state will allow you to keep one dollar in assets for each dollar you have spent on your long-term care plan.

For Family Caregivers: Family Medical Leave Act and Family-Friendly Leave

The Family Medical Leave Act allows you to take up to twelve weeks off annually to help care for a family member without putting your job at risk. Family leave loans are available to help sustain you during these periods.

If you think you may need to care for an elderly relative, be sure to check the provisions of the 1993 Family Leave Act on taking leave for this purpose and contact a leave specialist in your agency.

Department of State employees can contact a department leave specialist in the Office of Employee Relations HR/ER/WLD about paid and unpaid leave at 202-261-8160.

FMLA covers those who have worked with their firm for at least 12 months, have clocked over 1,250 hours, and has at least 50 employees within 75 miles of your location. If your employer denies or interferes with your FMLA request, let them know of the federal mandates and consider calling a lawyer.

Note:

Websites, web pages, contact information and phone numbers commonly change. If you find that a phone number referred to herein is disconnected, or a web address is no longer valid, please let me know. My contact information is at the end of this book.

Thank you!

9. What Do You Need to Know About Senior Mobile Home Parks and Communities?

"I have learned that even the smallest house can be a home."
– Henry David Thoreau

Senior Mobile Home Parks

Buying a mobile home in a senior community or park is a hybrid option so to speak. You own the home yet will rent the space or property on which the home sits. Many seniors purchase a mobile home as their sole residence or as a part-time home.

Senior mobile home parks function like age-restricted Home Ownership Associations. The minimum age is typically set at 55 years old. Common spaces like pools, spas, and club houses are maintained by the park staff. Individual lots are maintained by mobile homeowners who must adhere to rules and regulations established by the park and agreed to in a housing contract.

Locations

You can find senior mobile home communities across America, though coastal real estate is popular. Most senior mobile home parks are in Florida, Arizona, California, and Washington State. Florida boasts over 350 parks.

Full Time or Snowbird?

Being able to escape cold winters and hot summers may be ideal, which is why most senior mobile home communities are set in areas that stay warm yearlong. However, this lifestyle is cost prohibitive for many.

Before making the decision to become a snowbird, you must take a realistic assessment of the costs. Owning or renting two homes is more expensive than one, but that is just the beginning. You may also have to pay property taxes in both states. Separate income tax and inheritance and estate taxes may also affect your financial situation.

Living full time in a senior mobile home community also comes with its pros and cons. You will reduce the amount of travel you have each year, which is especially useful if you own a pet. You will avoid the hassle of winterizing your home each year. You will not have to change your mailing address or cancel your subscriptions.

However, summer heat and humidity can be dangerous, and year-round living means you will miss out on the vacation-like feeling that snowbirds enjoy.

What to Look For

Do your research before becoming a resident of a mobile home park. The Florida Bar Association suggests that you run free public record searches for "red flags" including:

- Check if park owners commonly evict tenants
- See if the park is dealing with any legal issues that would prevent you from buying, including "liens" and "judgements"
- Contact the DMV and verify that the seller of the mobile home is actually the owner
- Check for back taxes and hidden liens

Legal issues are not the only thing that need to be addressed. Look for compatibility with you and your lifestyle before investing in a community. Ask to see the rules and regulations, park prospectus, and community. Here is a list of preliminary questions to ask:

Thoreau's Senior Living Options Planner

1. What is the preferred method of transportation around the park? Are golf carts allowed?
2. Are there guest restrictions? Who is allowed to visit the park? How long can they stay before the park charges you a fee?
3. How many cars are allowed on my lot? How much does guest parking cost?
4. What amenities do you have? Ask the park how active members are in your favorite clubs and activities.

Schedule a park visit before signing an agreement. See if you can attend a social event to check for like-minded people within the community. Talk to them about any questions or concerns you have.

Consider reaching out to past owners to see how and why they left the park.

Financing

Financing is always difficult but becomes even harder when borrowing on a mobile home. Traditional banks often won't lend to mobile home buyers.

If you are planning to buy your mobile home new, you may find that your retailer can direct you towards a funding source. Ask them for their recommendations and non-affiliated lenders.

There are also specialized mobile home lenders. You may need to check with your park manager for recommendations.

The Federal Housing Administration (FHA) and the Veterans Administration (VA) both have loan opportunities available for mobile homes. There are several criteria that you must meet. Call your local offices for more information.

Thoreau's Senior Living Options Planner

What are All the Costs?

When setting a budget, you need to be aware of all the costs associated with renting and maintain your mobile home. Here is what you should include:

Mobile home rent or mortgage: In most mobile home communities, you will rent the land and buy your home. Calculate your average rent or mortgage costs. If you are buying, remember to include interest.

Leased land: Each month, you will pay rent to the park. Prices will vary based on the lot size, amenities, activities, and location. Check to see what utilities will be included in your lot rent so that you can set aside additional money for services not covered by the park.

Irregular expenses: You will need to make repairs and upgrades to your mobile home. Consider purchasing insurance and setting aside money each month to ensure a stable living situation.

What is Typically Included in Lot Rent?

Read your lease agreement carefully to find out what is included in rent and what services are optional. Though parks vary, here are a few typical services include in lot rent:

Garbage pick-up: This fee may be included in your lot rent or listed as an extra fee on your bill. In either case, this is a bill you'll be paying.

Utilities: Mobile homes will provide utilities but how you are billed varies. Some parks divide the energy and water bills equally between all residents, while others bill residents individually. Sometimes, a park may offer a flat rate.

Upkeep: Your park may offer free gardening and maintenance for your mobile home.

Thoreau's Senior Living Options Planner

Amenities

Here is a list of typical amenities offered at senior mobile home parks across the country:

Clubhouse

Library

Pools

Spa

Fitness center

Tennis courts

Walking trails

Billiard room

Line dancing

Community luncheons

Potluck dinners

Ice cream socials

Coffee socials

Holiday parties

Bazaars

BBQs

Hobby clubs

Water aerobics

Shuffleboard

Bocce ball courts

Pickleball courts

Horseshoes

Thoreau's Senior Living Options Planner

Craft classes

Table tennis

Bingo

Card games

Poker tournaments

Do Mobile Home Communities Have Security?

In general, mobile home communities do not provide security.

If you are looking for additional security, you may have to pay extra to be part of one of the gated senior mobile home parks. However, this isn't your only option. Neighborhood watches can be an effective way to deter criminals. Safes for your valuables and security systems are other options. Some people even purchase "fake" security systems. These are cameras and signs that signal a security system even when one isn't there.

Carports, Garages, and Storage Sheds

Some manufactured homes come with built-in garages, though many do not. You may be able to purchase your own carport or storage shed to place on your lot depending on the amount of land you have left and the terms of your lease.

If you need additional storage, check with your park to see what options are available to you. Many park owners sell and lease sheds to tenants.

Taxes

When purchasing your home, you will pay a sales tax.

You will also pay annual property taxes on your mobile home. These rules are complicated and vary by county and state.

No matter where you are located, the property tax will be based on the value of both the land and the home itself. Some counties will give one tax bill to the landowner and another to the homeowner, while others will issue just one bill.

Here are a few examples of taxes in different states:

Florida: You will pay a 6% sales tax on the purchase of your mobile home as of this writing. You may also be responsible for county sales taxes.

Each year, you will have to purchase a mobile home decal. This is a registration tax, and the price depends on the size of your vehicle.

Any improvements on your property such as sheds, porches, or skirting will be subject to a tangible personal property tax.

California: You will pay a 7.25% sales tax on the purchase of your mobile home as of this writing or a use tax if you bought your home out-of-state.

Each year, you will be expected to pay either your local property tax or an annual vehicle license fee. Which tax you are subject to will depend on the year your home was originally purchased.

Arizona: The Arizona sales tax rate is 5.6% as of this writing, but you can expect to pay local sales taxes in addition when you purchase your mobile home.

Your home will be subject to personal property taxes each year. The cost of this will vary depending on your county, city, mobile home park, and the year that your home was built.

Call the county assessor to get an idea of the figures.

What About Maintenance?

Just like your family home, a mobile home needs routine maintenance and inspection. Here are a few ways you can keep your new home in good shape:

Level: Check that your mobile home is level each year. The structure can begin to sink without proper care, causing leaks, cracks, and issues with the doors and windows.

Roof: Many mobile homes have flat roofs which need to be treated regularly. Check local regulation as some states require you to recoat or reseal each year.

Skirting: Your skirting protects your home from pests, provides ventilation, and acts as an insulator. Keep your skirting in good repair and replace as necessary.

Set aside 1–3% of the cost of your home for repairs each year.

Hidden Costs

When taking out a loan for a mobile home, pay attention to the interest rate your bank is offering. As mobile homes are considered "personal" property rather than "real" property, interest rates are often higher than for a single-family home.

Another difference between traditional real estate and mobile homes is appreciation. While a well-maintained single-family home will appreciate over your lifetime, your mobile home is more likely to depreciate.

Insurance

Insurance for mobile homes is like homeowner's insurance. You will be able to choose a standard policy or one that is suited to your needs. While you aren't required to purchase coverage by law, your mortgage lender or senior mobile home park may require you have proof of insurance.

A standard policy will include dwelling coverage, personal property coverage, and liability.

Dwelling coverage will help rebuild and repair physical damage to your property by covered peril. Many policies do not cover fire damage.

Personal property coverage will provide protection for stolen or damaged goods. Liability will protect you if someone is injured on your lot.

You may also obtain coverage for garages or sheds, and additional living expenses in case you are unable to stay in your mobile home due to damage.

Emergency Services

Find out how far away police, fire, ambulance services, and the hospital are from the considered location. Some municipalities also publish average response times to specific areas.

Selling

If you own your home free and clear, you can sell your property on the open market, ask your park manager for help, or enlist a real estate agent. Check to make sure your realtor has a special RE license to sell personal property if you choose to contract with them.

If you still have a mortgage on your home, you will need to pay off your lien and add yourself as the lien holder. You can do this by finding a qualified buyer. They will be able to pay off your lien with a down payment. Then you can transfer ownership to them.

Selling mobile homes can be difficult. Since your senior mobile home community functions like a home ownership association, your buyer will need to be approved by the community. This usually means they'll have to pass a background check including their criminal record and credit report.

What Happens If I Pass Away?

As with other property, you can designate ownership of your mobile home to whomever you choose after your passing. Depending on the value of the property and the rules of the state, the property may go through probate or pass immediately into the hands of your relative after a title transfer.

Thoreau's Senior Living Options Planner

10. Is Moving in with Family the Right Option for You?

"The child may soon stand face to face with the best father."
– Henry David Thoreau

Moving in with Family Forms

Completed ✓	This chapter contains the following checklists, forms, questionnaires, and/or worksheets:
	Practical and Lifestyle: What to Ask Yourself Before Moving in with Your Family Form
	Practical and Lifestyle Questionnaire for Host Family Members
	Family Living Space Questionnaire
	Safety, Disability and/or Mobility Considerations Questionnaire
	Living with Family Relationship Worksheet for You
	Living with Family Relationship Worksheet for Your Family
	Household Rules for Living with Family Form
	Home Preparation Costs Planning Form
	Living Expenses Planning Form

This section will help you evaluate your option to move in with family. The questionnaires and forms also aid in addressing concerns of everyone involved and establishing parameters to help make your experience joyful and organized.

Moving in with family can be an opportunity to bond in a multigenerational experience. Having family around can help you avoid the depression that can come with isolation, receive aid with daily living, and keep a watch out for changes in your health needs.

However, due to family dynamics and history, finances, personalities and unresolved issues, without planning this can be the recipe for disaster.

Asking questions and addressing issues before moving in can help make the transition go smoother and enrich the living experience. The following forms and worksheets have been designed to help you and your family consider issues and items and help you plan.

1. Practical and Lifestyle Aspects
2. Living Space
3. Relationships
4. Financial Considerations
   a) Preparation Costs
   b) Living Expenses

Practical and Lifestyle Aspects of Moving in with Family

This category includes the practical considerations of moving in with family members. For example:

Would you be relocating to a new town, city or even climate?
Relocating to a different town or state will require you to acclimate to new surroundings, locate services such as the local pharmacy, doctors, bank, grocery stores, faith-related community, senior facilities, the library, recreation center and others. There might also

be adult day care centers, meals, counseling and therapeutic activities in the area.

Will you need to arrange any in-home services?
If respite care, a caregiver, or home health professional is needed, these services should be arranged beforehand or soon after moving in. Establish who pays for these services and how.

Will you have your own transportation?
You might still drive and will have a vehicle that needs parking. Otherwise you can become dependent on family members for rides or will need to check out local transportation.

Will your social life be disrupted?
If you are moving far you will want to establish a social network in your family's community. This can include joining local organizations and/or finding a church or faith-based community.

Thoreau's Senior Living Options Planner

Practical and Lifestyle Aspects: What to Ask Yourself Before Moving in with Your Family Form

Yes/No	Questions to Ask Yourself
	Does moving in with my family require me to relocate a long distance from my current home?
	Will I be moving to an area with a different climate? If so, how will that affect your daily life and activities? _____ _____ _____ _____
	Will moving in with my family change my social life? If so, what will you do to reestablish a social network after you move? _____ _____ _____ _____ _____ _____ _____ _____ _____ _____

Thoreau's Senior Living Options Planner

Yes/No	Questions to Ask Yourself
	Will moving in with my family take me away from any activities such as gym recreation, bowling league, exercise, or other clubs and organizations? If so, list what you can investigate in your new location: _____ _____ _____ _____ _____ _____
	Will moving in with my family members require me to relocate and take me away from friends or people I love? If this is the case, how can I stay connected with those people? _____ _____ _____ _____ _____ _____ _____ _____ _____

Thoreau's Senior Living Options Planner

Yes/No	Questions to Ask Yourself
	Will moving in with my family change my current mode of transportation? If so, what will you do to replace your form of transportation and keep you from being solely dependent on family members for rides? _____ _____
	Will moving in with my family take away any of my independence? If so, will I feel resentful or appreciative? _____ _____
	Will moving in with my family place me in any unfamiliar situations that make me uncomfortable (such as around children, a hectic environment, constantly meeting new people, etc.)? _____ _____

Thoreau's Senior Living Options Planner

Yes/No	Questions to Ask Yourself
	Will I be moving any pets in with me? What special considerations for my pets are needed? _____ _____ _____
	Do I expect to be happy living with my family members? If not, why? _____ _____ _____ _____
	Meal Planning Do you have specific foods you eat or a special diet? _____ _____ _____ Who will prepare meals, and will you eat with family? _____ _____ Who will pay for food and how will this be divided? _____ _____ _____ _____

Practical and Lifestyle Questionnaire for Host Family Members Form

Yes/No	**Living with Family: Lifestyle Questions for Family or Host**
	Does anyone smoke tobacco or marijuana? If so, are there specific smoking rules and what are they?
	Does anyone involved have a pet or pets? If there are pets, are those pets safe for everyone that will be living in the home and any visitors?
	Who is responsible for which pets?
	Who will be allowed to feed the pet(s)?

Thoreau's Senior Living Options Planner

Yes/No	Living with Family: Lifestyle Questions for Family or Host
	What are the specific parameters for the pet(s)?
	Will your (father, mother, relative) be permitted or advised not to answer the door when no one else is home?
	Do you have an alarm system?
	If you have an alarm system will your (father, mother, relative) and/or any required health care helpers be given the code and password? If so, keep a list of anyone this is given to. Change the code and password when any caregiver quits, is terminated or is no longer needed.
	What keys will your (father, mother, relative) need?

Thoreau's Senior Living Options Planner

Yes/No	Living with Family: Lifestyle **Questions for Family or Host**
	Are there any areas that will be considered off limits for your (father, mother, relative)? _____ _____ _____ _____
	Does your relative have a vehicle they will be bringing?
	Where will this vehicle be parked? _____
	Are there parameters for visitors? If so, what are they? _____ _____ _____ _____ _____ _____

Thoreau's Senior Living Options Planner

Yes/No	**Living with Family: Lifestyle** ***Questions for Family or Host***
	Meal Planning Does your parent or relative require specific foods or a special diet?
	Who will prepare meals?
	Will your family members eat together or at the same times as your parent or relative?
	Who will pay for food?

Thoreau's Senior Living Options Planner

Living Space

Moving in with family members will require planning. In addition to the space requirements, there might also be special needs for mobility or vision issues for example. Seniors can require special adaptations. Some of these changes are not expensive but will require time and planning for installation.

Note: *This section is mostly for host families or household members.*

Consider where your parent/relative will stay in your home and if anyone will be displaced from their room or inconvenienced. If needed and within your budget, consider a room addition.

Some home health agencies will perform home evaluations for senior and special needs living for safety and mobility. Evaluate the available space for privacy and mobility and avoid stairs when possible. See the lists at the end of this section for more considerations.

Moving

When moving a parent into your home, he or she will have clothing, personal items, and depending on the length of stay expected and space available, maybe furniture and personal items.

This is often the time your parent or relative will need to downsize their belongings. Thoreau's Downsizing Planner for Seniors will help with planning a successful downsize and move. Thoreau's Downsizing Planner for Seniors is available through Amazon at:

https://www.amazon.com/dp/B079SJNFPM

Privacy

Privacy is a consideration for your family and your relative that will move in. This includes bedroom and bathroom privacy and possibly a private entrance to the area. If caregivers are entering your home, you and your family will want to maintain your privacy with these people also.

You might need to declare certain areas off limits and even install interior door locks for those rooms, especially if your relative has any cognitive challenges that might cause him or her to wander or become disoriented.

Home Prepping

To prepare your home for a senior relative, consider their needs for:

- space
- privacy
- safety
- living accommodations

Stairs – If your relative has any challenge with stairs, consider an electric stair lift. While they are expensive, they can be less than the cost of adding a room on a first floor if none is available.

The chair lifts provide a safe alternative to staircases. The lifts are electric motorized chairs that attach to a rail that still allows use of the stairs by other household members.

Otherwise make stairs as safe as possible with non-slip surfaces or low pile carpeting, nightlights, and a strong banister or handrail.

Bedroom

Your relative should have a private bedroom that provides enough space for belongings, wardrobe, and any needed safety, mobility, and health equipment needed.

Bed height is another important factor for seniors and mobility. When knees are higher than hips while in a sitting position on the edge of the bed, the bed height is too low. If feet are not touching the floor the bed height is too high.

Bathroom

The bathroom should be close to your relative's bedroom and on the same floor. Use non-slip mats on bathroom floors and if needed in bathtubs and showers. Taller commodes are available and appreciated by most seniors. There are also lids with removable arms.

Consider installing a walk-in tub. Add a stool for seating and install safety rails near the commode and in the shower or bathtub. There are safety rails that can double as towel bars. Towel bars are not designed for people to stable themselves or prevent a fall. Consider replacing them with secured safety bars.

Clutter

Provide adequate storage and organizational space for your relative's belongings to help them stay clutter free. Realize they might need some assistance to stay organized.

Emergency Intercom

Installing an emergency intercom in your guest's bedroom so they can alert you if needed is a great idea.

Nightlights

Keep hallways, bathrooms, and doorways illuminated with nightlights.

Electrical Cords

Electrical cords can be a trip and fall hazard. Tape cords down if needed and run them out of the way behind furniture.

Medication

Store medications in a daily pill organizer in the bathroom, bedroom, or kitchen. Make sure all medication is labeled and kept out of reach and secured from accessibility by children.

Living Areas

Like beds, chairs should be the right height. You can add cushions to raise seat height when needed. Make sure all chairs and other furniture is secure and not wobbly. Remove throw rugs and check all thresholds for hazards.

Lighting

Lights need to illuminate enough and be working. Add more floor or ceiling light if needed. Install the 'Clapper' in areas such as the bedroom so the senior can get into bed with the light on and then shut the light out. Use motion-sensor lights outdoors for entry and exit areas.

Railings and Banisters

Make sure secure railings and banisters are installed in stairways, bathrooms and anywhere else needed. All steps and stairways should always be well lit.

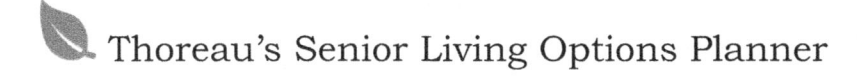

Kitchen

Keep items that your relative will use within their reach.

Tools

Keep tools and chemicals in a secure place. If your relative has dementia, these items can cause injury.

Outside

If your parent or loved one is at risk for wandering, keep doors closed and locked and install alarms. You can also investigate a Bluetooth tracking device if the situation warrants.

Complete the following 'Safety, Disability and/or Mobility Considerations Questionnaire.'

Note: For estimating the costs of home prepping, there is a 'Home Preparation Costs Planning Form' in the 'Financial Considerations' section found later in this chapter.

Living with Family: Space Questionnaire

Yes/No	Living with Family: Living Space
	Questions for Host Person or Family
	Will you have a local home health agency perform a home evaluation of your home prior to having your relative move in? _____ _____
	Do you have room in your home to provide the privacy your parent or relative is comfortable with, and to maintain your family's privacy?
	Do you have a private bathroom for your new resident?
	Is there a separate entrance for your relative?
	Who will provide the needed furniture?
	Will your home accommodations be sufficient for the next one to three years?
	Is any remodeling required to build accommodations such as a bedroom, bathroom or private entrance? If the answer is 'yes,' who will pay for this and how? _____ _____ _____

Thoreau's Senior Living Options Planner

Yes/No	Living with Family: Living Space
	Questions for Host Person or Family
	How long is any remodeling expected to take until complete? _____ Expected Completion Date: _____ Expected Move-In Date: _____

Thoreau's Senior Living Options Planner

Safety, Disability and/or Mobility Considerations Questionnaire

Yes or No	Living with Family: Safety, Disability and/or Mobility Considerations
	Questions for Host Person or Family
	Does your new resident need to and is he or she capable of navigating steps or stairs safely?
	Can your (father, mother, relative) easily and safely 'lock and unlock' and 'open and close' all doors in your home?
	Can your (father, mother, relative) easily navigate and exit your home in an emergency from any location?
	Can your (father, mother, relative) easily reach all interior and exterior light switches, door handles, locks, and faucets in your home?
	Can your (father, mother, relative) smell natural gas?
	Can your (father, mother, relative) feel when water is too hot?
	Can your (father, mother, relative) hear all alarms, alerts, doorbells, and phones in your home?
	If your (father, mother, relative) needs a walker or wheelchair, is your home completely accessible?
	Will your (father, mother, relative) be permitted to set any temperature controls and if so, can he or she read, reach, and adjust all temperature controls?

Thoreau's Senior Living Options Planner

Yes or No	Living with Family: Safety, Disability and/or Mobility Considerations
	Questions for Host Person or Family
	Will areas need to be wheelchair accessible?
	Do any different door handles need to be installed?
	Will handrails for assistance be installed in the bathroom? Near commode and in shower area. _____ _____ _____
	Are handrails needed anywhere else in the home such as entry and exit areas? If so, where? _____ _____ _____ _____ _____ _____ _____
	Will a raised toilet seat or taller commode be installed? When the senior's knees are higher than hips while in a sitting position, the commode height is too low. If feet are not touching the floor the height is too high.

Thoreau's Senior Living Options Planner

Yes or No	Living with Family: Safety, Disability and/or Mobility Considerations
	Questions for Host Person or Family
	Hall and Doorway Wheelchair Clearance Will any halls or doorways need to be widened for wheelchair (or walker) clearance?
	Will special locks, door chimes and/or other alert and prevention devices be installed?
	Auto Shut Offs for Stove Tops, Coffee Makers, etc.
	Interior and Exterior Lighting
	Temperature Control
	Are laundry facilities easily accessible?
	Hazard Review: Dangling Cords, Poisons, Slippery Surfaces, Unsteady Chairs, Throw Rugs, Electrical Cords, etc.
	Hot Water Maximum Temperature Set to 120 Degrees F
	Is the bed height correct? When the senior's knees are higher than hips while in a sitting position on the edge of the bed, the bed height is too low. If feet are not touching the floor the bed height is too high.
	Will an emergency intercom be installed?
	Will a third-party emergency alert system be used?

Thoreau's Senior Living Options Planner

Financial Considerations

Financial Considerations for Your Family

Having an elderly relative move into your home can require renovation costs and added daily living expenses. Depending on your parent's mobility and other needs, you might have to install safety features and even add or remodel rooms. These costs can add up fast.

If a walker or wheelchair is required, doorways need to be at least 36 inches wide, some furniture might need to be relocated or removed, ramps installed, and door handles made lower.

If you or a family member leave a job or reduce work hours to take care of your elderly relative, there might be a significant loss of income. In this case, some people change to telecommuting or start a job or other income they can produce from home.

Other financial factors will depend on your parent's specific situation. At this time, social security benefits will be reduced by one third if you are not paying your children or family members any rent. SSI deems free room and board as 'in-kind support and maintenance.'

There are also daily living expenses, transportation, and health costs. AARP reports that the average cost of an in-home health aide is more than $20,000 a year.

How Moving Elderly Parents into Your Home Can Affect Your Taxes

Tax law is perpetually changing, so you should consult with your accountant or tax preparer for current information. As of this writing, here are a few ways your tax liability could be affected:

As of this writing, if you claim your elderly parent as a dependent, his or her income limitation is $3,950 a year (not including social security payments). In order to qualify as a dependent, you must also have paid more than 50% of your parent's expenses for the year.

There might also be qualifying tax deductions for money you pay for dentures, hearing aids, wheelchairs, walkers, medical transportation and increased utility bills and grocery expenses.

See IRS Publication 501 for regulations about dependents.

In the case where your parent pays you rent, you need to declare that as income on Schedule E.

Insurance

Because health and medical care can be costly for seniors, if you are moving in with your adult children you will need to discuss your insurance coverage. As with all subjects regarding moving in, express your fears and expectations and discuss your finances. While this might be awkward at first, this can open the door to easier conversations and mutually beneficial solutions.

Thoreau's Senior Living Options Planner

Home Preparation Costs Planning Form

Description	Amount
Room Addition	$
Remodeling	$
Bathroom Addition	$
Bathroom Fixtures/Handrails	$
Bathroom Accessories	$
Stair or Hallway Handrails	$
Stair Chair Lift	$

Thoreau's Senior Living Options Planner

Description	Amount
Moving or changing interior and exterior light switches, door handles, locks, and faucets in your home	$
Moving or changing door handles/locks	$
Moving or changing faucets	$
Installing any intercom, alarms or systems	$

Thoreau's Senior Living Options Planner

Description	Amount
Interior or Exterior Lighting Installations or Changes	$
Wheelchair Accessible Remodeling	$
Wheelchair Ramps	$
Interior and Exterior Lighting Installations or Changes	$
Total Estimated Home Preparation Costs	$

Thoreau's Senior Living Options Planner

Living Expenses

Living expenses include food costs, personal hygiene items, transportation, possible utility cost increases and any other daily living costs. Medical or assistance expenses include those covered by insurance and services that are not covered such as a home caregiver.

You will need to make decisions such as:

- Who will pay for your guest's food?
- What transportation will you need to provide?
- Will you need to buy your guest personal hygiene items?
- Will your parent or relative require in-home care?
- Will you or a spouse need to reduce work hours or quit a job to care for your parent or relative?
- Can you afford the extra expenses?
- Will anyone else (such as a sibling) contribute to expenses?

Write down and express your expectations about care, chores, meals, and any other costs. Moving your parent or relative is not always only about finances, however, be aware that expenses are commonly more than anticipated.

Thoreau's Senior Living Options Planner

Living with Family Monthly Expenses Worksheet (for Families)

Living with Family Monthly Expenses Worksheet Questions for Your Family
Meals and Diet
Does your family member have special diet requirements and if so, what is the estimated monthly cost of these meals? Monthly Cost: $ _____ Who will pay for this food? _____ _____
Otherwise how much will your family member contribute to groceries monthly? Monthly Contribution: $ _____
Rent
Will your family member be paying rent and if so, how much? Monthly Rent: $ _____
Internet and Phone
Does your family member have his or her own cell phone? Yes _____ No _____ Who will pay for this phone? _____
Will your family member have any specific Internet or cable needs? Yes _____ No _____ Monthly Cost: $ _____

Thoreau's Senior Living Options Planner

Living with Family Monthly Expenses
Questions for Your Family

Transportation

How many times on average each week does your family member need to go somewhere that requires transportation?

_____
_____
_____
_____

Does your family member have his or her own vehicle and driver's license? Yes _____ No _____

If 'Yes,' who will pay for gas, car maintenance, and insurance?

_____
_____

If 'Yes,' is easily accessible parking available for your family member's vehicle? Yes _____ No _____

If 'No,' what forms of transportation will be available?

_____
_____
_____
_____
_____

Thoreau's Senior Living Options Planner

Living with Family Financial Worksheet
Questions for Your Family

Utilities

Will your family member need any additional utility services or increase your utility usage and cost in any way?

If so, how much for each monthly?

Utility _____ Monthly Amount $_____

Utility _____ Monthly Amount $_____

Utility _____ Monthly Amount $_____

Utility _____ Monthly Amount $_____

Utility _____ Monthly Amount $_____

Total Monthly $_____

Living with Family Monthly Expenses Worksheet
Questions for Your Family

Will your family member need to hire help in the form of home care, nursing, or aid?   Yes _____ No _____

If Yes: Estimated Monthly Cost: $ _____

Who will pay for this care?
_____
_____

Thoreau's Senior Living Options Planner

Your Monthly Expenses When Living with Family

Your Monthly Rent and Food Expenses When Living with Family	
Description	**Monthly Amount**
All Utilities Average Monthly Cost	$
Your Share of Housing Cost (Mortgage, Rent, etc.)	$
Home Maintenance Expenses	$
Monthly Insurance Expense (Property, Renter's)	$
Groceries	$
Sundries	$
Medical	$
Other:	$
	$
	$
	$
	$
	$
	$
Total Living Expenses (All Above)	**$**

Vehicle Ownership Expenses

Description	Monthly Amount
Average Monthly Maintenance	$
Monthly Fuel	$
Monthly Loan or Lease Payment	$
Monthly Auto Insurance	$
Auto Taxes, License, Registration (Monthly Cost)	$
Carwash and/or Detail	$
Parking Costs	$
	$
	$
	$
	$
	$
	$
	$
Total Monthly Vehicle Expenses	$

Thoreau's Senior Living Options Planner

Services and Amenity Monthly Expenses	
Description	**Monthly Amount**
Gym Membership	$
Golf or Country Club Membership	$
Laundry Services	$
Cleaning/Maid Service	$
	$
Note: If you do not own a vehicle, estimate monthly transportation costs here.	$
Other:	$
	$
	$
	$
	$
	$
	$
	$
	$
Total Amenity Monthly Expenses	$

Thoreau's Senior Living Options Planner

Add all three totals from above "Your Monthly Expenses When Living with Family" to estimate your total living expenses.

TOTAL of Your Monthly Expenses When Living with Family	
Add all three totals from above three 3 forms Description	**Monthly Amount**
Total Monthly Rent and Food Expenses	$
Total Monthly Vehicle Expenses	$
Total Amenity Monthly Expenses	$
Your Total Monthly Living Expenses When Living with Family	$
Your Monthly Income	$
Minus Your Total Monthly Living Expenses When Living with Family	- $
Total Monthly Over or Above Amount	$

Relationships

When you live with people that you have not lived with in decades, old patterns of behavior can show up. If you and your parent used to fight about a household issue, that might come up again. Or if one of your siblings is around more to help with your parent, you might find yourself revisiting childhood fights. Simply being aware of these patterns can help you avoid them and defuse the situation.

Meeting with a professional that specializes in family relationships can help.

For adult children having a parent(s) move into their home:

- Set ground rules and expectations for you, your family and your parent.
- Recognize that your parent is giving up some independence and that you might well be in the same situation one day. Think about how you would feel and empathize.
- Assure your parent that you will not tell him or her what to do or criticize.
- When your parent expresses a concern, listen, and repeat the concern back to your parent to be sure you understand.
- Avoid discussions of politics, values, or belief systems if you do not agree.
- Make everyone's privacy a priority with clear boundaries.

If you have children living in your home, set a positive tone with them from the start.

Sometimes a senior's behavior can scare or even embarrass children. Especially if the senior is suffering from health issues. Tell your children they are not to blame for and of your relative's (or their grandparent's) potential behavior.

Thoreau's Senior Living Options Planner

Living with Family Relationship Worksheet for You

Yes/No	Questions to Ask Yourself Before Moving In
	Will moving in with my family reduce my monthly expenses?
	Will I have the privacy I need?
	Does my family have a healthy way of addressing conflicts?
	Do I enjoy spending long periods of time with my family?
	Are there unresolved issues between my family and me or between other family members that could interfere with peacefully living with my family? _____ _____ _____ _____
	Are all parties willing to work to resolve these issues? How can these issues be resolved? _____ _____ _____ _____ _____ _____

Thoreau's Senior Living Options Planner

Yes/No	Questions to Ask Yourself Before Moving In
	Is there any pattern of personality conflict between any family members and me? If the answer is 'Yes,' are there triggers or specific things that set these conflicts off? If so, what are they? _____ _____ _____ _____ _____
	What can be done to avoid conflicts with my family? _____ _____ _____ _____
	If I disagree with anything my adult child does, am I comfortable discussing it? _____ _____ _____ _____
	Am I comfortable with all members of my family including any children or grandchildren? _____ _____ _____ _____
	If there are children in the home, do I have a preestablished relationship with them?
	Am I allowed to correct the children?

Thoreau's Senior Living Options Planner

	Are there any conflicts of authority over the children?
	Are the children comfortable with me moving into the home? (If they are not, this might need to be addressed with a professional before considering the move.)
	What boundaries would be beneficial to establish? _____ _____ _____ _____ _____ _____ ____

Yes/No	Questions to Ask Yourself Before Moving In
	What do I expect from each of my family members regarding any type of assistance? _____ _____ _____ _____ _____ _____
	Do I expect my family to provide rides or any transportation services and will I pay them to do this?
	Do my family members ever ask me for money?
	Can my family afford their current lifestyle?
	Will moving in with my family create any financial burden or hardship on them?

Thoreau's Senior Living Options Planner

Can I have visitors to the home? If so, are there limitations or boundaries such as who can visit and when?

_____

_____

_____

_____ _____

Notes

Thoreau's Senior Living Options Planner

Living with Family Relationship Worksheet for Your Family

Yes/No	Questions Your Family Needs to Ask
	Will having my parent (or relative) move into my home increase my monthly expenses?
	Will all family members have the privacy they need?
	Do I and my family members enjoy spending long periods of time with my parent?
	Are there unresolved issues between my parent and my children?
	Does my family have a healthy way of addressing conflicts?
	How can these issues be resolved? _____ _____ _____ _____
	Are there unresolved issues between my parent and my spouse or any other household residents?
	How can these issues be resolved? _____ _____ _____ _____

Thoreau's Senior Living Options Planner

Yes/No	Questions Your Family Needs to Ask
	Is there any pattern of personality conflict between my parent and myself or anyone else in the house? If the answer is 'Yes,' are there 'triggers' or specific things that set these conflicts off? If so, what are they? _____ _____ _____ _____ _____
	What can be done to avoid these conflicts? _____ _____ _____ _____
	What boundaries would be beneficial to establish to avoid conflicts? _____ _____ _____ _____ _____

Thoreau's Senior Living Options Planner

Yes/No	Questions Your Family Needs to Ask
	If I (we) disagree with my parent, am I comfortable discussing it?
	Are all members of the household comfortable with my parent?
	Are my children safe and comfortable in the presence of my parent?
	Is my parent allowed to correct the children?
	Are there any conflicts of authority over the children?
	What boundaries would be beneficial to establish with the children? _____ _____ _____ _____
	How does my parent feel about moving in? _____ _____ _____
	Are family meals customary?
	Does my parent expect to have family meals?

Thoreau's Senior Living Options Planner

Yes/No	Questions Your Family Needs to Ask
	How do each of my household members feel about my parent moving in? _____ _____ _____ _____
	Does my parent expect to attend events with the family or family members and is this OK?
	Does my parent expect to go on vacation with the family and is this OK?
	Will my parent be expected to babysit (or pet sit) at any time?
	Will any household members need to change their work or school schedules to accommodate my relative? If so, who and how? _____ _____ _____ _____ _____
	Will my household income be affected by changes in work schedules? If so, estimate how much: $ _____

Thoreau's Senior Living Options Planner

Yes/No	Questions Your Family Needs to Ask
	Does my parent or relative have any special considerations that everyone needs to be aware of such as: • reduced cognitive functions • loss of memory • depression • medication effects • challenge with balance or mobility
	Does my parent expect me and/or my family members to provide him or her with transportation?
	If so, is providing transportation OK and under what circumstances? _____ _____ _____

Thoreau's Senior Living Options Planner

Household Rules for Living with Family Form

House Rules
What boundaries would be beneficial to establish?

Thoreau's Senior Living Options Planner

House Rules

Thoreau's Senior Living Options Planner

	Living with Family

Thoreau's Senior Living Options Planner

	Living with Family
	Accessibility
	Supervision
	Responsibilities

Thoreau's Senior Living Options Planner

	Living with Family
	Living Space
	Transportation
	Visitors

Thoreau's Senior Living Options Planner

	Living with Family
	Meals: Diet Requirements
	Medications

Thoreau's Senior Living Options Planner

Notes About Living with Family

Thoreau's Senior Living Options Planner

Notes About Living with Family

Conclusion

"Make the most of your regrets; never smother your sorrow but tend and cherish it till it come to have a separate and integral interest. To regret deeply is to live afresh." – Henry David Thoreau

Thank you so much for purchasing Thoreau's Senior Living Options Planner. *I am so grateful for you.* I hope this planner helps you organize and make the best decision for you and/or a loved one.

If you or a loved one needs to downsize to make a move, this book is a partner to <u>Thoreau's Downsizing Planner for Seniors</u>, which you can find on Amazon.

To order more copies of this book or give one as a gift, you can also find this book on Amazon.

If you see anything we can improve or spot a typo in this book, please let us know. You can contact us at:

>phil@tweetside.com

If you found this book useful, please leave a review on Amazon.

Thank You and I Wish You the Best Always!

Philip Baker

Made in the USA
Monee, IL
21 December 2021

86823317R00129

Manford of Morning Glory Mountain

The Circle is Drawn

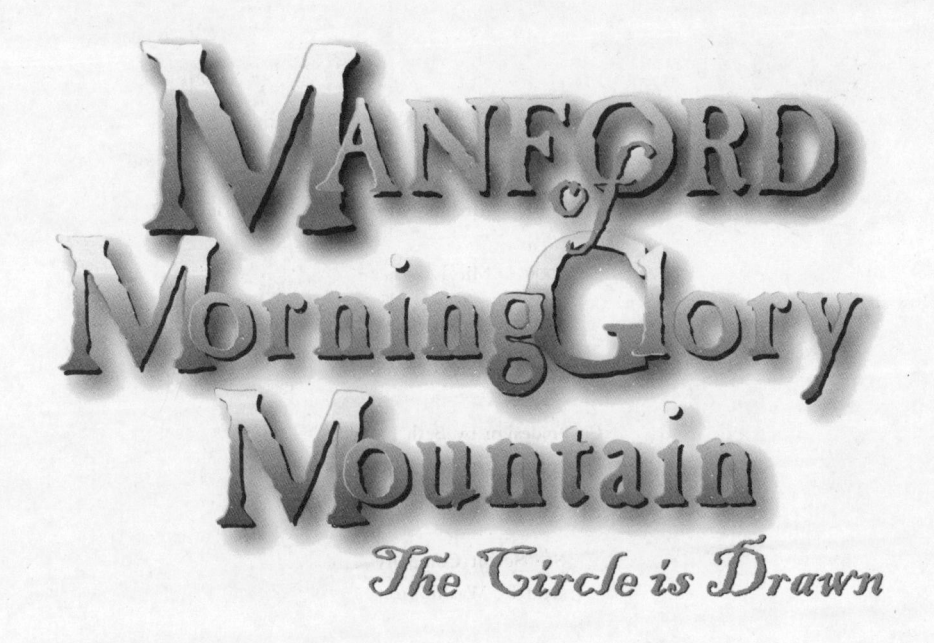

Mic Lowther

Illustrations by Jeff White

Manford of MorningGlory Mountain
The Circle is Drawn

Book 1 of the Manford of MorningGlory Mountain Series

2006 © Mic Lowther
All rights reserved.

Illustrations by Jeff White

Cover design by Beth Farrell
Text design and layout by Beth Farrell

Sea Script Company
Seattle, Washington

ISBN: 0-9672186-4-0

Library of Congress Card Catalogue Number: 2006920020

First Printing January 2006

No part of this book may be reproduced or utilized in any form or by any means,
digital, electronic or mechanical, including photocopying and recording,
or by any information storage and retrieval system without
permission in writing from the author.
www.manford.com

SEA SCRIPT COMPANY
1800 westlake ave n. ste 205   seattle wa 98109
tel 206.748.0345   fax 206.748.0343
info@seascriptcompany.com

WHO IS MANFORD?

I write about success. I write about winning. I write about things that work. I don't think failure and disappointment are the natural outcome of things. Out of this comes Manford, the young, enthusiastic, I've-got-an-idea, adventuring moose who bounds through these pages never for a moment thinking that something can't be done.

Manford's story began in the 1990s while on a backpack trip in Alaska with my friends Vicki, Doug, and Ken (The Usual Suspects).

"This is Manford," Vicki said, pointing to a small stuffed, plush moose hanging from her pack. "He'll be going on adventures with us from now on."

We took turns reading stories around the campfire on our trips. Over time, we went through *The Velveteen Rabbit, Winnie-the-Pooh, Alice in Wonderland, Wind in the Willows*, and I got to wondering if Manford could be the star of his own campfire story. I created a few friends for him to pal around with, gave them whatever names came to mind, wrote one story to read to Vicki on her birthday, and figured that would be the end of it.

"Write some more," she said.

I did, putting the characters in a variety of situations that either Vicki or I or one of the other Suspects thought up. Then a curious thing happened. Manford and his friends started going on their own adventures. Whole stories would occur to me fully formed as if the characters were off on their own and I was just along to write things down.

I wrote thirty-six stories in five years on whatever subject seemed interesting at the time. Some are silly. Some are hilarious. Some are serious and thoughtful. Many are educational, such as explaining why a butterfly flutters, how to follow trails and use a compass, the good and bad of forest fires, the history of potato chips, how a gold processing mill operates, making dyes from plants, how eclipses happen, and much more. Sometimes I would stop in mid-chapter to read a whole book on whatever subject had come up so I could tell the story accurately.

These stories are collected in two volumes, beginning in spring and wrapping around to spring again. The title of Book 1, *The Circle is Drawn*, refers to Manford gathering his circle of friends and exploring the world around him. The title of Book 2, *Riches for the Finding*, refers to discovering treasure in various forms—silver and gold and jewels, or knowledge and learning and new skills.

I invite you to join the fun, exploration, and discovery with Manford and his friends in *The Circle is Drawn* and *Riches for the Finding* and look forward to his next adventures in upcoming *Manford of MorningGlory Mountain* books.

For Vicki

Books in the Manford of MorningGlory Mountain Series:

The Circle is Drawn
Riches for the Finding

CONTENTS

Chapter 1: New in the Neighborhood.............3

Chapter 2: Surprises in Small and Large Packages...19

Chapter 3: In WhiteFlower Meadow.............35

Chapter 4: Watcher at MorningGlory Crossing...53

Chapter 5: Uphill, Fog, and Dancing Bears.......71

Chapter 6: The Place with No Trees.............87

Chapter 7: Happy To Be Me..................105

Chapter 8: A Certain Smelly Something.........121

Chapter 9: Eyes in the Forest..................137

Chapter 10: Good Neighbors, Unite!............155

Chapter 11: Secrets Revealed..................173

Chapter 12: Improving the View...............189

Chapter 13: Florida-by-the-Pond..............207

Chapter 14: Message in the Dust..............223

Chapter 15: Rescue at Eight, Black Tie Optional...239

Chapter 16: Journey to Long Ago.............257

Chapter 17: Of Rain and Flood and Darkness....275

Chapter 18: Ahead of His Time...............291

Chapter Notes...............................305

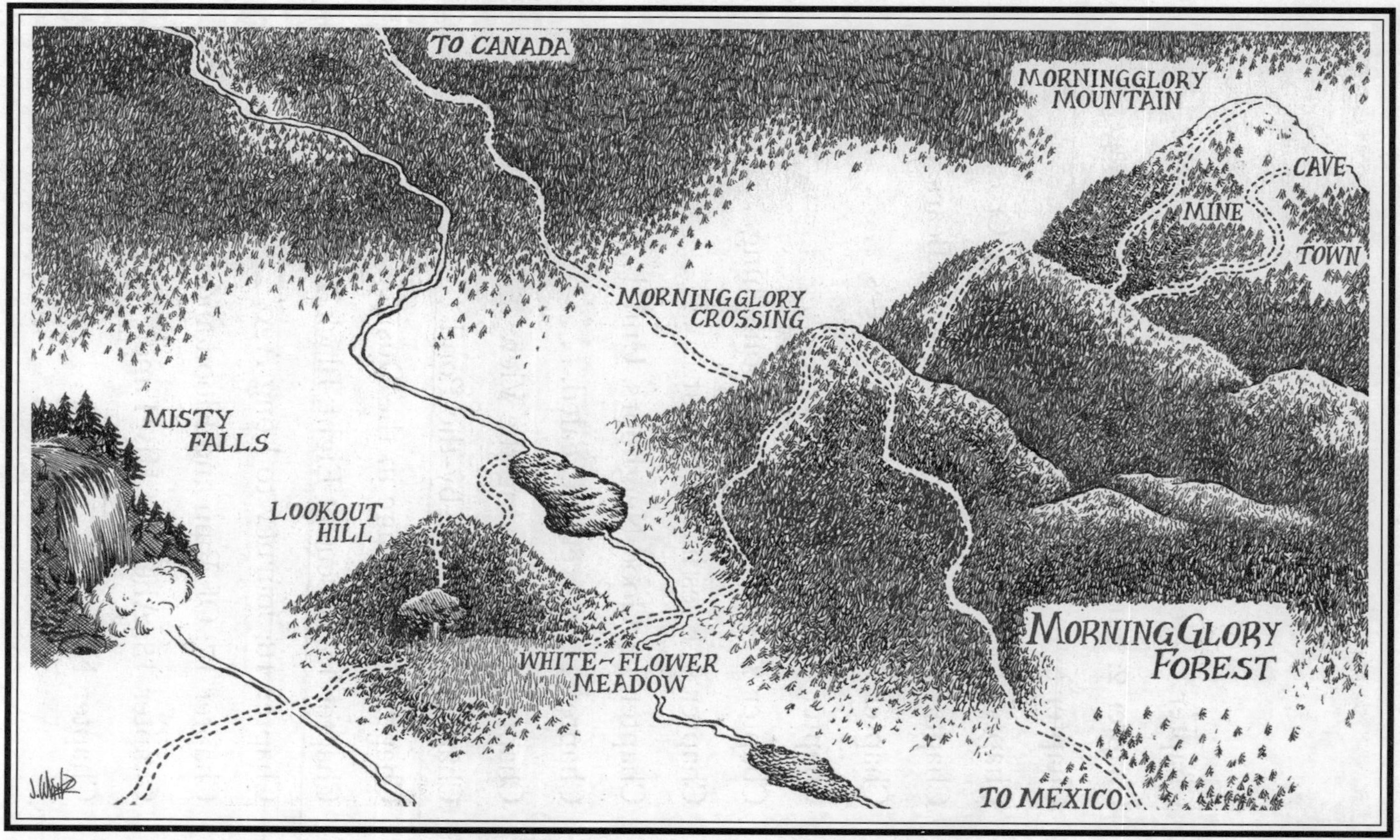
TO CANADA
MORNINGGLORY
MOUNTAIN
CAVE
MINE
TOWN
MORNINGGLORY
CROSSING
MISTY
FALLS
LOOKOUT
HILL
WHITE-FLOWER
MEADOW
MORNING GLORY
FOREST
TO MEXICO

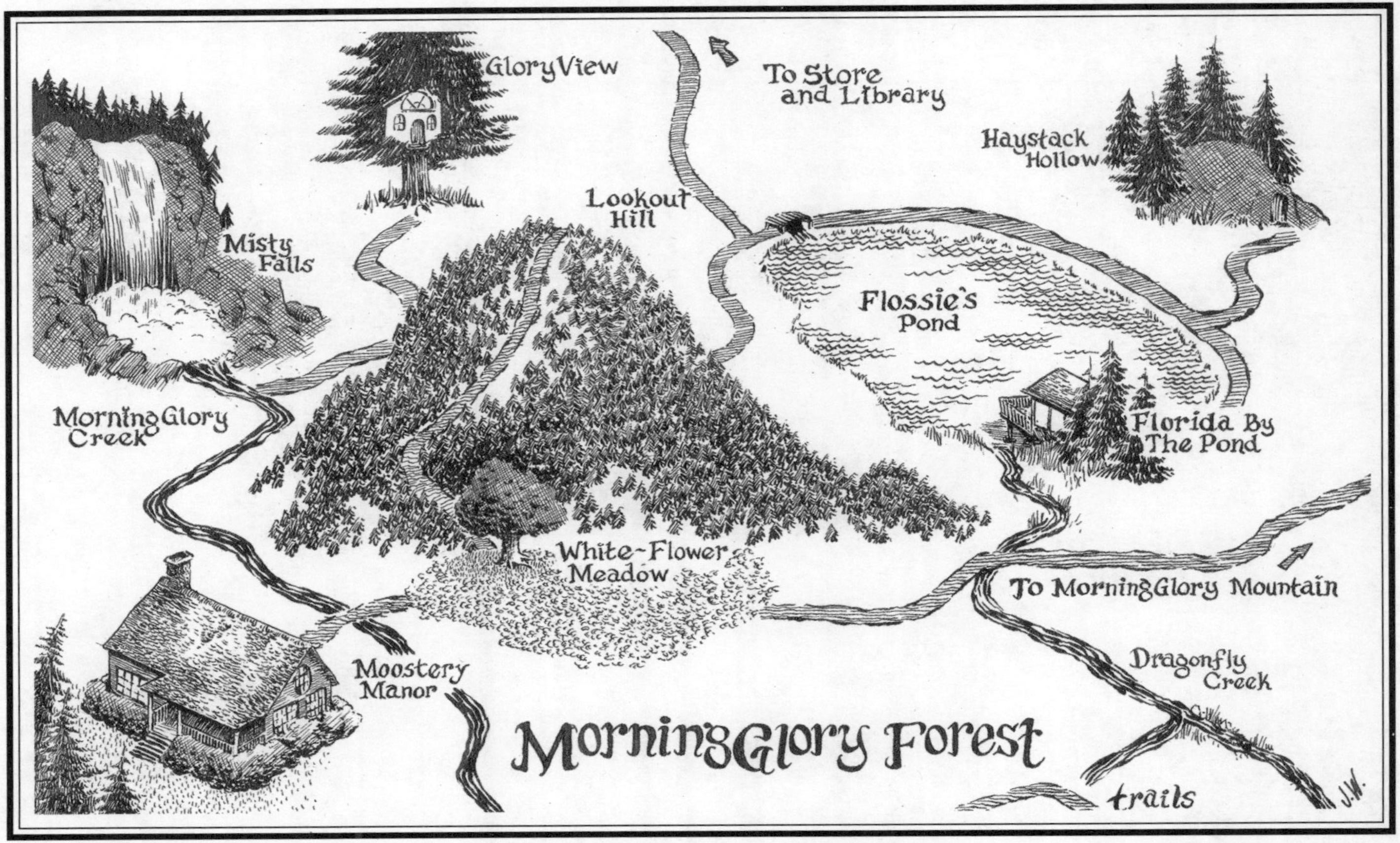
Glory View
To Store
and Library
Haystack
Hollow
Misty
Falls
Lookout
Hill
Flossie's
Pond
Morning Glory
Creek
Florida By
The Pond
White-Flower
Meadow
To Morning Glory Mountain
Moostery
Manor
Dragonfly
Creek
Morning Glory Forest
trails
J.W.

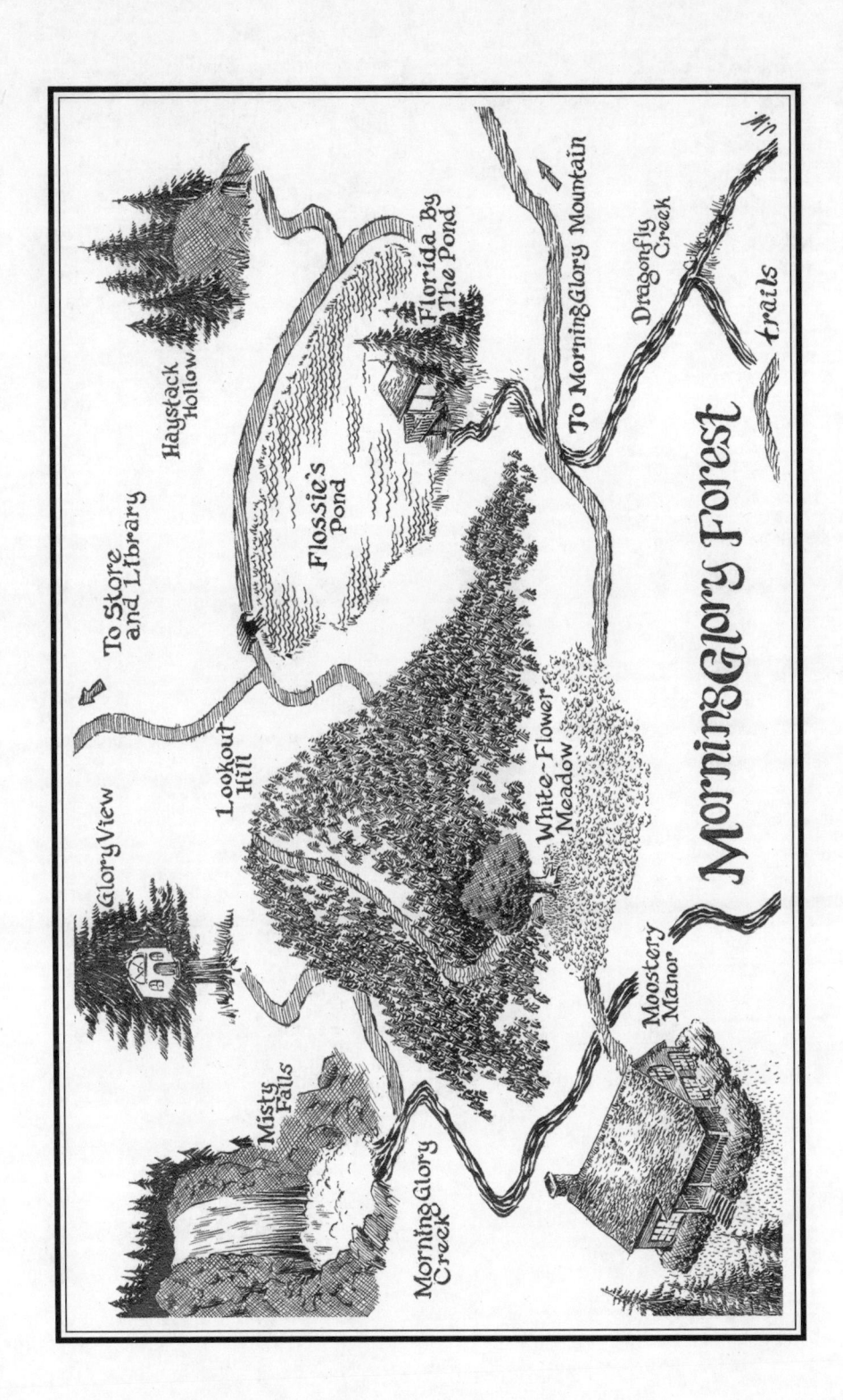

Manford of Morning Glory Mountain

The Circle is Drawn

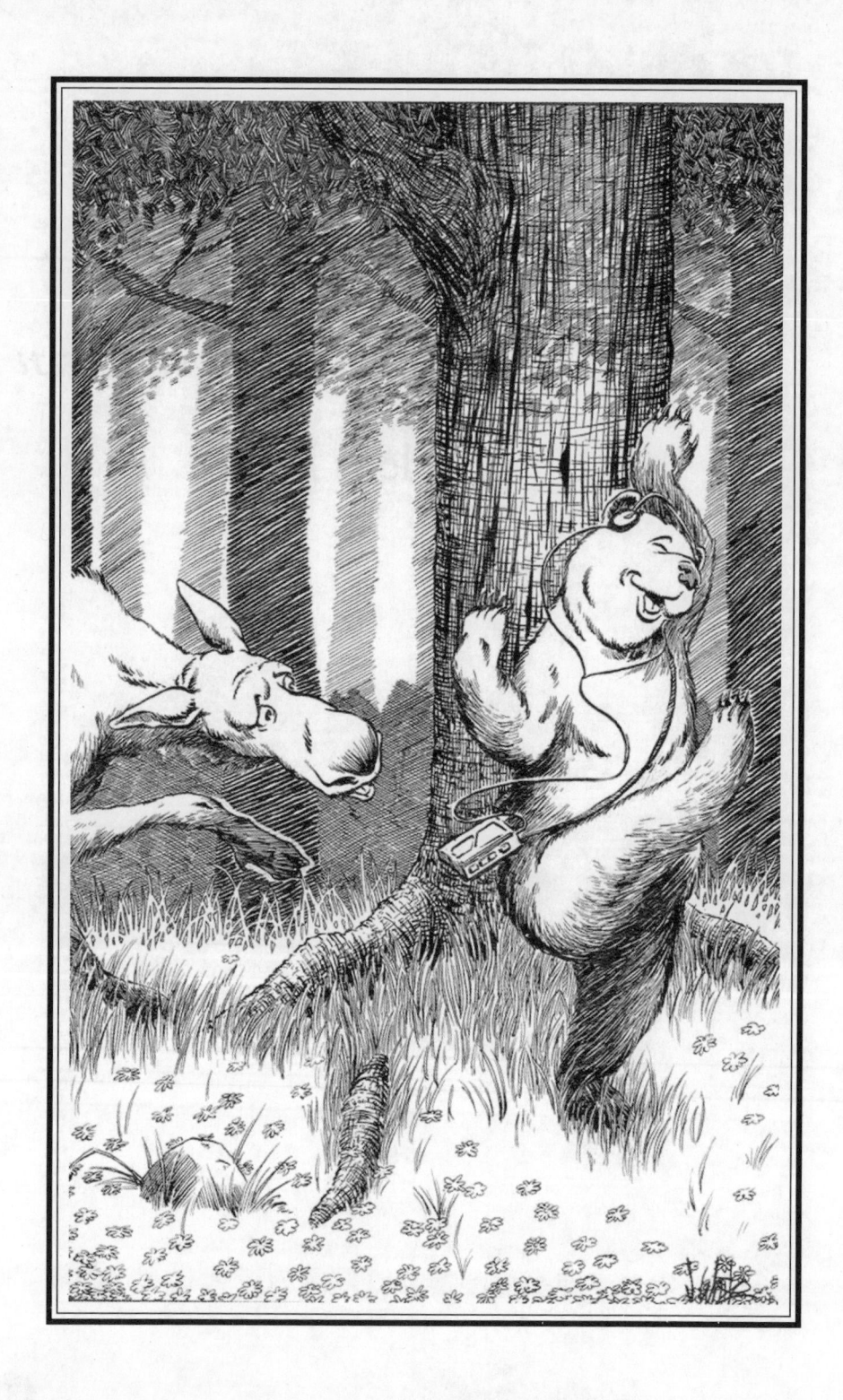

1

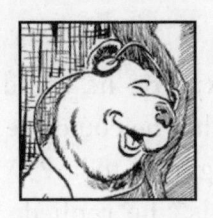

New in the Neighborhood
In which we meet Manford and Manford meets new friends

The sun struck the top of MorningGlory Mountain first at The Place With No Trees. Light moved slowly down the mountain then, down rocky cliffs to where only short trees grew, down to spruce groves wet with morning dew, then to the forest of beech and noble fir at the base of the mountain itself. A gentle wind blew, rustling leaves and breaking the early stillness. It was morning. It was spring. It was time to go exploring.

Manford had been awake for hours. From his bedroom window, he'd watched the sky grow brighter as dawn slowly came, until now the sun shone in to warm his soft, fuzzy nose.

"Time for breakfast, Manford."

That was his mother calling. They had moved to MorningGlory Forest just the week before and had already settled into their familiar routine. "Time for breakfast, Manford," his mother would always say. It sounded so comforting first thing in the morning.

They'd finished unpacking and putting things away, filling the shelves of new cupboards and closets with tidy stacks and rows of belongings.

Today he could explore; he could look around his new neighborhood to see what he could see.

"What are you going to do today?" Manford's mother asked.

"Explore the woods," he replied. "I want to see what's around us."

"Maybe you'll find some new friends."

"I hope so."

"You're having a birthday in a couple of days," his mother went on. "If you meet someone nice, invite him or her to your party."

"Oh, I will. Should I tell them to bring presents?"

"That wouldn't be polite, dear. Just let them think of it on their own."

"But what if they don't think of it?"

"Having new friends is present enough."

"I suppose," Manford said. His mother was always so logical.

"Now remember to be home early," she said. "Your father will be on TV tonight and you won't want to miss that."

"Okay," Manford said, and he skipped out the front door and into the woods.

Now there's something you should know about Manford before we go much further. Skipping out the front door may be easy for you, but for Manford, it's not so simple. Manford is a moose, you see, and he has four feet.

Manford walked north along a worn path through the woods, looking up and down and around at everything. He saw huge trees with great, overhanging branches. Sunlight streamed through them, soft yellow-green light that made bright patches on the forest floor. Flowers of red, yellow, white, pink, and purple offered frequent spots of color. Fresh grasses, spiky horsetails, and new green ferns waved gently in the slight breeze. He nibbled at leaves and blossoms as he went. Some tasted good, others—phooey!—didn't!

He stopped to listen. A bird chirped to his left. Soon, another answered in the distance to his right. A woodpecker drilled a tree trunk behind him.

"Hello," Manford said. Those who saw him only looked at him and flew off.

He came to a creek and turned to follow it upstream. The bottom was rocky and slippery but Manford waded along sure-footed, stopping at times for a drink. The water made soft sounds as it splashed over rocks and washed against the mossy bank.

The land rose up beside the creek as he walked along. He was led into a canyon. The sounds of the water grew louder until a rainy, splashing sound came from where the creek led around a bend. Manford grew more and more curious and followed the creek still farther. Around the bend, he saw where the canyon ended just ahead at a tall cliff. A lovely waterfall spilled lightly from it.

He walked closer, looking up at the misty stream of water rushing over a ledge far above and falling down, down, down, into a large pool at the base of the cliff. He waded around the edge and under the falls, letting the water splash over his head and back and down his long, skinny legs, thinking how cool and good it felt.

Then he noticed the cave behind the waterfall. It had a large, arched door, a mailbox fastened to the rock wall next to it, and a fuzzy mat on the step for wiping feet. Ivy grew around and over the doorway, framing it in a pleasant leafy green. There was a sign on the door:

Misty Falls
Millie & Veronica
Welcome

Manford saw a large, brass knocker below the sign and banged it three times. No one came. He banged it again, harder.

The door drifted open slightly.

"Hello, anybody home?" he said, pulling the door open farther. No answer. He looked inside, neither saw nor heard anyone, so pushed the door shut.

I wonder who they are,' he thought as he walked through the falls and pool and back the way he'd come.

He backtracked to where he'd first entered the creek. He left the water there and headed northeast along the forest path. Trees surrounded him. They looked like they went on and on in all directions. '*So much to explore,*' Manford thought. '*It'll take all summer.*'

He came upon a large meadow about mid-morning. Soft grass grew over most of the thirty-acre clearing, along with white, many petaled flowers he knew to be daisies. He saw a broad branching tree across the meadow that made a round spot of shade on the ground.

Sounds came from the direction of the tree. They weren't water splashing or gurgling sounds; not wind blowing or leaf fluttering sounds, either; not even bird chirping or insect buzzing sounds—not woodsy sounds at all. This was different. This sounded like music, rock-and-roll music, playing very loud.

There was something moving in the shade of the tree. Manford walked closer, the music got louder, and the moving form took on a shape. Moose are nearsighted, you see, and have to get up close.

'*It's a bear,*' he decided, when he was near enough to figure it out. '*Yes, a bear. It's listening to that music and. . .dancing.*'

"Hello," Manford said. The bear danced on, not hearing him above the loud music. Manford walked closer and said, "Hello" again. The bear kept dancing and didn't even look his way.

He walked closer, till it seemed the bear might reel right into him, and shouted, "Hello!" one more time. The bear looked up, startled, and paused for a moment.

"What did you say?" it asked in a loud voice.

"I said, HELLO," shouted Manford.

"Oh, hello." It started dancing again.

"What's your name?" yelled Manford.

"What?" said the bear, pausing again.

"I asked your name," said Manford. "You don't suppose you could turn that music down, do you?"

"Name?" asked the bear. "I'm Veronica. Who are you?"

"I'm Manford. Really, could you turn that music down?"

"What?" said Veronica. "Just a minute, I can't hear you. I'll turn the music down." She did so and the music faded away.

"You said your name was Shortbread?" asked the bear.

"No, it's Manford."

"Manford. . .hmmm, I haven't heard of you. You must be new to MorningGlory Forest."

"I moved here last week with my mom," said Manford. "She thought it was a nice neighborhood."

"It is. There's lots of space."

"Is that your home at Misty Falls where the sign says, 'Millie & Veronica'?"

"Uh huh, how did you know that?"

"I followed the creek there. Who's Millie?"

"That's my mom."

"She wasn't home," Manford said. "I knocked but nobody answered."

"No," said Veronica, "she's traveling with the circus again."

"Circus?"

"Sure, haven't you heard of Millie, the Dancing Bear? I thought everyone knew about her."

"I'm only one year old," said Manford, "or at least I will be in a few days. There are lots of things I haven't heard of, I suppose."

"Probably," said Veronica, "but don't feel bad. I just turned two."

They sat down in the shade of the tree. Veronica plucked a white daisy and placed it behind her ear. Manford nibbled the grass.

"Does this place have a name?" he asked.

"Which place?"

"Where we're sitting."

"This is WhiteFlower Meadow," Veronica said.

"It's named after the daisies, I'll bet," said Manford.

"Is that what these flowers are?"

"Yes."

"Well, the one who named it didn't know that. They were just white flowers growing in a meadow."

"Who named it?"

"I did," said Veronica.

"Did you name MorningGlory Mountain, too?"

"No, that was already named. The forest around us is MorningGlory Forest and the creek you followed to my place is MorningGlory Creek."

"Why didn't you call this MorningGlory Meadow?"

"We had enough MorningGlorys as it was," said Veronica. "Besides, there aren't any morning glories here, just. . .what did you say these were?"

"Daisies."

"Daisies, Daisy Meadow. . .hmmm."

"You were dancing to music when I got here," Manford said. "Did you learn that from your mom?"

"Uh huh."

"Are you going to join the circus, too?"

"Someday, maybe. My mom learned from her mother, who learned from her mother, and so on. I come from a long line of circus bears."

"Why do you keep her name on the door if she's gone?"

"Because she's famous," Veronica said. "She has her posters hung all over inside. She also still lives there. She'll be home at the end of summer."

Veronica offered to show Manford around. The two new friends left the shade of the tree to follow a trail leading north from the meadow.

"I'd like to see her dance sometime," said Manford. "Is she ever on TV?"

"She has been."

"My dad's going to be on TV tonight."

"He is?" Veronica asked. "Why is that?"

"My dad's in show business, too," Manford said. "He dances with the ballet in New York."

"You mean The Great Bucknikov, the world's only ballet dancing moose? *He's your dad?*"

"Sure is," said Manford proudly. "Have you seen him?"

"Yes, I have," said Veronica. "He's spectacular! I'll be sure to watch tonight, too. How did he ever get into ballet in New York?"

"It's a strange story and I don't understand it all. Maybe my mom will tell you sometime."

"I want to hear that."

"Oh," Manford said, suddenly remembering, "I'm having a birthday party the day after tomorrow. Want to come?"

"Sure," said Veronica, and the two continued their walk through the forest, Manford giving directions about what time to come and how to find his house and trying very hard not to say anything about presents.

They followed along the trail, stopping to look at things around them and to sample the foliage as they went. They climbed steadily uphill, but in a short while the path flattened out in an open, grassy area. Manford stopped.

"Is this the top?" he asked.

"It's the top of Lookout Hill," said Veronica, "but the real mountains are over there. Look."

Manford looked to the east and saw three mountains much larger than the small hill they'd climbed. The farthest one was huge, far taller than the others. It rose to meet the clouds then passed on through them. It was the biggest thing Manford had ever seen.

"That's MorningGlory Mountain," Veronica said.

Manford stared. The mountain seemed to get bigger and bigger the more he looked at it.

"Have you ever been to the top?" he asked.

"No, I haven't," Veronica replied. "But there's a special place up there called The Place With No Trees. I've always wondered what it was."

"Oh, let's climb it sometime," Manford said enthusiastically. "We could take a picnic and climb up through the clouds and see everything around here. Want to?"

"Um, sure," said Veronica, but she sounded like she *wasn't* sure, like she wondered if it was really a good idea. "We'd need more than a picnic if we did," she said. "Climbing MorningGlory would take several days. You have to climb the two mountains in front of it first."

"Oh, fun," Manford bubbled on, "maybe after my birthday?"

"Maybe," Veronica said. "We'll see."

"There's a pond," Manford said, pointing below them. "Does *it* have a name?"

"I don't know whether it does or not."

The trail led them downhill through a series of twists and turns. Near the pond they crossed a bridge over another creek. Manford's hooves made clippy-clop noises on the wooden planks. Going for a swim seemed like a good idea. They ran and galloped down the last stretch of trail and plunged into the pond with a tremendous splash.

"Run for your lives! Run for your lives!" said a voice. There was a great squawking and flapping of wings.

"What was that?" Manford asked, poking up his head and blowing water from his nose.

"What was what?" Veronica said as she came sputtering

to the surface.

"*Bogies at ten o'clock! Bogies at ten o'clock! Run for your lives!*" the voice screeched again.

"That," said Manford.

"I don't know," Veronica replied. They looked around them.

"*Red alert, red alert! To your battle stations!*"

"Noisy thing, whatever it is," said Veronica.

"*Out of the pool, you two,*" the noise said again. "*Run along, run along.*"

"There's something pink in the top of that tree," Manford said, pointing toward the edge of the pond, "but I can't tell what it is."

"Can't see a thing," said Veronica. Bears are even more nearsighted than moose.

"Hello!" Manford yelled. "Come down so we can see who you are."

"Nothing doing," said the pink thing. "I'm staying right here until you two are gone. So, on your way, goodbye, leave me and my pond alone."

"Your pond?" said Veronica. "Since when?"

"Since yesterday, that's when."

"What happened then?"

"That's when I got here. I was the only one here so I declared it my pond."

"I just got here, too," Manford said.

"What *are* you, by the way?" the noise wanted to know.

"A moose," said Manford.

"That's what I thought. Your friend must be a bear."

"Right," said Veronica.

"I didn't know there were moose and bear in Florida."

"The noise is talking about Florida," Manford said to Veronica. "Is MorningGlory Mountain in Florida?"

"No," said Veronica, "Florida is three thousand miles from here."

"This isn't Florida," Manford said to the noise. "That's a

long way from here."

"Oh, dear," said the noise, "not again."

"Please come down," Manford said. "We won't have to shout if you come closer. And if you tell us who you are, we won't have to call you The Noise."

"You promise to be nice?"

"We promise," Manford and Veronica said at once.

The pink thing flapped its wings then and glided down to the edge of the water. It walked slowly toward them, stopped a safe distance away, then stood on one long, skinny leg and tucked the other leg under its body.

"I'm Manford," said Manford.

"I'm Veronica," said Veronica.

"How do you do," said the pink thing. "I'm Flossie."

"I'm a bear, as you observed," said Veronica. "What are you?"

"A bird," replied Flossie, holding her head high on her long neck. "A flamingo; *a pink flamingo*, to be exact."

"I've never seen anything like you before," Manford said.

"Really? There were thousands of others when I left. I wonder what happened to them. You're sure this isn't Florida?"

"Oh, I'm sure of that," said Veronica.

"Well, I *was* starting to wonder," Flossie said. "I haven't seen a palm tree anywhere around here and I don't remember any mountains like this in Florida."

"I'm confused," said Manford.

"Me, too, kiddo," said Flossie. "A week ago I was in Florida on a beach with so many other flamingos that all you could see was pink for half a mile. One night I couldn't sleep, so I decided to fly around for a while. Nothing looked familiar in the morning so I just kept going for days and days, looking and looking. I've been resting here since yesterday, wondering what to do next, hoping this was really Florida."

"It isn't," said Veronica.

"Just my luck," Flossie said. "I wonder why this keeps

happening to me?"

"Keeps happening?" Manford said.

"I did the same thing last year. I was flying along and lost my way then, too. I kept going until, eventually, I found palm trees and open water. I thought sure I was home. Trouble was there was all this cactus and desert. Turns out I was in Arizona."

"How did you get back?" Manford asked.

"I followed jet trails of airliners going to Miami."

"You must fly pretty fast," said Veronica.

"No, I could only follow one for a little while," Flossie said. "But there was always another one along soon. Maybe I can do the same thing this time."

"Why do you stand on one leg?" Manford asked. He'd been wondering about this ever since Flossie flew down from the tree.

"It's what flamingos do," Flossie answered. "We rest one leg while we stand on the other."

"I wonder if I can do that," said Veronica. She stood up on her hind legs, then leaned to one side and lifted one leg cautiously into the air.

"How's this?"

"Not bad," said Flossie. "Now tuck it under your arm."

Veronica brought the back leg slowly forward, lifted it, then lost her balance, tipped over, and hit the water with a great splash.

"Wow, you could surf on that wave," said Flossie, running toward shore. "Now you try, Manford."

Manford carefully lifted one front leg, then one back leg, and teetered unsteadily.

"Now what?" he said.

"That's not going to work," Flossie said. "Try standing up like Veronica did."

Manford heaved his front quarters into the air and balanced unsteadily on his back legs. He looked around, unsure about what to do next. His puzzlement lasted about six seconds, whereupon he keeled over backwards into the water with Veronica.

"*Man the lifeboats,*" Flossie shouted above the noise, "*Moose overboard!*"

Veronica and Manford were now splashing water on each other and at Flossie. The water just rolled off her delicate pink feathers.

"Drop by and see me again," Flossie said, unfolding her wings and getting ready to fly across the pond.

"Aren't you going back to Florida?" asked Veronica.

"I'm not in any hurry."

"I'm having a birthday party the day after tomorrow," said Manford. "Would you like to come?"

"Who's going to be there?" Flossie asked.

"Veronica, and you, if you like."

"Doesn't sound like much of a party with only two guests. Are we the only friends you have?"

"So far," Manford said, "but my mom will be there."

"Well, that's something," Flossie said. She paused, thinking a moment. "I have an idea. If I bring a friend and Veronica brings a friend, then you'll have four at your party, or six counting you and your mom."

"Sounds okay to me," Manford said.

"You'll get more presents that way," Flossie said.

"Mom said I wasn't supposed to talk about presents."

"Oh, yes, aren't mothers always that way. Don't worry, we won't say anything."

"Oh, no, not a thing," said Veronica. "What kind of presents would you like."

"Gosh, I don't know."

"Give us a clue," said Flossie, "what kinds of things do you like to do?"

"I like to go exploring and adventuring," said Manford. "I

want to climb mountains and see what there is to see."

"Edmund Hillary Lewis-and-Clark Moose; that's you?"

"Who are those people?"

"Explorers and adventurers," said Flossie. "You should read about them sometime. Do you have a friend to bring to the party, Veronica?"

"Uh huh, do you?"

"No, but I'll look for one. Well, it's been nice meeting you two," Flossie said. "See you later." And off she flew.

Manford and Veronica walked back along the trail. They stopped on the hilltop to look at MorningGlory Mountain once again then returned to WhiteFlower Meadow.

"Veronica. . ." Manford said.

"What?"

"What would it be like to see ten thousand flamingos standing on one leg?"

"I think it would look pretty strange," said Veronica. "Hmmm, if you gave one a push, do you think they'd all fall over?" They both laughed and sat down in the shade of the big tree.

Flossie, meanwhile, flew across the pond and into the woods. She was thinking. *'I'm not in Florida, that much is becoming fairly clear. But where am I? I forgot to ask. I only found out where I'm not. And what's more, thanks to my own bright idea, now I have to take a friend I don't have to a birthday party for a moose. Where will I find a friend on short notice? And what kind of present should I give to a moose? Flossie,'* she thought, *'you sure lead an interesting life.'*

She sat in a tree and looked around. *'It's quiet here'*, she thought.*' I'm not used to that. It was never quiet with those other flamingos around. And the air smells good, fresh and clean instead of like salt and fish. That's a pleasant change. The forest is different, not at all like the shore, but it has its charm. The neighbors are a little strange—moose, bears, who knows what all—but they seem friendly enough. Maybe I'll stay for the summer. Other birds fly north, if this is north. Why not me?'*

Below her, Flossie saw a trail leading through the trees. It was headed east, but Flossie didn't know that. She wouldn't know east from her great aunt Sally. But she was curious, so she dropped to the ground and followed it, stopping and looking and wondering as she went. She met no new friends. In fact, she met no one at all. *'Plenty of privacy here,'* she observed.

She saw a large mound off the path to her left after she'd gone about a quarter-mile. It was at the edge of a grassy clearing and was connected to the side of a hill. The mound was taller than she and maybe twenty feet around the outside. A path led to it. Out of curiosity, she followed.

The mound looked to be a dwelling. She walked around it and found an opening at ground level. A small amount of light came from within.

"Hello," she said loudly several times. There was no answer. She crouched low to the ground and poked her head into the entrance. A passage led inside. Occasional candles in holders on the wall lit the way. There was room for her to crawl inside. She did so, thinking she'd only look around.

The way led down to a large room with a fireplace, several chairs, and a couch. The furniture looked comfortable and recently used. There were pictures on the wall, small paintings of woodland scenes. Soft moss covered the floor.

'I should leave,' she thought. *'I should wait outside till someone returns.'* But she had to look around just a little.

Passageways led from the mound back into the hill to a kitchen with a huge pantry and a bedroom. She opened the pantry doors. Inside were bags and bags of potato chips—half a lifetime's supply, it appeared. She was puzzled.

Stairs led her to an upper level deep in the hill where she

found three more rooms. Two were bedrooms. The third, also with its supply of potato chips, looked to be a hobby room. It had a work table with paints and brushes and small jars of colored beads. Each room was neat and tidy. Each was lit with candles.

'Who lives here?' Flossie wondered. *'Perhaps the friend I'm seeking? I'd better go outside and wait.'*

She went into the main upstairs bedroom. The bed looked soft and inviting; she had to test it, just for a minute. Flossie lay down, sank into the covers and rested her head on the pillow.

'Florida can wait,' she thought. *'This is nice.'* And she fell asleep in moments, in the upstairs room, in the quiet house, with candles burning faintly in the hall.

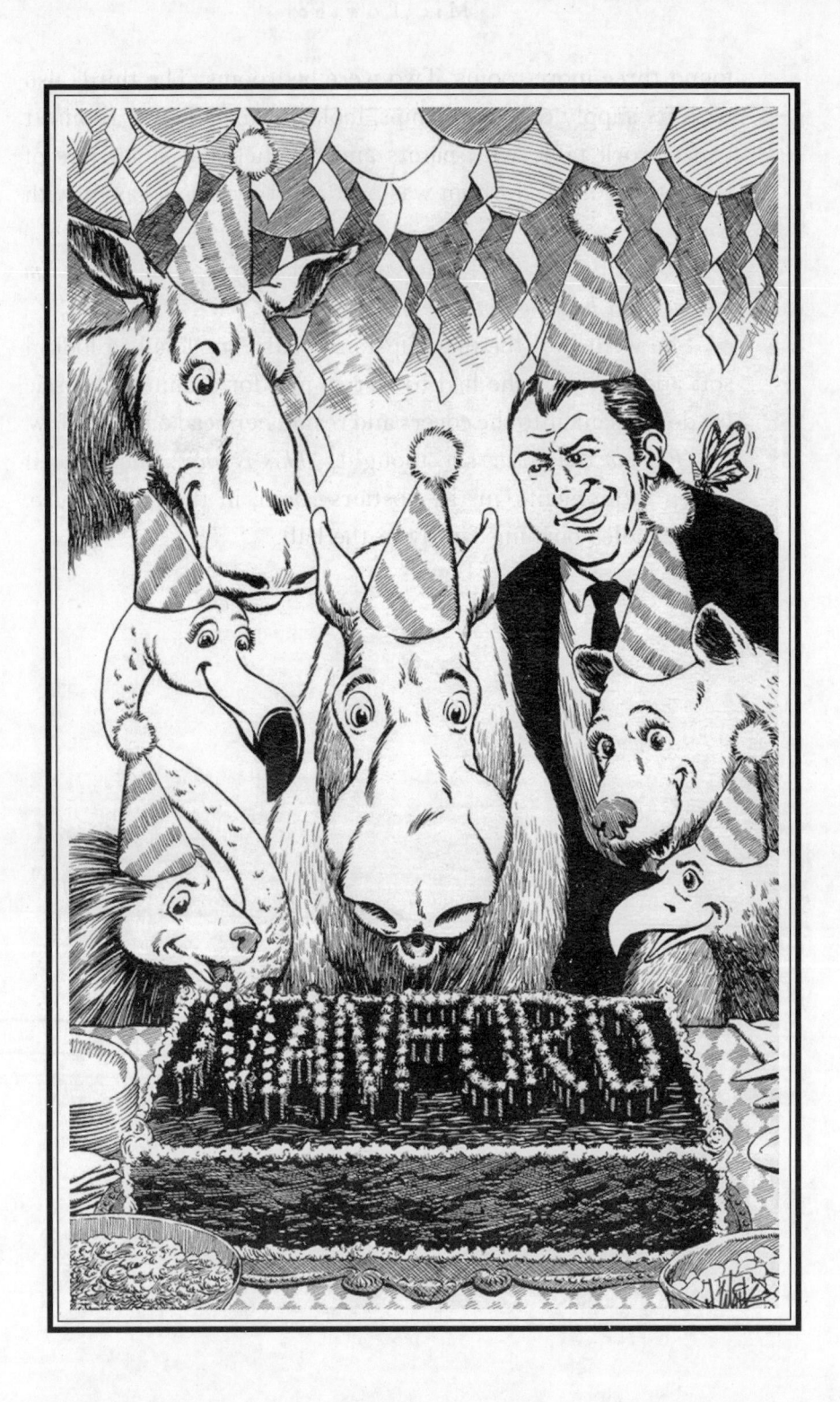

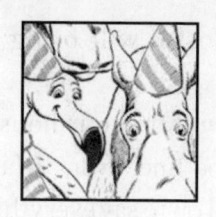

2

Surprises in Small and Large Packages

In which Manford has a birthday and a visitor

Manford lived deep in the forest. His house was large and painted white and had shingles and shutters of weathered gray. A path lined with rosebushes led to the wide front door. If you opened the door today, you'd find everyone inside very busy.

Manford's mother had been decorating since early morning. She'd strung colored paper streamers from the dining room chandelier to each of the corners of the room. Pleased with that, she'd strung more streamers to the middle of each wall. Then she'd blown up balloons and placed clusters of them about the room. Now she was arranging party hats, one at each guest's place at the table.

Manford was fussing. He went from one place to another, wondering if his guests would like the decorations; wondering if there would be enough food; wondering if everyone would enjoy the games he'd picked—fuss, fuss, fuss. He'd been with Veronica again the day before. They hadn't seen Flossie. It made him wonder.

"Do you think they will be on time?" he asked his mother.

"Do you think Flossie will bring a friend?" he asked his mother.

"Do you think they'll find our house?" he asked his mother.

"Everything will be fine, dear," Manford's mother said. She could always be counted on to say everything would be fine. "Instead of fussing," she went on, "help me bake your birthday cake."

"Okay," he said. "Is it going to be chocolate?"

"Of course, with chocolate frosting."

"I get only one candle," Manford said, sounding a bit sad. "Do you suppose my friends will think I'm too little if I have only one candle?"

"I was going to spell out your name with candles," his mother said. "Would you like that?"

"Oh, yes," he said, happy again.

Manford and his mother spent the next two hours baking a cake. It was chocolate, rectangular, and three layers high. He spread frosting between the layers, then over the top and down the sides. He put fancy swirls all over then his mother spelled M A N F O R D across the top with fifty yellow candles.

"See if you can blow all those out at once," she said.

They placed the cake in the center of the table. Manford was arranging plates and silverware when, at last, the doorbell rang.

"I'll get it," he said.

He found Veronica at the door. Perched on her shoulder was a large bird with feathers of dark brown turning to tan at the tips. Both were carrying presents wrapped with bright paper and ribbons. Veronica was laughing.

"What's funny?" said Manford.

"This sign over your door," Veronica said. The wooden sign, with elegant carved out letters said:

Mooster & Moosus B.W. Moose Welcome you to Moostery Manor

"What about it?" asked Manford.

"It sounds very moosterious, tee-hee."

Manford welcomed his guests inside and took them to the kitchen.

"This is my mom, Mary Moose," he said to Veronica. "And this is Veronica," he said to his mom.

"Pleased to meet you," they both said.

"And this," said Veronica, referring to the bird perched on her shoulder, "is the moostery guest." She started giggling again.

"My name," said the bird, "is Golly. I'm a golden eagle as you can tell by the color of my feathers."

"Welcome to our home," Mary Moose said politely. "What nice looking presents. Let's put them on the table."

"Golly lives in a tree," said Veronica as they went into the dining room. "It's above the canyon near Misty Falls."

"Is it a hollow tree?" Manford asked. He'd seen pictures of birds building nests in hollow trees.

"Oh, no," said Golly. "I have a house much like yours, except that it's much smaller and built among the branches of a large fir. I have a kitchen, sitting room, bedroom, study, and at the very top, a lookout. I call the house GloryView, because I have such a wonderful view of MorningGlory Mountain."

"Have you been to the top of the mountain?" Manford asked excitedly.

"Many times," Golly replied. "You must join me sometime. I'll show you the way."

"Oh, I'd like that. Veronica wants to go, too. Right, Veronica?"

"Maybe," she replied.

The doorbell rang again and Manford went to answer. Flossie had arrived with a small, black-and-gray companion who looked rather like a pincushion.

"Come in," Manford said.

"Thanks," said Flossie. "This is my new friend, Needlenose.

He says he's a porcupine." They had also brought gaily wrapped presents.

Manford introduced the new arrivals to his mother, Veronica, and Golly.

"Where'd you get a name like Golly?" Flossie asked.

"You've heard of goshawks, haven't you?" the bird said gravely.

Flossie nodded.

"Well, I'm a Golly eagle." Veronica started giggling again.

"That's a *very* old joke," said Flossie.

"I'm a *very* old eagle," Golly replied with a wink and a sly smile.

The group plunged immediately into friendly chatter, asking questions about each other and about where each lived. Veronica described her home in the cave behind Misty Falls. Golly told again about his tree house nearby.

Mary had set out dishes of nuts, popcorn, pretzels, and the like for them to nibble as they talked. Needlenose sat protectively near the potato chips and emptied the bowl almost as fast as it was refilled.

"I live in a burrow," he said, describing his home. "It was first owned by a bear. That's why it's so big, or so the real estate agent said. Foxes lived there after that, then about twenty families of woodchucks. There were others I wasn't told about, too. I can still smell them."

"Is it just one big room?" Veronica asked.

"Not any more. I had builders convert it to seven rooms on two floors."

"That doesn't even count the potato chip pantry," Flossie added. "It's as big as the kitchen."

"I *like* potato chips," Needlenose protested. "Besides, they keep me from eating the furniture."

"How do you know about it, Flossie?" Veronica asked.

"She's staying with me," said Needlenose. "I was out for the afternoon a couple days ago and found her asleep upstairs when I returned."

"I was going to stay only a few minutes," Flossie insisted. "I *intended* to wait outside."

"She sure was flustered when I woke her up," Needlenose chuckled. "She thought I was the Swamp Creature or something."

"Well, it *was* frightening," said Flossie, "not to mention embarrassing."

"Anyway, I have plenty of room so I invited her to stay."

"Where is this place?" asked Manford.

"Through the woods a short way on the far side of my pond," Flossie said. "It isn't marked. I couldn't tell if anyone lived there or not without going inside."

"You should put up a sign like I have at Misty Falls," said Veronica, "or like here at Moostery Manor."

"I have one at GloryView," said Golly.

"Maybe so," Needlenose said, thinking, "but I'd have to call it something."

"You could call it Needle Point," said Golly.

"But it's not pointed," Needlenose replied, "it's just a big mound connected to the side of a hill. Let's see...it's covered with grass...and there's a grassy field around it."

"It looks like a haystack," Flossie said.

"That's it...and it's hollow inside. I'll call it Haystack Hollow. And I can be the needle in the haystack!"

"I like it," said Veronica.

"Wonderful," Mary agreed.

Card games, board games, and guessing games occupied them through the afternoon. Flossie consistently won at cards. She'd played a lot while waiting in airports, she said, in her aimless travels about the country.

The video game proved the most popular. It had to do with searching for hidden treasure and everyone got to play at once. The game offered clues that led players from one place to another and then to somewhere else. Golly, wise old bird that he was, excelled at riddles and was good at unraveling clues.

They searched for treasure through a decaying mansion, a mine tunnel, a cave with many passages and rooms, a dark forest, down a fast river, across a mountainous desert, and through abandoned buildings in a mysterious ghost town. Danger and threatening creatures followed them all the while but each time they managed to escape. When they arrived at last where they thought they'd find the game's treasure, they found only another clue leading to even more adventures.

"Oh, noooo," said Manford.

"What a bummer," said Veronica.

"Silly game," said Flossie. "We should at least get something for making it this far."

"There's treasure here in the next room," Mary said from the doorway. "Manford, why don't you open your presents?"

"Good idea," he said, and everyone filed into the dining room to gather 'round the stack of brightly wrapped gifts.

"This one's from Flossie," Mary said, handing Manford a flat box wrapped in gray with a pink ribbon and bow. He removed the wrapping and pulled apart layers of tissue paper inside. There he found a peaked, gray felt hat with braided green cord around the brim.

"It's an alpine hiker's hat," Flossie explained. "You want to climb mountains and explore the neighborhood? You need an official hat to wear."

"Oh, thank you," Manford said, looking very happy.

"But a hat like that needs a feather," Flossie said, and she plucked a small one from her wing. "Here, now it's a personalized gift from me to you."

Manford secured the feather under the cord then tried the

hat on, placing it between his long, fuzzy ears.

"Looks great," said Veronica. "I suppose we'll *have* to climb MorningGlory Mountain now."

"This one's from Golly," Mary went on. It was small and square and wrapped in brown and white. Inside, Manford found a book. It had a pleasing flowered cover but no title, and its pages had no words. It was a completely blank book about an inch thick. There was a bottle of ink with it and a pen—a fine quill pen made from a stout brown-and-tan feather.

"If you're planning adventures," Golly said, "you'll need pen and ink and a journal to keep a record. As you probably noticed, the pen is from one of *my* feathers."

"Thank you," Manford said. "Mom has been teaching me to read and write so this will be useful."

"Excellent," said Golly. "If it's okay with her, I can help with your writing lessons."

"Of course," Mary said.

"Maybe I could learn to write stories," said Manford.

"Your adventures will make good stories," Golly said, "when you have some."

The next present was from Veronica, a soft, round package done up in crinkly, gold paper. Manford undid the wrappings.

"It's a scarf," he said. "How pretty!" It was black and brown with a gold-colored design and easily six feet long.

"It's made of bear fur," said Veronica. "Some of mine, some of Mom's, some she collected from other bears in the circus. I think it has lion and tiger fur, too. We had several made last time she was home and I thought you'd like one. It gets cold here in the winter, you know."

"Cold?" said Flossie with concern. "How cold?"

"I don't know. I sleep all winter and never notice. But it must get cold. There's still snow when I wake up."

Manford wrapped the scarf twice around his neck and let the fringed ends hang down to his knees.

"It will be warm, that's for sure," he said. "Thank you, Veronica."

"Here's a present from Needlenose," his mother said, handing him a square, flat box. "Oh, and look at the pretty bow!"

The box indeed had an unusual black-and-orange bow. In fact, the closer Manford looked at it, the more he thought it might be more than a bow. He was just about to touch it when it fluttered its wings and took off. It flew completely around the room then came to rest on Manford's nose.

"Hello," said what obviously wasn't a bow, "I'm Princess Columbine and I'm a monarch butterfly."

"Princess is a friend of mine," Needlenose said. "Flossie said she was supposed to bring a friend to your party so I brought one, too. She lives in the forest near me and comes by for a sip of soda now and then."

"Hello, Princess," said Manford, squinting down his nose to see her. "You're very pretty." Columbine was pleased to hear him say it.

Manford opened the box and discovered a flat necklace made of quills and beads. It had mysterious red and blue markings.

"It's an Indian ceremonial necklace," Needlenose said, " an Apache design, I think. I got the idea from a picture and I used *my* quills."

"It's most unusual," Manford said. "How do I use it?"

"You can wear it just for fun, I guess, but the real time to wear it is when you're looking for something lost. It has magical powers."

"How did it get those?" Flossie asked.

"I think it's the markings," Needlenose said. "I haven't actually tried it."

"Thank you," Manford said. "It's really nice. I'll try it first chance I get."

"The last one's from me," Manford's mother said, handing him a box wrapped in blue with two yellow bows. Manford opened it.

"It's a backpack," he said. "Did you make it?"

"Yes, I did, and you're set for big adventures now: a hiker's hat for your head, a scarf to keep your neck warm, a backpack to carry supplies, a magic necklace to help you find things, and a journal to keep a record."

"They're wonderful presents," Manford said. "Thank you, everyone."

"Now it's time for lunch," Mary went on. "That is, if any of you are hungry."

"We're hungry, aren't we?" asked Manford.

"Yes!" they all replied.

Mary carried bowls and dishes of good smelling things from the kitchen as the partygoers gathered at the table. She'd made a variety of treats—hot things and cold things, leafy things and meaty things—figuring that whatever kinds of animals came to the party, there would be something each liked. For Manford, she'd baked his favorite, willow leaf pie. They were about ready to eat when the doorbell rang once again.

"Who could that be?" Mary said.

"I didn't invite anyone else," said Manford.

"It's a man," said Needlenose, looking out the front window, "a big man, dressed kind of funny. He doesn't look very friendly."

"*Hit the decks*," screeched Flossie, looking out over top Needlenose. "*Under the furniture! It looks like Al Capone.*"

Mary opened the door.

"Um, good aftanoon, Missus Moose," the man said. He wore a black, pinstriped suit with a white carnation on the lapel, a black shirt and white tie, and a black, straw hat with a white band. He wore sunglasses and was smoking a big cigar.

"Da name's Johnny," he went on. "Mind if I come in? I have a little somethin' here for your birthday boy." He reached into his inside jacket pocket, but stopped as Flossie covered her head with her wings and dove under the dining room table. The other animals hung nervously in the doorway. Mary Moose smiled as she welcomed the man in.

"You're just in time for lunch," she said. "Manford, Veronica, Flossie, Golly, Needlenose, and Princess Columbine, I'd like you to meet Johnny. He'll tell you who he is."

"Pleased ta meet all of youse," Johnny said, tipping his hat and looking round the room. "Scuse me, miss," he said to Flossie, still under the table. "I didn't mean to make ya noivous." Seeing they awaited his explanation, he continued.

"It's like dis, see. I'm da guy who represents Manford's dad, The Great Bucknikov. I get him parts in ballets and other stage performances all over da woild. I'm the one what helped make him a star."

The animals seemed relieved and gathered round Johnny to hear what else he had to tell.

"Bucky wanted ta come home for his little Manford's birthday, see, but he can't. He's got a big gig in New York. So he sends me. All da way from New York to find Manford and his mom somewheres in da woods. It wasn't easy, I'll tell ya dat.

"He sent you dis present, little fellow," Johnny said, reaching again into his coat pocket and handing a videotape to Manford. "Hope ya don't mind I didn't wrap it. I was in kind of a hurry to get here on time."

"What is it?" Manford asked.

"It's a tape of his greatest performances. He thought you'd want to see 'em, especially those what wasn't on TV."

"I saw him on TV the other night," said Veronica. "I think we'd all like to see it."

"That's right," said Golly.

"If ya don't mind," Johnny said, "I am kinda hungry. Why don't we talk some more whiles we have lunch and watch da tape later."

The animals returned to their places and Mary set a place for Johnny. Soon the table buzzed with questions for the big man. How had he found them? Why was he wearing black? What was Manford's dad like? Princess Columbine fluttered across the table and came to rest on Johnny's white carnation, probing it for sweets while she flexed her wings.

"Mr. Johnny," Veronica said, "could you tell us how you met Manford's dad and how he got into ballet?"

"Sure," Johnny said, munching a hot dog piled high with ketchup, mustard, onions, and relish. "Would youse all like ta hear it?"

"I would," said Columbine. Heads nodded round the table.

"Please, do tell it," Mary said. "It's a wonderful story."

"Well, it kinda went like this:

"A few years ago, me and some pals went off to da woods in Alaska to go huntin'. We split up after a while and each of us took off alone. I had a big gun and was ready for anythin', but all I heard for hour after hour was quiet. Quiet makes me noivous.

"About the time I figured nothin' was ever gonna happen I heard a loud voice.

"'Help, please help me.'

"I looked around, didn't see nothin' at first, then I spotted a moose through the trees. I took aim and got ready to shoot, then I heard da voice again.

"'Don't shoot! Please don't shoot me.'

"I looked at the moose real hard. This had to be some kind of trick me pals was playin', but none of 'em was around.

"'Is that you talkin' to me, moose?' I said. 'If this is a gag, you're gonna be moose cheese in a minute.'

"'Yes, it's me. Please put down the gun. I need your help.'

"'So whadaya want?' I said, lowering the gun.

"'Take me to New York.'

"'Right, what for?'

"'I want to dance in the ballet.'

"'Pretty funny, moose,' I said, taking aim again. 'Now, listen, I don't like the sound of this. Foist of all, how are you talkin' to me anyway?'

"'Lots of animals can talk. Not many people are good at listening.'

"'Izzat so. Well, how do ya even know about New York and the ballet?'

"'I saw it on TV.'

"'Uh huh, who is this really?'

"'It's the truth,' the moose went on. 'When campers park their Winnebagos in the campgrounds, I watch TV through the windows. I've seen New York and I've seen the ballet. It's so beautiful, so graceful; I want to be a ballet star.'

"'Sure,' I said, putting down my gun. 'I just walk into New York and make you a star. Pretty likely.'

"'I've seen people like *you* on TV, too. You can be very persuasive.'

"'True, true, but what makes you think New York *wants* a ballet dancing moose?'

"Then he told me, and I knew that he was right.

"'You got a name, moose?' I said.

"'Buckwheat.'

"'Okay, Buckwheat, you got yourself an agent. Meet me in a town called Sundown in the Catskills in three weeks. I'll take you to da city from there. And don't get turned into a hatrack along the way.' The moose nodded and faded outa sight.

"'*Buckwheat,*' I said to myself, '*what a name! It'll never do for the ballet. It's gotta be somethin' else, somethin' foreign with a bit of mystery. Like Buckyev, maybe. . .how would that work? Nah—wait, I got it, Bucknikov. That's it, The Great Bucknikov!*'

"I went to New York to set up an audition. No one was interested at foist. In fact, dey all laughed in my face. But they didn't laugh long. I *can* be *very* persuasive.

"The audition took place in the dead of night. I figured it

would be best to keep it secret but word leaked out. Everybody who was anybody in ballet wanted ta see my Bucky's audition.

"So da music began. The first ballerina came on stage doing a Bourrée—that's stepping sideways real fast—across the stage and up to footlights. Then the second ballerina came on from the other side and did da same thing.

"Then came Bucknikov, standing on his back legs, doing turns around and around, across the stage and back again, ending with his head bowed low.

"The ballerinas were excited to see him. The first ran toward him doing a Grand Jeté—a big jump—landing on one side of his antler. Then da second ballerina did likewise and landed on the other side. Bucky lifted them majestically into the air. We practiced a bit in the Catskills, ya see.

"Then came da finale, what Bucky told me would make him a star. The ballerinas slid down his neck and sat on his back. Then he began to rotate his antlers like a helicopter. Whup, whup, whup, whup then faster whup-whup-whup-whup until he lifted himself and the ballerinas up off da stage and flew out into the auditorium, over the audience, round and round. The ballerinas grabbed baskets of flowers we'd stashed in the rafters and scattered them over da crowd. Everyone stood up and cheered.

"Opening night was a sellout. People stood in line to pay $200 a ticket to see Bucknikov, my Bucky. And he's been sold out every night since.

"Everybody loves Bucky now. New York loves him, the ballerinas love him, and I love him. And Bucky loves his little Manford, too. That's why he sent me all da way from New York to bring youse his best wishes on your birthday."

Manford beamed. Tears rolled down Flossie's beak. Golly and Princess Columbine shouted "Bravo." Needlenose swished his tail, sending quills flying to break balloons in the streamers overhead: *Pop! Bang! Pow! Pow!*

"I just love that story," Mary said, dabbing her eyes with her kerchief. "It's better every time I hear it. Sigh! Well, are we ready to light the candles?"

"Yes," came a chorus of voices. She and Johnny started at opposite ends of the cake and lit the fifty candles that spelled MANFORD.

"Ready to blow 'em out?" Johnny said when they'd finished.

"Guess so," Manford said. He moved closer to the cake. He made a wish, then took a deep breath, deeper...deeper...deeper, until his eyes started to bulge and his ears stood straight up on his head. Then he blew out a long puff of breath that started dousing candles at the *M* and continued to the *F* in the middle. Still going strong, he kept blowing, blowing, blowing on to the *R*, on to the *D*, where the last candle finally winked out. He blew so strong and steady that the candles all leaned over at an angle and the frosting had begun to ripple and pile up at the far edge.

Led by Johnny's booming voice, the guests sang *Happy Birthday, Happy Birthday* to Manford. Manford smiled, said thank you to his new friends; then, all the way to the tip of his nose, he blushed.

And blushing isn't easy for a moose.

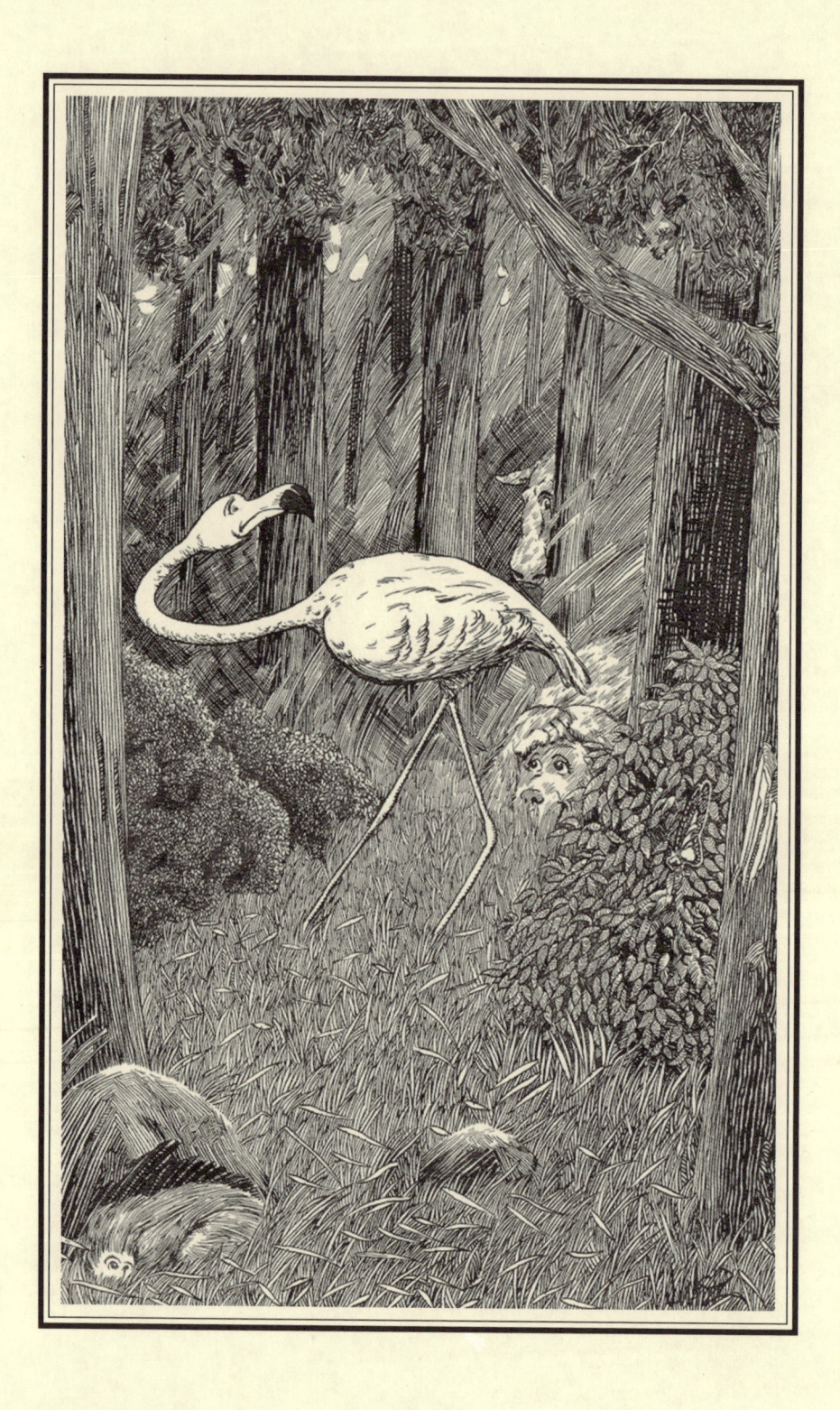

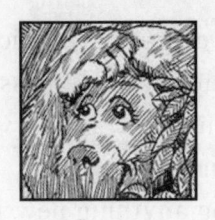

3

In WhiteFlower Meadow
In which new neighbors play games and plant a garden

Manford regarded himself in the mirror. He looked so wonderful wearing the hat Flossie had given him. He looked like an authentic hiker of the Alps. He wasn't really sure what Alps were, but they sounded like they ought to be mountains; big mountains, probably. He'd ask his mom about them next time they did lessons.

'If I look so authentic,' Manford thought, *'I should be exploring. I should be out seeing more of the neighborhood.'* He left the house. He followed the path through the woods, crossing MorningGlory Creek and going on to the meadow where he'd first met Veronica. She wasn't there. No one was there. He saw only trees and grass and daisies. *'Explore the meadow; that's what I'll do,'* he told himself. He started walking around its edge.

He looked deep into the woods on his left. He saw...trees. He looked out across the meadow on his right. He saw grass and white daisies. He walked and stopped, walked and stopped, looking all around him, seeing what there was to see: trees and grass and daisies.

Rounding the big tree where Veronica had danced, he walked along the top of the meadow. He passed the trail that led to Lookout Hill; he'd been there. Today, wearing his new hat, he wanted to see something new.

But he wasn't seeing anything new. Everything around him looked the same: trees and grass and daisies. He kept going, looking here and looking there. Exploring was tedious business sometimes, it seemed, not always one new discovery after another.

'Whoa, here's something,' Manford said to himself. A trail led out the east end of WhiteFlower Meadow. He hadn't known about that. He set off to follow it, heading into woods again. The trail was flat and well used. Trees were still growing new leaves and the undergrowth was sparse. Birds chirped and squirrels scampered through the brush. He would remember these things to write in his journal.

Manford had walked nearly half a mile through the woods when he came to a patch of open ground fifty feet long and thirty feet deep. The trail crossed a creek just beyond it. He went to the water's edge.

'What creek is this?' he wondered. *'Not MorningGlory. That's behind me.'* A trail led along the creek, crossing the path he was on. *'Now, I have a choice of new things to explore,'* Manford thought. *'Hmmm, I think I'll go left. No, don't be saying left. It should be, um, north.'* Explorers sounded more authentic saying north.

The water flowed swiftly, growing noisier as he followed upstream. He walked a quarter-mile then climbed a steep grade where the creek rushed toward him over large rocks. It sounded like a waterfall as it hurried by. He climbed farther, looking ahead through the trees to see where the water came from. He saw a pond. *'Hey, I've been here,'* he thought. *'This is where we met Flossie. This is the far end of her pond.'*

Manford crossed the creek where the pond flowed into it

and he walked along the shore, soon coming to a short stretch of beach. *'Do ponds have beaches?'* he wondered. *'There are no waves washing in, and no palm trees, but it's flat and sandy and next to the water. That's good enough.'*

He walked all along it leaving hoof prints. He lay down in the sand. The sky was cloudy overhead and a breeze gently rustled in the trees. *'Yes, this is the life!'* he thought. *'Exploring a new neighborhood is fun.'* He closed his eyes to take a nap but was too full of excitement to stay still. He got up and waded deep into the water to wash off the sand, then walked back to shore to continue his trek around the pond.

Soon, he found another path leading east and decided to try that. After passing through more forest he came to a clearing. Flossie was there, sitting atop a large, grassy mound.

"Hello," said Manford.

"Hello," Flossie replied. "That hat looks good on you."

"Thanks. I'm wearing it today because I'm exploring, or maybe I'm exploring today because I'm wearing it—one or the other. Is this where you stay with Needlenose?"

"This is his little bungalow. It's quite comfy, really."

"Isn't it strange to live underground?"

"I suppose. Other birds live in trees or on the ground, in roofs of buildings or holes in the sides of cliffs. Some even live in birdhouses. Flamingos live at the shore. Sleeping in a bed under a hill is not what we do. But it's fine for now; Needlenose is good company."

"He hasn't put up a sign yet to say this is Haystack Hollow."

"Oh, my, no," Flossie said. "He's much too picky just to hammer something together and be done with it. He has to find the right piece of wood and the right style of type and then carve it just so. He'll be at it for a while."

"On the contrary, my feathered friend," said Needlenose, emerging from the burrow, "it's almost finished. Once I find a post and pound it into the ground, Haystack Hollow will be officially marked."

Princess Columbine flew from the burrow just then.

"Hello, Manford," she said.

"Do you live here, too?"

"No, I'm just visiting. I live wherever I happen to be at the time. What are you doing today?"

"Exploring."

"That's why he's wearing that goodlooking hat," Flossie said.

"What have you discovered so far?" asked Needlenose.

"I found a trail from the end of the meadow to a creek. Then I found a path from there to the other end of the pond. After that I found Haystack Hollow."

"And it's barely past breakfast," said Flossie. "You've been busy."

"We were going to the meadow," said Needlenose. "Want to come along?"

"Sure, but let me take you there," said Manford. "I'll show you my new discoveries."

Columbine fluttered along ahead as the group went back around the pond and across the creek, south along the creek to the trail crossing, then west past the bare spot to the meadow. They found Veronica listening to music and dancing around the tree when they arrived. They settled down nearby to watch.

Veronica was concentrating, paying close attention to what she was doing; not exactly dancing with her eyes closed, but not exactly seeing much of anything, either. She spun and twirled and moved her legs this way and that, keeping time to the music. Many minutes passed. When she finally noticed she had an audience, she moved closer to them and danced an even fancier routine. She bowed when the music ended.

"That looked very good," said Needlenose.

"Thank you," Veronica replied.

"Do you practice every day?" Manford asked.

"I do when I think I might really join the circus someday. When the circus doesn't seem like such a hot idea, I do something else. I guess I dance mostly for fun."

"Sounds like a good reason to me," said Flossie.

"But I've had enough of it for now," Veronica continued. "Now that we're all here, what shall we do?"

"We could play games," said Manford.

"What kind of games?" Needlenose asked.

"How about hide-and-seek?"

"Good idea," said Veronica.

"I'll play," said Columbine.

"Now hold on a minute," said Flossie. "That's fine for you, you have colors that blend with the surroundings. How is somebody pink like me supposed to hide?"

"If you get far enough away, we won't be able to see you," Veronica said.

"If I get far enough away, I'll get lost."

But hide-and-seek was what the others wanted so Flossie went along with the idea.

"I might as well be 'it'," she said. "Okay, run along while I count to fifty, but don't go *too* far away." She stood behind the tree and closed her eyes to count while the others went to hide. When she finished, there was no one in sight.

"Here I come, ready or not," Flossie said. *'Such an intelligent thing to say,'* she was thinking. *'They're ready, but I'm not. Now what do I do? They're probably hiding right under my nose.'*

She walked around the edge of the meadow staring intently into the woods. Nothing moved. She kept walking, sticking one long, spindly leg slowly out in front of the other. She stopped and looked again. Still, nothing moved. *'Surely I can find something as big as a moose or bear,'* she said to herself. *'Maybe they look like rocks when they scrunch down and keep still.'* She saw a rock that looked suspicious. She walked through the trees to it and looked closely. Nope, just a rock.

She crossed the meadow. The new spring grass and daisies were growing but they weren't deep enough yet to hide anything big. She kept looking, behind rocks and trees and up in tree branches. She found no one.

'Where are they hiding?' she kept wondering.

Where, indeed? Let's put on our special glasses and take a look. Columbine is in plain sight on the tree where Flossie did her counting. With her wings folded flat, Princess looks like a dead leaf or part of the bark.

Veronica is in the woods not far away, rolled into a ball next to a tree. She does look like a rock; too bad Flossie picked the wrong one.

Manford is standing very still in dense trees. His color is dark and the trees throw soft shadows across him until he almost disappears.

This is how animals use their coloring to escape danger. You can see why playing hide-and-seek with them isn't such a great idea.

Flossie heard something crunch. She walked into the woods, looking from tree to tree. Needlenose had accidentally crushed some dead leaves. He held his breath and squeezed tightly under a rock. Flossie walked by, not seeing him then continued on around the meadow.

She'd found no one after fifteen minutes of looking. What's worse, whenever her back was turned, the hiding animals moved to new positions.

"Okay, enough of your camouflage tricks," Flossie said. "C'mon out. I'll never find you." Animals burst from the woods all around her.

"Bunch of show-offs," she said. "If I tried to hide, you'd find the spot of pink right away." The others were laughing.

"Now it's your turn to pick a game, Flossie," Manford said.

"All right, I will, hopscotch."

"How do you play that?" asked Veronica.

"I'll show you." Flossie led them to a bare patch of ground near the big tree. Grasping a rock with her foot, she drew a pattern of squares on the ground: one square, then two, then one, then two again, until she'd drawn ten squares which she numbered one to ten. She tossed the rock into square one then started to explain.

"The idea is to hop through these squares to the end, then turn around, hop back, pick up the rock, and hop out."

"Hop?" said Manford.

"That's right. When the squares are one wide, you hop on one foot. When they're two wide, you land on two feet. You have to hop over the square with the rock in it. Let me demonstrate." Flossie gracefully hopped over square one, then, with small assists from her wings, one- or two-footed her way to the end. She turned around and hopped back, picked up the rock with one foot, and hopped out.

"Next, you toss the rock on square two and do it over again," she said. "You win if you keep going like that all the way to ten. You're out if you land in the wrong place, or with too many feet, or toss the rock on the wrong number."

Flossie continued her demonstration. She did everything right until she tried to toss the rock to square seven and it rolled into eight.

"What happens now?" Manford asked.

"Someone else gets a rock and starts."

"Can we use the same one?"

"No, the one I threw stays there."

"Do we have to hop over it, too?" asked Veronica.

"Uh huh," Flossie said, "that's the advantage of going first. Why don't you try, Needlenose?"

"I don't hop," he replied.

"Oh, come on," she said.

"Sorry," he said, "porcupines do amazing things, including eating a hiker's boots or the door off an outhouse, but we don't hop."

"I can hop," said Columbine, "but I can't throw the rock."

"I'll do it for you," said Needlenose. As Flossie had done, he tossed the rock into square one. Columbine fluttered over it to land astride the line between squares two and three, half of her feet on either side. From there she easily flew from square to square and returned. Needlenose continued to throw for her until he missed square six and the rock rolled into seven.

"Too bad," Flossie said. "How about you, Veronica?"

"Okay, I'll try it." Veronica dropped a rock in square one, jumped and landed with two feet in squares two and three, then hopped her way to ten, avoiding squares where rocks remained. The ground shook when she jumped and she left deep footprints in the dirt.

"Good going!" said Flossie. "Now, hop your way back."

Standing on one foot, Veronica attempted to turn around for her return. She tripped and went sprawling, erasing most of the diagram. "I think we can safely say that you're out," said Flossie. "Shall I redraw it for you, Manford?"

"You'd have to draw two squares, then four for me," he replied. "I have too many feet for this."

"I guess we're each good at some things but not others," Flossie said. "I'm too pink to hide in the woods; most of you don't hop."

"How about a game we can all play?" said Needlenose.

"Like what?" said Veronica.

"Blowing bubbles. I'll bet we can all do that one way or another."

"Super," Manford said, "I'm sure I have the stuff at home. I'll go get it."

Rain clouds were gathering when Manford returned a while later. Only Golly was in the meadow. He was expertly jumping through hopscotch squares someone had redrawn.

"Where did everyone go?" Manford asked.

"Down to the pond," Golly said. "I got here as they were leaving and said I'd wait for you. I've been playing this interesting game. It takes good coordination to do it right."

"It also helps to have wings," said Manford.

They walked to the pond and found the others on the sandy beach. Manford had brought a bottle of soapy water and several small wire hoops. He dipped a hoop to cover it with soap film then blew into its center. A trail of bubbles big as ping-pong balls came out and rose to drift on the wind. Light sent wavy patterns of orange, green, and violet dancing over them. Each reflected rounded images of the pond and the sky. Some popped right away. Others flew across the water and into the trees. Manford dunked the hoop again and sent more bubbles flying.

"It also works this way," Flossie said, taking another hoop. She dipped it and waved it in the air. Bubbles surrounded her, floated around and over her, then traveled with the wind. They stood and watched them float away.

"Here's how you make big bubbles," Needlenose said. He held a hoop and blew into it ever so slowly. The soap film pushed gently outward then began to grow. It became a huge bubble that wobbled and dripped on the hoop and looked like it would burst at any moment. Still it grew bigger until it finally took flight when Needlenose was about out of breath. Big as a soccer ball, it rose slowly and drifted halfway across the pond before it popped.

"Good one!" said Veronica. "Now it's my turn." She dipped the hoop several times and blew bubbles big and small. Some of them hung in the air around her. She used the hoop to catch them before they floated away.

"Hey," she said, "if you catch them, you can blow them into more bubbles."

"Look at this," Golly said, when it was his turn, "when two

bubbles stick together, the side they have in common is flat." The others gathered round to see several sets of two, three, and four stuck together bubbles.

"When many bubbles join," he went on, "they share many flat sides. What do you suppose would happen if seven bubbles stuck together?" Everyone thought about that a moment.

"If one was caught in the middle, it would be a cube," said Needlenose. "It would have six flat sides." They blew and trapped bubbles, trying to make this happen. But even in clusters of twenty bubbles or more, they never found one completely enclosed.

"Columbine hasn't had a turn," Manford said. "Want to try this, Princess?"

"I don't think I can make enough air," she said.

"Sure you can," Manford said, holding a hoop for her. "Come up next to it and fly like a hummingbird."

Columbine hovered before the soapy hoop and fanned her wings. The film pushed slightly outward and a bubble began to grow. The Monarch Princess flew for all she was worth, creating a tiny breeze that made the bubble bigger and bigger and bigger. When it finally let loose, it was big as a watermelon. It sagged and drooped and stretched as the wind began to push it, then gathered itself into roundness and floated happily on.

"Wow, Princess, what a bubble!" said Manford.

"That was really something," said Flossie. "Look, it's still going." The bubble was halfway across the pond before it burst.

"This is fun," said Veronica; "let's make some more." They went on taking turns with the bubble hoops to make tiny bubbles, giant bubbles, and stuck together bubbles that sailed away on the wind.

The breeze stopped at one point. The bubbles Needlenose was making sank to surface of the pond. Instead of breaking when they hit, they bobbed lightly atop the water.

"Look, they float!" said Columbine.

"That makes sense, I suppose," said Flossie. "Bubbles are wet. It must take something dry to pop them."

"I just noticed something else," Golly said, pointing to a large bubble he'd made. "If you look into a bubble's center, you see a stretched out image of the sky and trees ahead of you. But there's something odd about it. Do you see what it is?"

The others looked from one bubble to another.

"I see a picture of the trees across the pond," said Needlenose. "Wait...oh, cool! It's two pictures, really: one right side up, then the same thing upside down. It looks like the trees are growing both up and down."

"That's what I thought, too," said Golly. "The bubble must work like some kind of lens. One image must be from the front side of the bubble, the other from the back."

"I'm seeing something else," said Veronica, looking into a bubble that hung before her.

"What?" said Golly.

"Us."

"I see us, too," Manford said. "We're reflecting in it like a mirror. And there are two of each of us, too."

"Probably for the same reason." Golly said.

Rain began falling then, turning quickly from a sprinkle into heavy drops that made patterns of ever-widening circles on the pond. Flossie and Veronica sent dozens more bubbles flying.

They didn't pop. Falling raindrops passed right through.

"Whoa, I never expected that," said Manford.

"Me, either," Needlenose said. "Look, the bubbles bounce around when raindrops hit them, then the extra water flows around the sides and drips off the bottom."

"That's amazing," said Veronica. "I wonder if the same thing happens when it snows."

Bubbles began to collect on the wet sand at their feet, sparkling with color in the light like a carpet of jewels.

"I guess Flossie's right," Golly said. "It takes something dry to pop a bubble."

"What a weird game," said Flossie. "We start out to blow bubbles and turn into a bunch of scientists."

The shower ended about the time the soapy water was gone.

"What should we do now?" Manford asked.

"How about jumprope?" said Flossie.

"Too much like hopscotch," said Needlenose; "some of us can't jump."

"Instead of a game," Golly said, "maybe you'd like to help me with something."

"Sure," Veronica said, "what kind of something?"

"When I flew over, I was looking for a place to plant a garden. You could help me do that."

"What do you want to grow?" asked Manford.

"I bought some wildflower seeds from a catalog. They looked pretty so I thought I'd try to grow them. Maybe you'd like to plant something, too."

"I could plant potatoes and make my own potato chips," Needlenose said.

"I could plant berries," said Veronica. "I never get enough berries."

"First we need a place to put it," Golly went on. "The trees are too thick where I live. A garden there wouldn't get enough light."

"How about here in the meadow?" said Columbine.

"No, I don't think so," Golly said. "The meadow is nice the way it is. A place off by itself would be better."

"There's a place down the path that might work," Manford said. "I found it this morning when I was exploring. C'mon." He led them to the open area near the creek. Golly recognized the spot. He walked around on it for a while, looked up now and then, and pecked in the dirt a few times.

"It's more than I need for a few wildflowers," he said, "but it is a good place. It'll get plenty of sunlight and rain, and trees will only shade it part of the day."

"What do we do now?" Manford asked.

"Poke holes in the ground and drop in seeds, I guess," Golly said.

"No, this is a much bigger project than that," said Flossie. "You need to turn the dirt over first."

"Do what?" said Needlenose.

"The dirt is packed down from years and years of rain pounding on it. You need to loosen it up and get air into it so the plants can grow roots more easily."

"I can dig," said Veronica.

"Good. Dig this whole clearing back to where the trees begin. Needlenose, you and Manford follow behind and smooth down the dirt as she goes."

Veronica moved dirt like a backhoe. Facing the woods, she methodically dug a long trench along the edge of the trail. Then she moved forward and dug another trench, heaping dirt into the one behind. She continued in this fashion across the entire area. Needlenose and Manford followed, smoothing the ground.

"Very nice job," Flossie said when they'd finished. "Now let's get some seeds. We should probably plant them in rows up and down."

"Rows?" said Needlenose.

"Yes, is that a problem?"

"Golly's planting wildflowers. You can't plant wildflowers in rows."

"Why not?"

"Because they're wild. They should grow here and there and wherever they want, but not in rows."

"Oh," Flossie said, "I suppose you're right."

"What kinds of flowers are you going to plant, Golly?" Veronica asked.

"I have scarlet bugler, which are red; butter-and-eggs, which are yellow; and globemallow, which are orange. Their pictures in the catalog were very colorful."

"Sounds good," said Flossie. "What are the rest of us going to plant?"

No one seemed to know. They stood thinking in silence, looking at one another.

Suddenly, with the sound of the rushing creek in his ears, the soft brush of breeze on his back, and the smell of fresh earth in his nose, Manford got that twinkling 'I've-got-an-idea' look in his eyes and said, "I've got an idea!"

"What?" the others replied all at once.

"Let's plant a picture."

"Let's *what*?" said Columbine.

"Let's plant different colored flowers that make a picture when they grow."

"What kind of picture?"

"How about one of MorningGlory Mountain?"

"I get it," said Veronica.

"Wow," said Needlenose, "that *is* a good idea."

"Excuse me, but how is that different than planting things in rows?" Flossie asked.

"This is art," said Needlenose. "Rows aren't art. Here, I'll show you." Needlenose shuffled into the freshly dug dirt and began to rough out a drawing with his paws and tail. He made three mountains, two short and one very tall. He drew clouds drifting across them. At the base of the mountains, he sketched in forest.

"Is this what you had in mind?"

"I think so," said Manford.

Needlenose drew a line around the outside of the picture.

"We'll put some kind of border around it," he said, marking

that area with the number one. "What should we plant there?"

"Strawberries," said Veronica. "I'll bet we could get strawberry plants at the store."

"Good," said Flossie, "you won't have to trample through the whole garden to eat them that way."

"Manford, what are you going to plant?" asked Columbine. "Willows?"

"Lettuce," Manford said, "both red and green."

"Perfect," said Needlenose. "We'll put another border of that just inside the strawberries." He drew a second line inside the first and marked that area two.

"My wildflowers can be the forest at the base of the mountain," Golly said. "That's where they'd grow anyway. They'll feel right at home."

"Absolutely," said Needlenose, and he marked that area three. "Now, we need something to make mountains."

"Pansies," said Flossie. "Pansies with brown and red faces will look like mountains when they grow."

"Excellent," Needlenose said, marking the mountains four. "How about the clouds?"

"White petunias," offered Golly.

"Of course," said Needlenose. He marked the clouds five. "We have only sky left to do. Any ideas for sky?"

"Columbines," said Columbine. "They're blue."

"That works," said Manford.

"I don't want to sound too radical about this," Needlenose said, marking the sky six, "but there's another blue flower we could use."

"What's that?" asked Veronica.

"Morning glories."

"Sounds kind of themey," Flossie said.

"We ought to have morning glories growing somewhere," Veronica said, "especially with so many things around here named after them."

"Okay, Manford," said Needlenose, "here's your plant-by-number picture. How do you like it?"

"It's wonderful," Manford replied.

"Then let's go shopping for seeds and meet back here tomorrow."

The next afternoon found them planting from seed packets and flats of small, growing plants. They planted columbines and morning glories for sky. Golly poked holes in the loose ground with his beak. Flossie followed holding packets while Columbine sucked tiny seeds from them with her straw-like mouth and shot them into the holes. Needlenose finished off by filling in dirt behind them.

Petunias for clouds went in next, then pansies for mountains, all by the numbers. Golly scattered his wildflower seeds to make forest. Manford planted lettuce for the inside border, then Golly poked holes so Veronica could place her strawberry plants around the outside edge. To finish, Needlenose smoothed the picture over by brushing it with his tail.

"It will look nice when it grows," said Columbine.

"That was a good idea, Manford," said Needlenose.

"Thanks," our young moose replied.

"I'll check it from the air as summer gets on to see how it's doing," Golly said.

"Gee," said Veronica, "you were only going to poke a few seeds in the ground and look what it turned into."

"Indeed," replied Golly.

"You should have known that was too simple," said Flossie.

"Yes, it reminds me of something my grandfather used to say."

"What was that?"

"'*Anything worth doing is worth overdoing.*' It was our family motto, he always said."

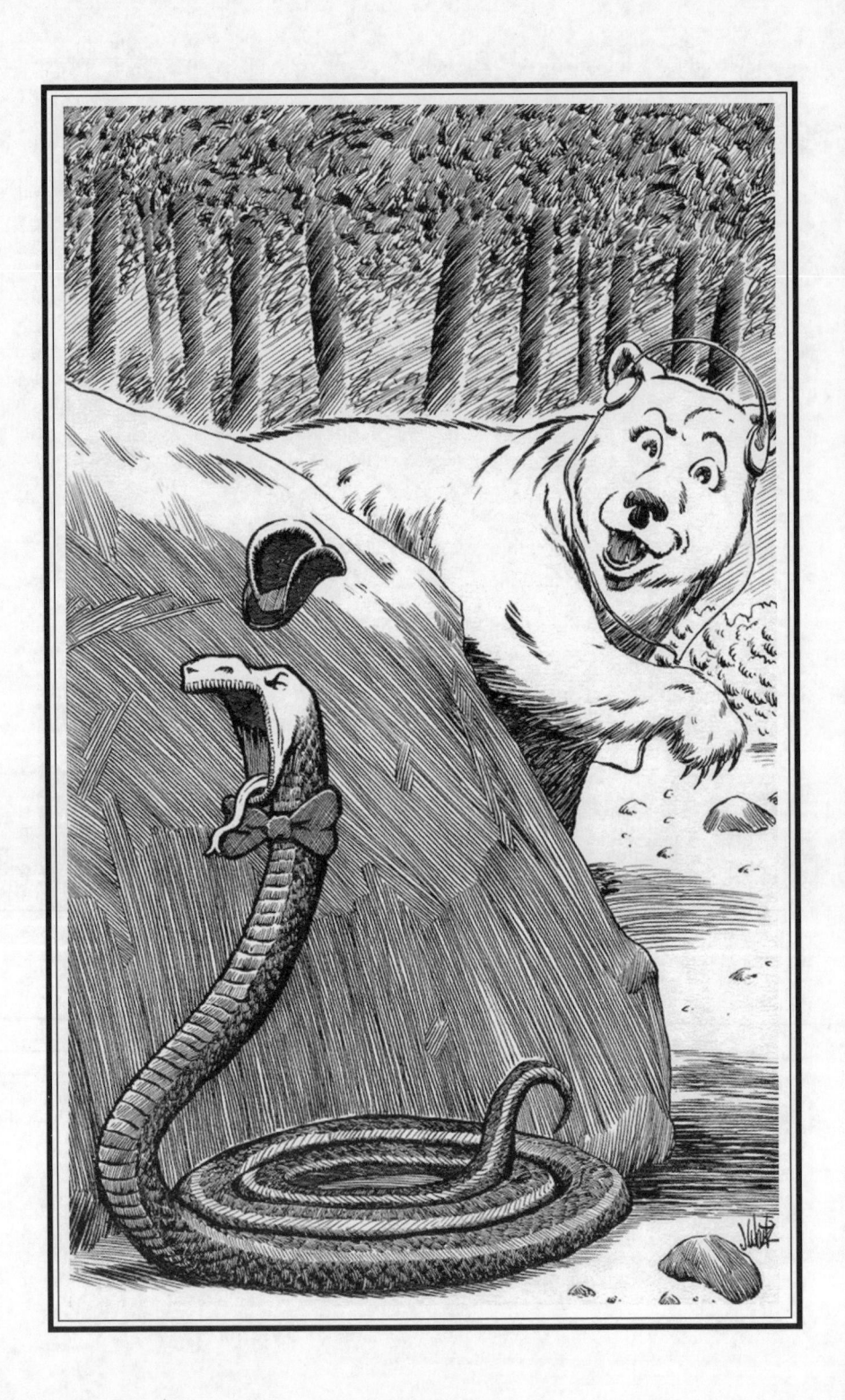

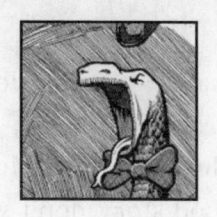

4

Watcher at MorningGlory Crossing

In which we hear voices

AAAAAA BBBBBB CCCCCC

Manford was practicing his penmanship under Golly's watchful eye.

"Make the letters round," Golly said. "Can't be sloppy about letters if you want us to read what you write."

"Like this?" Manford said, showing what he'd done.

"Better, but practice those Bs more. They're not round enough yet."

B B B B B B. Manford wrote more Bs, making them round, trying to keep them on the lines; looking forward to the day he could tell of his adventures in his journal.

"Golly," he said, "when I get good enough, I'll need adventures to write about."

"You've already had several," Golly replied. "You went exploring and met Veronica and Flossie. You could write about that."

"That was already covered in Chapter 1," Manford said.

"True. What about your birthday party and meeting Mr. Johnny, or is that old news, too?"

"Uh huh."

"Hmmm," Golly said, "I guess you do need some new adventures."

"We could climb MorningGlory Mountain," Manford said. "That would make a good story, don't you think?"

"I do, but you should ask your mother about it first."

"Mom," Manford called out at once.

"What is it?" Mary Moose replied.

"Is it okay if I climb MorningGlory Mountain?"

"By yourself?" she asked, coming into the room.

"Um, no. You'll go along, won't you Golly?"

"Yes, indeed" Golly said. "I offered to show you the way, remember?"

"Veronica will want to go," Manford continued, "and so might Flossie and Needlenose. We should ask them."

"How about Princess Columbine?" Mary asked.

"Oh, yes, this will be a great adventure; everyone should go. You, too, Mom. Want to join us?"

"I don't think so, but I'll help you get ready."

"Mom knows a lot about wilderness trips," Manford said to Golly. "She used to be a guide."

"That sounds interesting," Golly said. Mary smiled and returned to what she was doing.

After Manford's lesson, he and Golly went to find the others. Veronica was dancing under the tree in the meadow again.

"Sure, I'll go along," she said. "It's even starting to sound like a good idea."

They found Flossie in her pond.

"Climb a mountain?" she said. "Why would I want to do that?"

"To see what's up there," Manford said.

"To see what things look like from up so high," added Veronica.

"Everything looks small and flat, take my word for it,"

Flossie said.

"But we want to see for ourselves," Manford went on. "It's more fun to do things than to just wonder about them. And we'd like you to be along, too."

"Well, that's very thoughtful of you. What about Needlenose?"

"We haven't asked him yet, but we will."

"I'll go if he does, I suppose. How long will this journey take?"

"Three days to get to the top for those who are walking," Golly said. "You and I can travel much faster, of course."

"If I don't get lost; I get lost on long trips, you know."

"I'll show you the way," Golly said.

Needlenose and Columbine were sipping soda atop Haystack Hollow when the group arrived. They agreed at once to join the expedition, though Columbine said she'd rather ride than fly.

"I get faint flying at high altitudes," she told Manford. "I'll ride on your new hat, if you don't mind."

They discussed what supplies to take and agreed to meet in the meadow next morning. Manford returned home. His mother helped him gather his equipment and baked him a willow leaf pie.

"This will taste good when you get to the top," she said.

Manford went to bed early. He dreamed of mountains, tall mountains with peaks in the clouds. . .brightly glowing clouds.

Veronica was waiting in the meadow next morning when Manford arrived. She was wearing a headset and tape player and had brought a basket of blueberries.

"There's nothing to eat on top," she said, "no trees or even bushes. I brought these for a treat when we get there."

Manford wore his backpack and hiker's hat. He carried the

scarf from Veronica in the pack, along with the necklace from Needlenose, the journal from Golly, and his willow leaf pie.

Golly arrived, circling slowly round the meadow and landing nearby.

"It's an excellent day for an adventure," he said. Indeed, the sun was behind a thin layer of clouds and there was little wind. It would be calm and cool for hiking.

"I saw Flossie and Needlenose getting ready when I passed over," he said. "They'll be along soon." He had brought no equipment, figuring he could find what he wanted to eat along the way and quickly fly home for anything else if necessary.

Flossie flew in a while later, a large canvas bag hanging from her feet. She settled slowly toward the ground, allowed the bag to come to rest, then landed and stumbled over the cord tied around her feet.

"I feel like a sky crane," she said.

"Potato chips, I'll bet," said Veronica. "Is that what's in the bag?"

"You got it," she replied. "Flossie's Flight Service: ten bags of potato chips for Sir NeedleNibbler; a few tins of sardines for me."

Needlenose eventually came shuffling up the trail, Princess Columbine fluttering from flower to flower ahead of him. Mary joined them then, also.

"Did you decide to go with us after all?" Golly asked her.

"No, but I wanted to talk to you all before you left."

"Certainly," Golly said, and he and the group gathered round to listen.

"Please be careful on this adventure," Mary said. "There's nothing to be afraid of in the woods but you can get into trouble if you're not paying attention. Stay together. Don't some of you get too far ahead and leave others lagging behind. Stay on the trail. You can get hurt or lose your way taking short cuts. Help each other. If one of you has a problem, stop and fix it right away. Don't ignore things and let them get worse.

"If you've looked at your mountain lately," she went on, "you can see there are still patches of snow toward the top. Snow sometimes makes bridges over creeks or covers deep crevasses. Be certain they're solid before you cross them. And finally, get plenty to eat and drink along the way and be sure to keep each other warm."

"Thank you," Golly said, "those are good things to remember."

"Absolutely," agreed Flossie.

"Have a good trip," Mary said, and she left them to return home.

Golly gave directions, "The trail to MorningGlory Mountain is that way." He pointed to the east end of the meadow. "I'll fly ahead over the trail, and Flossie, you fly behind me. The rest of you can follow along watching for us."

"I can't fly very far at a time with this bag," Flossie said.

"That's okay," Golly said. "Fly for a while, rest where the hikers can see you when they catch up, then fly on again. We'll relay up the mountain this way and not get lost."

Thus the journey began at mid-morning as Golly and Flossie started out ahead. Manford, eyes bright with excitement, led the hikers. Princess Columbine rode gaily atop his hat. Needlenose moseyed along in the middle. Veronica carried her basket of blueberries and brought up the rear. She sang and danced through the woods, listening to music on her tape player.

The trail was level for a time, taking them past their plant-a-picture garden, across the creek, then directly east through thick forest. It was easy to follow, particularly with Golly flying overhead and Flossie marking the trail in bright pink always just a short way ahead. The sun stayed behind clouds most of the time but occasionally shone through, making crisp shadows and bright patches of light on the trees and ground.

They began treading uphill within an hour. Manford walked eagerly ahead, showing no sign of strain. Needlenose, not a fast walker to begin with, started to drag. Veronica slowed her prancing pace to keep from stepping on him. The trail leveled out for a time then started uphill again. The distance between Manford and the others widened.

"Wait for us," Veronica shouted, but Manford didn't seem to hear. Soon he was far ahead. They could no longer see him when they rounded bends in the trail. Manford met Flossie waiting in the trail.

"Where are the others?" she asked.

"Um, I don't know. They're coming, I suppose."

"Weren't you listening to your mother's safety talk? Let's wait for them, okay?" Needlenose and Veronica arrived a few minutes later.

"Give it a rest, Manford," Needlenose said between huff-and-puff breaths. "I can't keep up with you."

"Yeah," added Veronica, "what's the rush?"

Golly flew down to see what was happening.

"I'm too slow," Needlenose said. "Manford gallops ahead like he's headed for the pot of gold and this bear keeps singing and dancing and rumbling along behind me. Any minute I'm going to get squashed."

"I'm being careful," Veronica said.

"Look here, compadres," said Flossie, "it's very simple. Golly, you carry the blueberry basket. That'll keep you from soaring around like you had nothing to do.

"Veronica, let Needlenose ride on your shoulder. He's heavier than the blueberries but you'll never notice.

"Manford, watch behind you. Don't be trotting ahead if you can't see Veronica. Okay, everybody?"

"Good idea, Flossie," said Golly.

"I like it," added Needlenose.

They departed again after a short rest. Golly and Flossie took their loads of supplies, Manford and Veronica their passengers. The trail now led steadily uphill. Occasional breaks in the trees showed solid, green valleys slowly receding below. MorningGlory Mountain was still far ahead; in fact, they weren't even climbing it yet. They had two other mountains to cross before that part of the adventure could begin.

They stopped for lunch around noon in a rocky clearing and browsed among bordering trees and undergrowth for things to eat. Princess Columbine found bright colored blossoms and sipped their nectar. Manford munched happily on leaves and tiny twigs. Flossie tossed down a sardine or two and Needlenose ate potato chips. It was too early in the season to find berries, so Veronica ate whatever was handy. Golly wasn't hungry, he said, but joined the others to sip water from puddles formed in hollows in the rocks.

After lunch they went on, climbing continuously. Manford and Veronica, being strong youngsters, didn't grow tired, but Flossie made them rest anyway. Her continual take-offs and landings were tiring, she told them, and besides, she wasn't as young as she used to be.

The day grew warm in the woods. Clouds scattered before the sun and the faint wind did little to relieve the heat. The walkers moved onward, keeping a constant stream of chatter going as they went. Veronica sang and skipped to music from her tape player, but occasionally passed the headphones to Needlenose so he could listen, too.

They stopped to rest atop the first mountain in mid-afternoon. Another trail crossed there extending north and south. A sign marked the junction:

MorningGlory Crossing
←Canada 148
Mexico 2490→
MorningGlory Mountain↑

"What trail crosses here?" asked Manford. "It looks terribly long."

"It *is*," said Golly. "It follows the mountains up and down the whole West Coast."

"Maybe we should hike that one sometime, too."

"Yeah," said Needlenose.

"If you don't mind," Flossie said, "let's do one adventure at a time."

"WHO GOES THERE?" said a tremendously loud and official sounding voice.

"Who said that?" Manford asked.

"Beats me," said Needlenose.

"It's loud, whoever it is," said Veronica.

"WHO GOES THERE?" the voice said again.

"I don't see anything," Flossie said, edging nearer to Veronica. Princess Columbine, who had flown to the sign, returned quickly to the safety of Manford's hat.

"Neither do I," said Golly.

"I think it came from over there," Veronica whispered. She pointed about ten yards beyond the sign.

"AT THE RISK OF REPEATING MYSELF," the voice boomed once more, "WHO GOES THERE?"

"There are six of us," Golly said to the voice, "three who fly; three who walk. We are journeying to MorningGlory Mountain. Who are you?"

"I AM THE WATCHER OF MORNINGGLORY CROSSING," came the thunderous reply. "YOU MUST HAVE MY PERMISSION TO PASS."

"It's coming from behind that big rock," Veronica said to Manford. "I'll go look. You guys keep talking." She crept softly along the trail.

"O Crossing Watcher," Golly continued, "how do we get your permission?"

"THREE QUESTIONS MUST BE ANSWERED."

"Go ahead," Golly said.

"THE FIRST IS THIS: WHAT IS SEEN BOTH DAY AND NIGHT, SOMETIMES HIDDEN, SOMETIMES BRIGHT?"

"A riddle," Golly said. "Oh, good." He thought a moment then replied, "The moon."

"CORRECT. NOW QUESTION TWO. . ."

Veronica reached the rock just then and slowly peered around the edge. She began to laugh.

"Is that you making all that noise?" she said to something the others couldn't see.

"A BEAR!" the voice suddenly cried. "OH, MY GOODNESS, HELP! A BEAR!"

"It doesn't seem to like bears," Flossie said. "That's something."

"I won't hurt you," Veronica said. "Here, come along and tell us what this racket is about." She reached behind the rock and lifted up a long black snake for everyone to see.

Flossie shrieked at the sight of it and ran in horror toward the bushes. The bag tied around her feet tripped her again and she landed on the ground in a heap. She buried her head under her wing.

"If you please," said Veronica, setting the creature in the center of the trail, "just who, and what, are you?"

"MY NAME IS SSAM," it replied warily, but still in a loud voice. "I'M A GARTER SNAKE."

Ssam was two feet long, black with green and yellow stripes running lengthwise, and wore a black bowler hat and bow tie. He seemed uncomfortable, suddenly being stared at by creatures many times his size.

"You can come out, Flossie," Veronica said. "This fellow won't hurt you."

"Is it poisonous?" she asked, her trembling voice muffled by her wing.

"NO," said Ssam, "I'M COMPLETELY HARMLESS."

"Then do you suppose you could turn the volume down to about three?" Flossie said. "You have the loudest voice I ever heard."

"Yes," Princess Columbine said, "why must you talk in all capital letters?"

"I'M MUCH HARDER TO IGNORE THIS WAY," Ssam boomed on. "BUT I COULD TALK IN SMALL CAPITALS IF YOU LIKE or *even italics*."

"A regular volume would be fine if you could manage it," said Golly. "So tell us, how were you made Watcher of MorningGlory Crossing?"

"I appointed myself," Ssam said, talking normally now. "No one said I couldn't."

"Why?"

"Snakes aren't popular creatures, you know. No one gives us a chance to make friends. So, instead of hiding and running away and being looked down on all the time, I decided to take a position of authority and gain some respect."

"The black hat and bow tie are uniform of the office, I presume," Golly said.

"Oh, yes," said Ssam. "One must look the part, you know."

"Do those who pass answer your questions?" Veronica asked.

"Most usually try because the questions are easy. If they refuse and just walk by, I thunder out a dreadful curse on them. It makes them nervous, that's for sure. Those who answer wrong I just let go, but I don't give them the password."

"Password?" said Columbine.

"Yes," said Ssam, "only if my questions are answered correctly do I give it out."

"Then we must still answer the other two," said Golly, seeming delighted at the prospect.

"I have a better idea," Ssam said. "Take me with you. I'd like to see the top of MorningGlory Mountain but it's too long a journey for me."

"I guess we can take you along," said Golly. "Does anyone object?"

No one did, though Flossie looked fearful about having a snake in their midst.

"Where will he ride?" she asked.

"In my pack," Manford said to Ssam. "There's a soft place on top of my scarf. I'll leave the flap open so you can see out." Thus, the six became seven, adding one who crawled to those who walked and flew, all bound once more for MorningGlory Mountain.

Downhill they traveled now as the trail zigzagged along a steep slope. Veronica and Manford marched back and forth with their passengers; Golly and Flossie passed overhead. Views of the countryside diminished as they dropped into thick forest but they saw many more flowers. Columbine fluttered from her perch often to explore some colored blossom, then beat her wings furiously to catch up as Manford pushed on.

They heard the sound of rushing water in the distance. It grew louder as they descended till soon the trail ran round a bend and crossed a stream. The travelers waded into the water to take cool drinks and wash their faces and to listen to the water's pleasant sound. Then they continued on their way.

"What's question two, Ssam?" Manford asked.

Ssam paused to take a deep breath, then said, "QUESTION TWO: I MARCH O'ER THE LAND AND INTO THE SEA. I AM MASSIVE AND ANCIENT. WHO CAN I BE?"

"My ears!" Manford cried in pain.

Columbine was blown off her perch and lay dazed on a tree branch. Needlenose's quills stood straight out.

"Awesome!" said Veronica. All forward progress stopped.

"Sorry," said Ssam, "but I must present my questions properly."

"How can something so small talk so loud?" Veronica asked.

"Through lots of practice. I figured no one would pay attention to me if I had a squeaky little voice. It's been very effective, I must say."

"That's certain," said Princess Columbine. She beat her wings limply, flying a wandering path back to the peak of Manford's hat. "Please warn us if you must do that again."

"So, what's the answer?" asked Needlenose.

"You tell me," said Ssam.

"What was the question again?" said Manford.

"I'll tell you," said Columbine, "it's permanently imprinted on my brain, 'I march o'er the land and into the sea. I am massive and ancient. Who can I be?'"

"Not the same effect at all," said Ssam. Columbine gave him an icy look.

"Land and sea," puzzled Manford. "Hmmm."

"Massive and ancient," said Veronica. "Hmmm."

"Hmmm," said Needlenose.

"While you're all hmmming, perhaps we should move on," said Ssam.

They did so and found Flossie sound asleep.

"What kept you?" she asked, when Needlenose shook her awake. They told her of Ssam's riddle.

"Hmmm," she said, "I *thought* I heard someone shouting. I'll have to think about that one." She flapped into the air in pursuit of Golly who, still clutching the basket of blueberries, was flying lazy circles high above them.

In time, the path again turned uphill. It was rocky in places and crossed open areas. They could see valleys and streams below and stands of trees on the mountainsides around them. The forest looked lovely with afternoon sunlight on the many shades of new green leaves.

"Clouds?" said Manford.

"What about the clouds?" said Veronica. "The clouds are

gone. It's sunny."

"Is that the answer to question two? Cloud shadows go over land and sea. Clouds are big, and they've been around a long time."

"No," said Ssam. "Nice try, though."

"Rivers, how about that?" asked Veronica. "Rivers flow across the land and into the sea. Rivers are big and old, too."

"That's true, but it's not the answer."

"Hmmm," said Veronica.

"Hmmm," said Manford.

"Is this a bumblebee convention?" asked Needlenose.

"Mountains," said Manford. "Is that it? Mountains march across the land and under the sea, too, I think. Where else would they go? And they're massive, and ancient. Is mountains the answer?"

"That's correct," Ssam said. "You kids are pretty smart."

"I knew it all along," said Columbine.

Golly was waiting for them when they reached a point where Flossie's pink plumage marked the trail.

"The answer is mountains," he said.

"I already guessed it," said Manford. "Did Flossie tell you the question?"

"I heard Ssam say it the first time," Golly said. "His voice really carries."

"He should give us earplugs," Columbine said, still sounding miffed.

"It will be dark soon," Golly said. "We've crossed the first mountain and are just starting up the second. It's probably time to make camp."

"Here?" Manford asked. The slope on either side of the trail was rocky and steep.

"You'll cross a small stream a short way ahead. There's a flat, grassy spot in a grove of hemlock trees there. That will be a good place."

They walked another half hour to the place Golly had mentioned. Making camp was easy. They had no tents or sleeping bags; they would just sleep in the grass.

They gathered dinner in the woods and drank from the stream. Veronica nibbled blueberries afterwards and Manford enjoyed a piece of willow leaf pie. Flossie ate sardines. Columbine sipped flowers. Needlenose ate potato chips.

Golly said he'd eaten earlier, finding fish in a pond while he'd waited for the group to make their way along. Ssam wasn't hungry, either. Snakes don't eat very often, he said, which is just as well because the less said about what snakes eat, the better.

Wind stirred branches in the trees and leaves rattled and whispered as darkness came. Insects chirped and buzzed, accompanied by soft sounds of the nearby stream. Stars shone in the clear night sky. The group sat in a circle and talked about events of the day, things they'd seen and done, their prospects for the days to come. Eventually, Manford brought up the afternoon's unfinished business.

"What's question three, Ssam?"

"Yes, the final question," Ssam said, taking a breath.

"Hold it," said Flossie, "give us a chance to cover our ears." She crawled into the bag she'd been carrying and pressed her head back firmly into the feathers between her wings.

Manford took out his long scarf and gently wrapped it around Princess Columbine.

"I wondered why it was called a muffler," said Needlenose, clamping his paws over his ears.

"I guess we're ready," Manford said.

"QUESTION THREE," Ssam began. "WHAT IS THERE WHEN NOT SEEN, SEEN WHEN NOT THERE, PRESENT WITHOUT NUMBER, GONE IN THIN AIR?"

"Hmmm," said Golly.

"There when not seen," puzzled Manford, "seen when

not there."

"I KNOW THE ANSWER," said a very small voice. No one heard it.

"Present without number," said Flossie, who had come out from her hiding place in the bag. "Sounds like flamingos to me."

"Gone in thin air," said Veronica. "That's Manford hiking at the front of the line."

"I KNOW, I KNOW," said the small voice again.

"Did you hear something?" asked Veronica.

"No," said Manford. "What was it?"

"Something far away, or very quiet."

"IT'S ME," the voice said. "I KNOW THE ANSWER."

"It's Princess," said Golly; "unwrap her." Manford did so. Columbine flew around in a circle then came to rest atop Ssam's bowler hat.

"Stars," she said. "That's the answer, stars."

"You're right," said Ssam. "What a brilliant princess you are." Columbine smiled sweetly and flexed her wings.

"I don't understand," said Manford.

"Stars are far away," said Ssam. "It takes many years for their light to get to us. When a new star is born, we don't see it until its light has traveled this far. That's *'there when not seen'*."

"I get it, I think," said Manford.

"Then if a star burns out," Golly said, "we still see the light that was on the way to us, *'seen when not there'*."

"Correct," said Ssam.

"And there are millions of stars," said Veronica, "that's *'present without number'*."

"Right."

"And *'gone in thin air'* is daytime, when you can't see them," said Manford.

"That settles that," said Flossie, "our science lesson for tonight."

"So, give us the password," said Needlenose.

"It's *Druid*, my friends. You earned it fair and square."

"Druid? What's a Druid?"

"People long ago who were fond of trees," said Ssam.

"You must be thinking of Dryad," Golly said. "Dryads are wood nymphs who live among the trees. The Druids were an order of priests in ancient Britain."

"You mean I've been giving out the wrong word?" said Ssam. "Oh, well, I guess it doesn't matter."

"What's the password used for?" asked Needlenose.

"I don't know; I only give it out. I've never had reason to use it."

"Maybe we'll find one," said Golly.

"Here's one," said Flossie, "we'll call this place where we've camped 'the Druid Room'."

"How far did we hike today?" asked Manford, changing the subject.

"Four or five miles, I'd say," said Flossie.

"Is that all? Gee, if we were hiking that other trail we crossed it would take us years to do it all."

"We're not going so far on this trip," Golly said. "We can take our time."

"How far will we go tomorrow?"

"Maybe more, maybe less. We'll see."

Manford, Veronica, Flossie, and Needlenose each chose a spot and lay down on the grass. Golly found a tree branch on which to roost and Ssam crawled into Manford's pack. Columbine settled on Veronica's broad, warm back. Darkness was fully upon them and they were soon fast asleep.

Manford was restless and nervous. He was dreaming, then he awoke and his eyes darted around him.

"Veronica," he whispered.

"What?" she said sleepily.

"I'm scared."

"Of what?"

"Well, I don't know, I've never camped out before."

"So?"

"What if something comes here in the night?"

"What kind of something?"

"Oh, a bear, maybe. Or. . ."

"Manford," said Veronica.

"What?"

"I'm a bear."

"Oh, that's right."

"If any bears come, they'll probably be my friends."

"I guess so," said Manford, "but I'm still scared."

"Look," said Veronica, "*people* are scared of bears, not us. And we have a moose, an eagle, a porcupine, and a snake with a voice that would raise the dead. Who's going to mess with us?"

"I guess you're right."

"You've been watching too much TV."

"Goodnight," said Manford.

"Goodnight," said Veronica.

But Manford dreamed again. . .of clouds that drifted across the tops of mountains. . .clouds with shifting, changing shapes. . .and voices that spoke to him.

"Manford," the dream voice whispered. "Manford. . ."

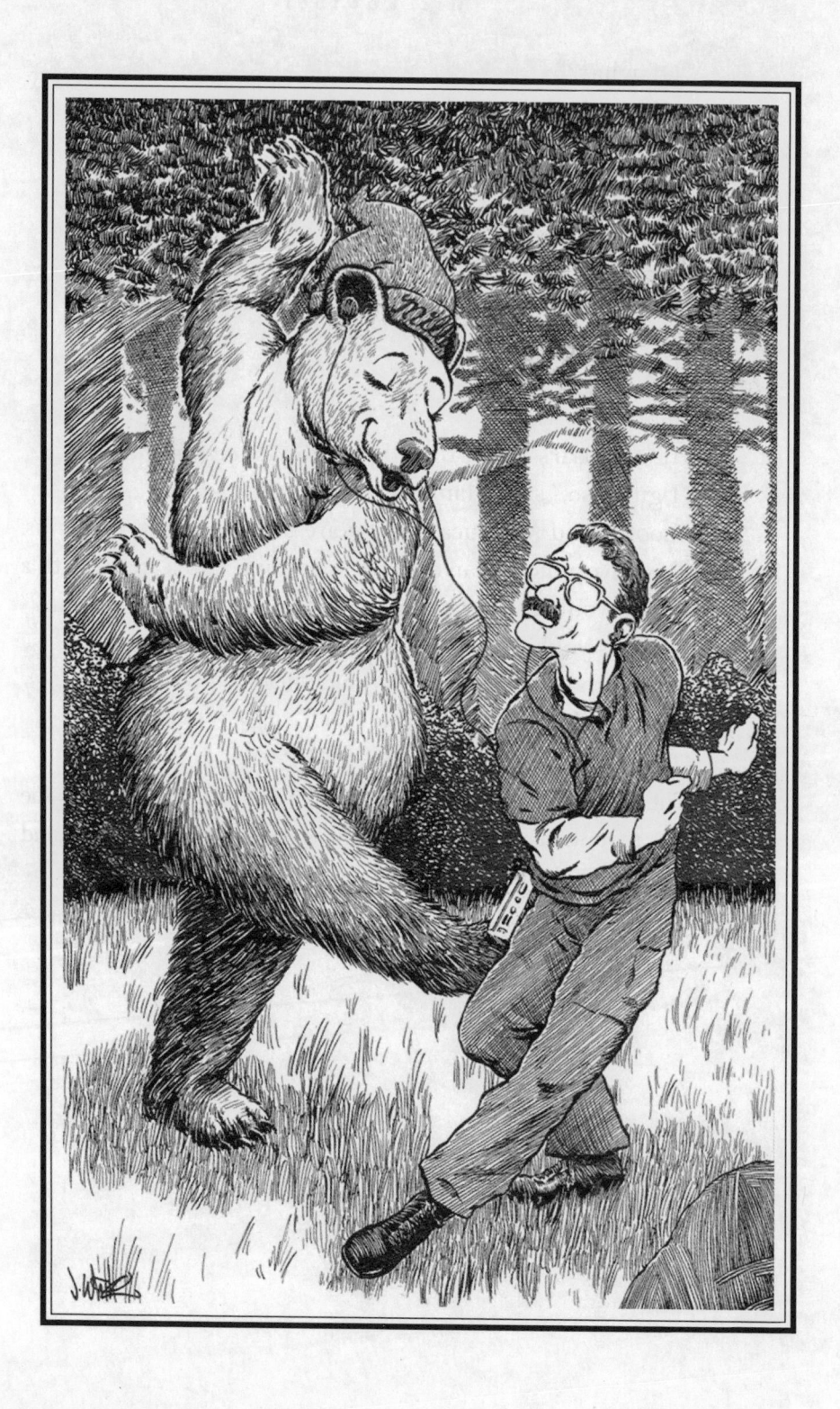

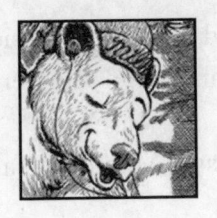

5

Uphill, Fog, and Dancing Bears
In which adventurers climb the great mountain and find a puzzle

"There's someone on the trail ahead of us," Golly said. It was already mid-morning. The night before, the travelers had talked of getting up early. Alas, it was no longer early and some were still sleeping. Golly had been scouting around while he waited.

"What kind of someone?" asked Manford.

"A man, I suspect. He's still asleep in his tent."

"That must be the one who passed me early yesterday," said Ssam. "He was very polite and not at all frightened. He answered my questions easily and never asked what they were about."

"How far ahead?" Veronica asked.

"He's camped near the top of this mountain," Golly said. "We may catch up with him today."

"We should introduce ourselves when we do," said Flossie. She began to imitate the others.

"'Hello, I'm Manford, the moose. My dad's a ballet star.'

"'And I'm Veronica, the bear. My mom's in the circus.'

"'Hi, I'm Needlenose, the porcupine. Want some potato chips?'"

The others laughed at her impressions and joined the fun.

"'I'm Flossie, the flamingo,'" said Veronica. "'I sleep standing on one leg.'"

"'I'm Golly eagle,'" said Manford in a deep voice. "'Make your letters round.'"

"'And I'm Columbine, the Butterfly Flower Princess,'" said Needlenose stuffily. "'When I grow up, I'll be Queen.'"

Columbine drew herself up and said in as loud a voice as she could muster:

"'ATTENTION ALL YE WITHIN 200 MILES OF MY VOICE. I AM SSAM, THE BLACK TIE GARTER SNAKE AND I'D LIKE TO ASK YOU SOME QUESTIONS.'" Ssam, the last to wake up that morning, smiled and bowed to Columbine.

"That would give this hiker something to wonder about," he said.

"No doubt it would," said Golly. "Now, if you're all thoroughly rested, I think we should be going."

"Yes," said Manford, "let's go."

Golly took off carrying the berry basket; Flossie followed with her bag of supplies. Veronica, wearing her headset again, took the lead on the trail this time. Manford followed, Columbine perched on his hat and Ssam peering out of his pack.

The path again led uphill. The hikers climbed uphill through trees, uphill through bushes, uphill through weeds and ferns. That's the trouble with mountains, you know: uphill. If it weren't for that, climbing them would be easy. The hikers climbed and rested, climbed and rested, looked up and looked down, and all the while kept thinking they would soon reach the top. They finally did about noon. Pleasant views awaited them there. Behind was the mountain they'd climbed the day before. Below, creeks meandered through sunlit valleys. And ahead...ahead of them stood MorningGlory Mountain, clouds drifting round it well below the top.

Manford and Veronica looked at the sights as they rested.

What they saw was fuzzy, as if scenes far away weren't quite in focus. Moose and bears are nearsighted, you'll recall. But MorningGlory Mountain was big, they knew that, fuzzy or not. And soon they were going to climb it.

They started downhill again. This might sound easier than going up but it isn't. Downhill starts off just fine but then your legs get tired and you want to go up again. That's how it is on the trail sometimes; something else always seems better than what you're doing. But if Manford or Veronica ever tired of uphill or down, they didn't complain. And none of it mattered to Needlenose; he was getting a ride. He called out directions as they moved along:

"Downshift to low!" on steep grades.

"Hard left (or right) rudder!" at bends in the trail.

"Warp six, Mr. Sulu!" when the trail was flat.

The way led across an open ridge at the bottom. The trail forked on the other side, splitting left and right around a barren, wind bent tree. Flossie was waiting for them there.

"We go that way," she said, pointing left. "That's where Golly headed and where most of the traffic has gone."

"Where does the other trail lead?" Manford asked.

"I don't know," Flossie answered. "Golly didn't say."

The climb of MorningGlory Mountain itself began at last. Veronica and Manford charged along with constant encouragement from their passengers. The grade was gradual at times, steep other times. Uphill again; there would be a lot more of it now.

The path led through forest once more. Leaves were green and new, flowers showed bright faces to the sun, moss and lichen made delicate patterns on tree trunks and rocks. It was late afternoon.

The trail crossed creeks and passed trailside waterfalls. It plowed through thick underbrush and crossed grassy fields. Rocks and fallen trees blocked the way in places and in others, the trail had been completely swept away by landslides and only a steep, gravel slope remained; each time the hikers made their way safely across.

The trail became steeper as they climbed. They walked several hours. Trees grew shorter and there were more openings to see what lay around and below them. They stopped to look and to rest, then went on.

The sun was setting. Manford watched the trail ahead, behind, and to either side for a place to camp. It was steep and rocky with no flat spots at all. Golly soared in for a landing as the sun disappeared.

"Where will we camp, Golly?" Manford asked. "I haven't seen a good spot."

"That might be a problem," he replied. "The only good place is about an hour ahead. It will be after dark when you get there."

"We can find our way in the dark," Veronica said.

"Finding the place isn't the problem," said Golly. "The hiker ahead of you is camping there. He's pitched a tent, built a fire, and moved in for the night."

"What will we do?" Manford asked.

"It's no worry for me," Golly said. "I can sleep in a tree. But unless you want to camp on this rocky sidehill, you'll have to join him."

"This should be interesting," said Flossie. "We'd better practice our introductions again." She and Golly flew ahead as the hikers talked about what to do.

"Maybe we should wait till he's asleep," suggested Manford.

"Maybe we should scare him away," said Veronica.

"Maybe he likes sardines and potato chips," offered Needlenose.

They thought about these and other plans as they walked.

The sky grew dark. The path became a dim shadow. In an hour they met Flossie and Golly waiting at a bend in the trail. They heard sounds of a creek nearby and saw where the trail led to a clearing. A campfire burned there, casting dancing, irregular shadows. Behind it, facing the trail, sat a man dressed in a blue jacket and pants. He had graying hair and was tossing small sticks on the fire.

"Any ideas?" Flossie asked.

"Let's just walk in and say hello," Manford said.

"It might work," said Veronica, "but you know how scared *people* get. He might start shooting. Then what?"

"Leave it to me," said Needlenose. "I'll handle it."

"How?" Flossie asked.

"Get closer so you can listen. You'll find out."

Needlenose shuffled forward along the trail before anyone could object. He made no effort to move quietly or circle the hiker's camp. He simply walked down the trail and into the clearing. He sat down at the fire. The others crept forward in the shadows.

"Hello, little fellow," the man said to Needlenose. "Making your nightly rounds?" He did not expect a reply.

Needlenose listened, paused a moment, then said,

"*Druid.*"

"Ah, The Voice got you, too, did it?" said the hiker. "I wondered what that password was good for. So, how is it you can talk to me?"

"Anything can happen on MorningGlory Mountain," said Needlenose.

"I suppose so," agreed the man. "If a mystery voice asks me questions and gives a password, why shouldn't the animals talk? What brings you here, my friend?"

"I'd like to sleep here tonight if you don't mind. It's the only nice place around."

"I'd be honored."

"I have a couple of friends. Could they come, too?"

"Sure, might as well have company."

Needlenose motioned for the others to come ahead.

Golly flew over the clearing and landed near the fire, carefully setting down his cargo. Then came Manford, hat on his head, pack on his back, smiling his best smile. Columbine fluttered round the fire and came to rest atop Needlenose's head. Veronica ambled in and sat down, and soon after came Flossie, dragging her bag of supplies.

"*A couple of friends*," the man said, laughing. "This looks more like half the creatures in the forest. Are there others?"

"Actually, yes," said Needlenose.

"I thought so. Well, my name is Turner. That's my first name; the rest doesn't matter out here. I've hiked around here before but have never been up this mountain."

"My name is Golly," said Golly.

"Yes, it would be," Turner replied, "the mythical Golly eagle. Pleased to meet you."

"Princess Columbine is my name," said the Royal Butterfly.

"I'm Needlenose," said the porcupine.

"Flossie, the flamingo here. Thanks for letting us move in."

"I'm Manford," said our adventuring moose. "It's our first time up MorningGlory, too."

"My name's Veronica," said the bear.

"Nice to meet you all," said Turner, "but you said there were others."

"ONE OTHER," said Ssam in his official voice as he crawled from Manford's pack. The others held their ears.

"And I think I know who..."

"SSAM: WATCHER OF MORNINGGLORY CROSSING."

"It's the riddle maker," Turner said; "a garter snake, I see. What a big voice you have, Ssam."

Each told something about his or her self and described parts of their journey so far. Turner had started hiking the week before. He had no particular destination, he said; he was just following trails that seemed interesting. He talked easily with them, as though sharing his campsite with a band of animals on expedition was the usual thing to do.

"Tell about some of your adventures," said Veronica.

Turner did. He often hiked parts of the longer trail they'd passed at MorningGlory Crossing, he said, and hoped to finish all of it some day. He'd walked in mountains and valleys, in deserts and canyons, in every kind of weather. He'd met many animals in his travels, some of them in interesting ways.

"There was one time I'll always remember," he said. "It was the oddest thing. No offense, Miss Veronica, but until this happened, I'd never been fond of bears. Bears had ripped up my pack and eaten my food. I'd awakened at night to find bears peering curiously into my tent. Bears got on my nerves.

"Smokey Bear, Yogi Bear, Winnie-the-Pooh, did I ever find harmless, *personable* bears like this in the woods? Not me. The only bears I ever met were up to no good.

"Then one day I met a bear that changed my thinking completely. It happened near here, though I can't remember quite where. One moment I was walking peacefully along minding my own business. The next moment I was face to face with you know what.

"I backed away from the bear, but it simply followed. I moved to the left then to the right; each time the bear cut me off. It wanted something, that much was clear, yet it didn't threaten. It only made sure I didn't get away.

"'Shoo, shoo, shoo. Out of my way, bear,' I said, 'I have places to go, things to do, miles to cover today.' The bear just sat there, unimpressed with my schedule.

"I settled down for a moment and looked the bear over. There was something different here. Its face had a puzzled, expectant look. Its eyes showed a deep, watery sadness like a puppy that wanted to play.

"Then I noticed the cap. The bear wore a ragged, red felt cap still strapped to its head. And there was a name printed there: *Millie*."

Veronica's eyes twinkled at the mention of Millie's name. The others looked at her in surprise, but no one said a word.

"Millie! Of course," Turner went on, "I recognized this bear! Millie had escaped from a circus wagon the year before. She'd never been found. Hope had been abandoned. She'd been mourned by circus goers everywhere.

"The booming voice of the ringmaster introducing her act suddenly came back to me." (He held his hands to his mouth like a megaphone):

"'LA-DEEES and GEN-tle-MENNN, EN-ter-TAIN-ment under the BIG TOP con-TIN-uuus. Please diRECT your atTENtion NOW to the CENter ring and welcome MILLIE, MILLIE the DANcing BEAR!'

"It was no wonder Millie looked sad. She missed the music. She missed the people. She missed the applause. Millie was lonely, and Millie wanted to dance.

"Well, I pulled my tape player from my pack. This one even had a double set of headphones—you never know when you're going to need such a thing. I put one set on, stretched the other set over Millie's ears and hit *Play*. She stood up at once, her eyes blazing with excitement.

"I bowed. Millie curtsied. She was surprisingly graceful at six hundred pounds. I put my hand on her waist, she put her paw on my shoulder, then we danced.

"Oh, Millie! I'd admired her from afar all these years, and here we were dancing. I wanted to tell her how lovely she looked, how becoming her fur wrap was, and that I noticed she was stepping out in the latest style: barefoot. But with the music in her ears and that dreamy look on her face, she wouldn't have heard me.

"We danced up hill and down—first slow dances, then fast dances, then exotic dances—on and on, hour after hour, across the meadow and through the woods until the batteries...in my tape player...died.

"Millie looked really disappointed.

"'Don't worry about a thing,' I said. I recharged them quickly on a currant bush then we were off again.

"We stopped to watch the sunset from a hilltop and then danced on by moonlight. I grew tired after a while, but not Millie, because anything that can run a steady thirty-five miles an hour doesn't get tired from a little dancing.

"At last we rested in a grassy clearing. Millie stopped to smell the wildflowers there. I braided a garland of daisies and placed them on her head. Then we danced on again—ten o'clock, eleven o'clock, twelve o'clock—until, at last, we reached the place that Millie called home.

"I felt a bit apprehensive here. *'This could get tricky,'* I thought. *'What if she invites me in for drink?'* But no, Millie wasn't that kind of lady. She just reached up with her cold, wet nose about as big as my fist and lightly brushed me on the cheek. And her eyes twinkled with delight as if to say, 'Thank you for a lovely evening.' Then she was gone.

"I waited outside, listening, and could have sworn I heard her humming. Then I walked up the trail, found my pack and put it on, and started into the night.

"'Good night, Millie', I said. 'I had a nice time, too. And you can visit my tent anytime.'"

Manford smiled and glanced at Veronica.

"What a wonderful story," said Flossie, a bit misty-eyed.

"It's true," Turner said, "all of it, isn't it, Veronica?"

"Uh huh. Millie's my mom. She told me about you."

"I thought there was a connection. Why else would a bear be wearing headphones? Where is she now?"

"Back in the circus. She got lonely for it again."

"Do you think she'd remember me if I visited her?"

"Sure. She'd even talk to you this time."

Campfire chatter continued. The animals asked more questions and Turner told more stories. To everyone's delight, he even danced around the fire with Veronica. At last, Golly flew off to a nearby tree, noting that it would be best to get some sleep. The others soon nestled down around the fire. Turner wished them goodnight and crawled into his tent.

Manford dreamed as before. He woke once, certain that someone had spoken to him, but all was quiet. He slept and dreamed again...

Morning brought fog; fog that rolled through the camp and looked to be solid all the way up the mountain; fog that clung to the ground and trees and made everything wet and fuzzy and gray; fog so thick it seemed you could carve out a piece and roast it like a marshmallow. Golly and Flossie were grounded. They had no instrument ratings so they couldn't fly until the weather cleared.

"The trail goes that way," Golly said, pointing up. "You hikers can go ahead if you wish. We'll find you later. Just remember what Ms. Mary said: Be careful."

"Will you join us, Mr. Turner?" asked Manford.

"I'll be along in a while, thanks," he replied.

Manford and Veronica, eager to be going, boarded their passengers and headed up the trail. Manford walked in front; it was his turn to lead today. The fog was solid around them but the sun glowed faintly overhead.

They walked back and forth on switchbacks for an hour, then two, and were still in the fog. The forest shrank to bushy spruce and hemlock growing about head high. They saw more rock around them. Small plants and berry bushes made patchy blankets of green. They climbed and climbed as the morning wore on, following turn after turn of the trail.

The sun began to seem brighter and the fog thinned to wisps of cloud blowing across their path. Pieces of sky showed through. Then they burst into the clear. Above them, MorningGlory Mountain rose into blue sky. Below, they saw white wherever they looked. Puffy, white fog, turned bright by the sun, covered the scene as if valleys had been filled with whipped cream. They watched as the fog shifted and changed, as it advanced and retreated on the mountain, as it billowed into ice cream and sno-cone shapes before them.

"I'm hungry," said Manford.

"There's not much to eat here," said Veronica, "and Golly still has my blueberries."

"There are no potato chips, either, without Flossie," said Needlenose.

"We could have some of my mom's pie," Manford said.

"The pie's for dessert," said Veronica. "There will be even less to eat on top. We'd better save it."

"How long before we get to the top?" asked Princess Columbine.

"It doesn't look far," said Manford. "The trail goes up this slope and levels off. Maybe the top's right up there." They climbed the slope before them and reached the place Manford had pointed out. Another uphill climb came into view.

"Guess not," said Needlenose. A strong wind suddenly began to blow. They climbed the next slope to find another beyond it, a rocky ridge with an extremely steep path. Patches of snow lay on the ground, bright white in the sun and faintly spotted pink and red in places where algae had grown. Tiny leaves and twigs scattered by the wind made deep indentations where the sun warmed them and melted them in.

The hikers climbed another slope, steeper and rockier. Gusts of wind pushed at them from above, making forward progress harder. Snow covered the trail for long stretches now and they had to step carefully across it.

"How many tops does this mountain have?" asked Columbine, holding fast to her perch.

"Lots, I guess," said Manford. The wind whipped at his hat, threatening to blow it and Columbine away. Manford's mother had added a chinstrap to the hat just before he left to begin his adventure. He fastened it and told Columbine to hang on.

They paused to look around. Snow lay deep in folds of the mountain and extended downhill in long chutes where avalanches had run. They saw melt water running in places, carving tunnels beneath the snow. Fog was breaking and scattering and they could see through it to the mountain far below. Needlenose pointed to something moving there. Golly and Flossie were finally in the air and on their way. It was mid-afternoon.

"We'll be easier to see if we're moving," said Veronica. "Otherwise we'll blend into these rocks and they'll never find us."

"I could get their attention," offered Ssam.

"Never mind," said Columbine, "they'll find us." They moved ahead once more.

The trail now seemed nearly straight up. They pushed forward against the wind and made their way slowly along the rocky, snowy path. Higher and higher they climbed. The wind blew them to a standstill at times, pushed them backward other times, but they hiked on. The top, if it really was the top, seemed just another little way, another few steps ahead.

The slope began to level. They struggled on to where they could see nothing but sky just ahead. And then they were there, standing on top of MorningGlory Mountain, standing on top of what had seemed so impossibly tall and far off three days before.

The summit was wide and, in the distance, slightly humped in the center. Huge rocks, some bigger than Manford and Veronica put together, lay about. The path sometimes went around them, sometimes over them, and sometimes, through narrow openings between them. Snow filled shaded hollows and covered large areas across the summit. Manford and Veronica wanted to stop and rest from their climb and look out from this lofty peak. They took shelter behind a large rock.

Golly and Flossie, meanwhile, were having trouble. It was all very well to be carrying berry baskets and potato chip bags on a still day, but the blustery wind created steering problems. As they neared the upper slopes where the wind blew strongest, the burdens hanging from their feet pulled against them when they tried to fly forward. Golly's basket seesawed back and forth, jerking him this way and that, at times spilling the contents. He flew close to the ground, landing often to regain his bearings and look back for a sign of something pink.

Flossie was being dragged all over the sky. The wind caught her supply bag each time she tried to fly, and with a cry of "Whooo-oooo-OOOHHHH," she'd be off, completely at its mercy. She gained ground, then lost it. She was blown to the left of the trail, then to the right. She tried flying near the ground but the bag caught in the rocks, snatching her from the air and bringing her down.

Turner, moseying along behind them, noticed Flossie's problems and went to her aid. He found her bruised and sobbing some distance from the trail.

"Care for a lift, Ms. Flossie?" he asked.

"Please," she sniffed, shaking dirt and leaves from her feathers.

"I'll tie your bag on the back of my pack. You can ride on top and look over my shoulder. You can't weigh much."

"That's the nicest thing anybody's said to me all day," Flossie replied. The two were soon underway.

"What's in the bag, anyway?" Turner asked.

"Potato chips for Needlenose," the flamingo replied.

"I should have known."

Above them, Manford, Veronica, and their passengers pushed on. They'd decided to cross the boulder field to look at the rounded area at the center of the mountaintop. Columbine held fast to the back of Manford's hat to avoid the wind. Ssam settled down to sleep inside the pack and await news of journey's end. Needlenose rode with delight on Veronica's shoulder, his quills blown straight back as though they'd been greased and combed.

Going was slow against the wind but they kept on. They reached the center of the mountaintop and climbed the humped ridge as the sun began to set once again. Standing on the edge, they were puzzled at what they'd found.

Before them lay an almost circular room sunk into the mountaintop and ringed with huge stones. It was fifteen feet deep and thirty feet across. The floor showed no sign of snow or rocks or anything that grew. It was covered with loose sand that was perfectly smooth. The trail led down through the stones and entered the room as though through a doorway. They descended, the circle of stones rising well above their heads. Inside it was warm and calm. Wind still blew across the mountain but had no effect inside.

"What sort of place is this?" Manford asked.

"I don't know," said Veronica.

And they walked around and looked at this curious place atop MorningGlory Mountain as the evening sky grew dark.

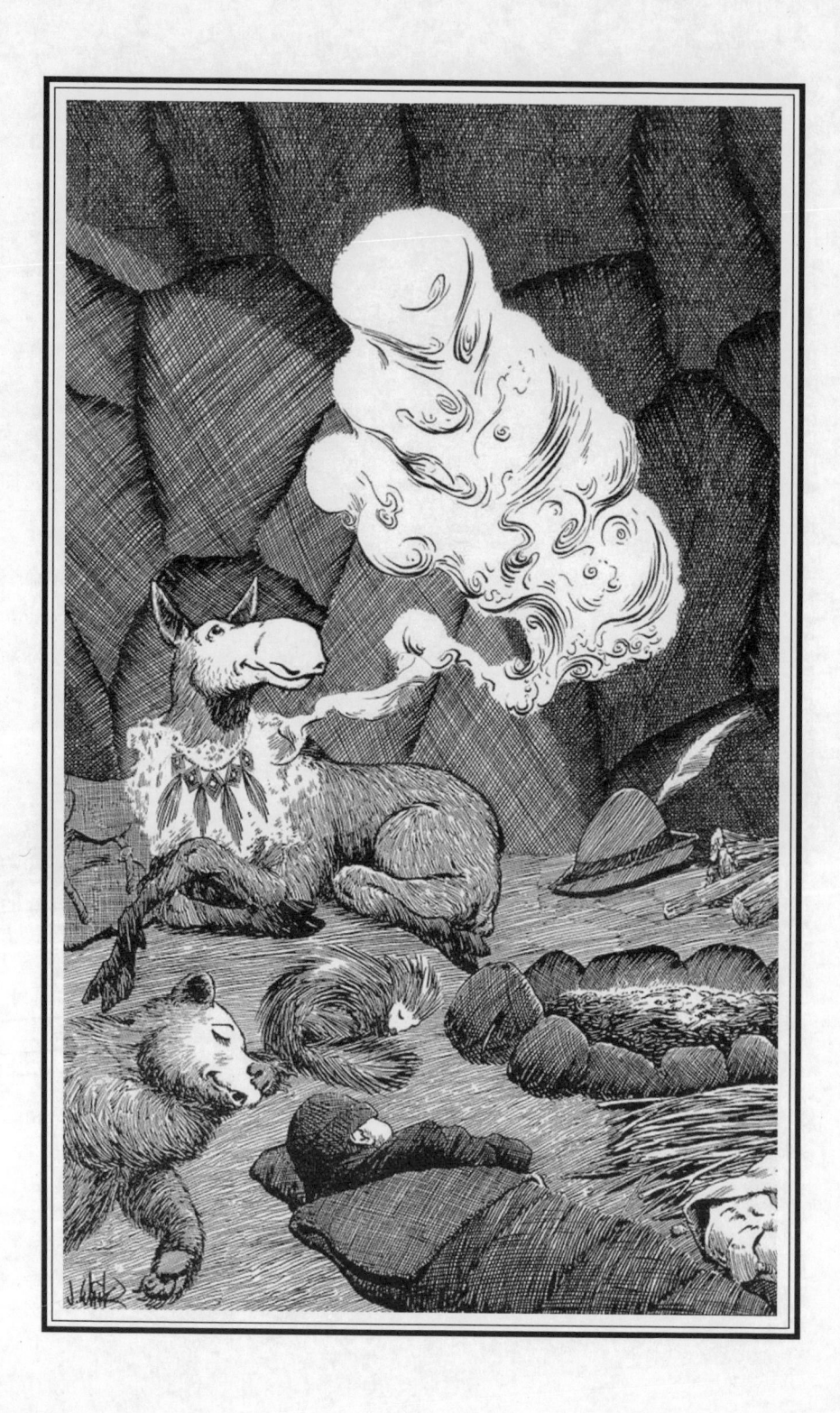

6

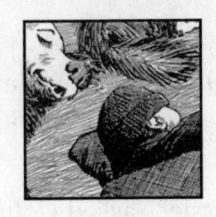

The Place with No Trees
In which legends come to life
and Columbine disappears

Soon, there were footprints all around the smooth, sandy floor. Moose prints from Manford who paced back and forth looking up along the ring of huge stones. Bear prints from Veronica who walked and sat down, walked and sat down, puzzled by what they'd found. And a curving, zigzag path left by Needlenose dragging his bushy quill tail from place to place.

"Whatever it is, it's a great place to camp," Needlenose said.

"You're right about that," said Veronica. "Soft sand, no wind—I like it."

"But where are the others?" asked Princess Columbine. "It's almost dark. They should be here by now. I hope they're not lost."

"Needlenose saw them coming up the mountain a couple of hours ago," said Manford. "I'll bet they're having trouble in the wind."

A dark shape swept low overhead and settled down for a landing inside the room.

"I thought I'd find you here," Golly said. His wing and tail feathers were ruffled. His head and neck looked like they'd been combed the wrong way.

"Rough weather, huh?" said Needlenose.

"It's great for flying kites, but we cargo planes had a tough time."

"Have you seen Flossie?" asked Columbine.

"I looked for her when I was near the top of the mountain. She's hitched a ride with Mr. Turner. Apparently, she had a terrible time."

"Oh, I hope she's okay."

They chose resting spots for the night while they waited. Half an hour passed. The sky turned pitch dark. They heard nothing more from MorningGlory Mountain than the blowing of the wind.

"We should have paid more attention to Ms. Mary," Golly said. "Stay together, she told us; that's just what we didn't do. Now it's pitch dark in a high wind and our party is still scattered. Not good. Not good at all."

"We should post a lookout," said Veronica. "Manford, you and Ssam go up and keep watch. Ssam can get their attention. Where is he, by the way?"

"Asleep in Manford's pack," said Needlenose. "He takes traveling very casually." Manford woke Ssam and took him to the ridge above the circular room.

"See anything?" Manford asked.

"No," answered Ssam, who was coiled about Manford's hat. Snakes don't see well either, particularly in the dark, so this was no surprise.

"Hear anything?"

"Just the wind."

"I guess we'd better wait." And so they waited, watching and listening in the dark.

"The wind has turned around," said Manford after a time. "It's blowing up the mountain now instead of down." They watched, they listened, but noticed nothing. More time passed.

"I smell something," said Ssam. He tested the air with his thin, red tongue.

"What is it?" asked Manford.

"I know I've smelled it before. Let me think."

"I still don't see anything," said Manford.

"Sardines," said Ssam, "that's what I smell. They must be nearby."

"Call to them," Manford said, placing his hat and Ssam on a rock. "They'll hear you if they're anywhere near." Ssam took a deep breath.

"FLOSSIE, TURNER, WE'RE HERE, COME THIS WAY," he shouted in a voice that filled the night.

Manford saw the fuzzy brightness of a flashlight wave in the distance.

"THIS WAY," Ssam continued. "WE'RE OVER HERE."

The flashes of light among the rocks grew brighter. Ssam kept calling; the light came closer, until Turner found where the lookouts waited.

"Thanks for the directions," Flossie said. "I think we would have heard you at the bottom of the mountain."

A round of cheers welcomed the last arrivals to camp.

"Let's eat," said Needlenose, "before I waste away to NeedleNothing." They shared what they'd brought as they talked and told about the day's adventures.

Flossie was grateful to Turner for her rescue from the terrible wind. Golly was glad they were together again and not wandering in the dark. Needlenose was happy his friends had returned, and grateful for his potato chips which he crunched loudly all the while.

"This place seems unusual," said Turner, "like it has some purpose. A sunken room with surrounding stones doesn't look natural."

"It's called The Place With No Trees," said Golly.

"I thought that meant the whole top of the mountain,"

said Veronica. "There are no trees anywhere up here."

"No *big* trees," Golly went on, "but there are grasses and small plants, and you can even find tiny trees if you look. But here, there is nothing."

"What does it mean?" Manford asked.

"I don't know."

"It doesn't seem likely anyone lived here," said Turner. "There's no food or water or firewood."

"Maybe Indians built it and had ceremonies here," said Needlenose.

"Maybe MorningGlory Mountain is a volcano and this is the crater," said Ssam.

"Maybe a rocket ship landed here thousands of years ago and blasted this hole," said Manford.

"I like the Indian theory best," said Flossie. "Now if nobody minds, I'm going to turn in. I'm cold and I've had a long day."

"Here, this will keep you warm," Manford said, and he took the long scarf Veronica had given him and wrapped it around Flossie. She nestled into it with a grateful smile. Columbine flew to her usual resting spot: Veronica's broad back. Turner rolled out his sleeping bag, crawled in, and wished everyone good night. One by one the others settled down around him in the dark.

They quickly fell asleep. The wind continued to whistle and sing as it passed overhead and among the rocks, but it was calm inside the room. Veronica dreamed of berry bushes full of ripe, sweet berries and smiled in her sleep. Flossie dreamed of Florida, sunshine, and ocean. Needlenose and Ssam slept soundly. Princess Columbine dreamed of precious jewels to decorate her wings and white flowers blooming in the night.

Manford dreamed of a wispy, white cloud. It was in the distance at first then it came nearer. It gathered and faded. It formed into odd and changing shapes. It drifted from place to place on the mountain, vanished for a time, then returned.

Manford shifted restlessly in his sleep. The dream cloud passed over where he slept and moved around the room's circular rim. It drifted to the floor. It passed smoothly around the room, traveling every inch of it in an orderly way. Then it stopped directly over him and changed shape again. It began to glow and pulse with soft light. It spoke quietly.

"Manford. . .Manford. . ."

Manford moved his head and shifted his legs in his sleep. His dream began to fade.

"Manford. . ." the voice said once more.

Manford stirred again, then lifted his head and opened his eyes in the dark. The dream was gone. The glowing cloud was still there.

"Welcome, Manford," said the voice. "Welcome to The Place With No Trees."

"What. . .who, um. . .who are you?" Manford asked.

"I am the Spirit of MorningGlory Mountain. This is my home, this mountain and this room where you sleep."

"Oh. . .um, are we disturbing you?"

"Not at all; I am pleased you have come. I seldom have visitors."

"Am I still dreaming?"

"No, I have been in your dreams these last days but you are awake now."

"Why are you talking to me?" asked Manford. "Why not one of the others, or all of us?"

"You have something I find interesting."

"Oh. . .what is that?"

"In your pack, the necklace of quills, that is interesting. Put it on."

"But Ssam's asleep in there. I'll wake him up."

"Be careful."

Manford opened his pack. The necklace was in a bag under the willow leaf pie. Ssam had crawled into one of the pack's inside pockets and lay sleeping, curled in a ball. Manford carefully pulled out the necklace.

"Needlenose made this for me, for my birthday," Manford said. He fastened it around his neck.

"He has given you a precious thing," said the spirit. "Care for it and use it well."

"He said it would help me find lost things."

"That is true, lost things and hidden things, some of great value. But it has power beyond that." The cloud extended a wispy arm to touch the necklace. It began to glow, too.

"What kind of power?" Manford asked in surprise.

"It will help you to see, to find what you are seeking."

"How do I use it?"

"You will learn."

"Oh...okay. I mean, I hope I do." Manford thought for a moment. "Um...did you want anything else?"

"I wanted to touch the necklace and tell you of its power. And also, sometimes it is pleasant just to talk."

"Should I wake the others? We could all talk then."

"No," said the spirit, "I will be leaving now."

"Can I ask a question first?"

"Yes."

"Who made this place, this room with stones all around?"

"I did. I find it pleasant here."

"Have you been here long?"

"I have always been here. Goodbye, Manford. Come talk to me again." The cloud rose, passed up and out of the room, and faded from sight.

"Goodbye..." Manford said. He gazed after his visitor for a long while, then settled back to sleep. The necklace still glowed softly around his neck.

He slept soundly and woke just after first light. Veronica was awake as well. They watched the sky grow lighter and waited for the first sunlight to reach The Place With No Trees. The wind had stopped.

"That's strange," said Veronica.

"What is?" asked Manford.

"Look at the floor around us."

"I don't see anything."

"That's just it. Our footprints are gone. The floor is smooth again, all around us and out to the edge."

"You're right," Manford said, noticing for the first time. "Maybe the wind did it."

"I don't think so," said Veronica. "Sand would have blown on us while we were sleeping. Besides, there was no wind in here."

"I wonder what happened," said Manford. He didn't know whether to mention his night visitor or not.

"Something mysterious, that much is for sure," said Veronica.

Manford made notes in his journal until the others awoke. Turner talked to each of them in his casual way as they set about getting ready for the day. Golly and Flossie noticed the smooth floor, but soon boot prints and quill marks tracked it again, along with marks of moose, bear, and birds.

There were no butterfly tracks, however. Butterflies don't leave heavy footprints, of course, even though they have six feet. Even so, had Columbine been wearing hiking boots that morning, or three pairs of tiny high heels, the sand would have shown no trace of her. There was no Royal Butterfly Princess that morning. Columbine was missing.

"Where's Princess?" Flossie said, suddenly noticing Columbine was gone. "She was sleeping on your back, Veronica. Did you roll over on her?"

"Oh, I hope not!" Veronica said, horror struck. They

searched the area where she had slept, sifting carefully through the fine sand. "I'd feel just dreadful if that had happened."

But Columbine wasn't there, nor did they find her anywhere within the ring of stones.

"I'll call to her," Ssam said. He shouted his loudest but they heard no reply.

They set out to look, each taking an area extending outward from the circular ridge. An hour of searching showed nothing. They returned to the room.

"Now what?" Flossie asked.

"I'm not sure," said Golly. "We have to keep looking, but where?"

"Manford's necklace," said Needlenose. "It's supposed to help find things. That might work."

"Yes, let's try it," said Veronica, looking at Manford. "Oh. . .you're wearing it. You had it on when you woke up this morning."

"Yes, I did," Manford said, "but I don't know how to use it. Were there any instructions, Needlenose?"

"No, I made it by copying a picture in a book."

"What kind of book?" asked Golly.

"It had pictures of things kept in a museum."

"Were there other pictures with it?"

"I don't remember."

"Think, Needlenose," said Flossie. "There might have been something important."

"I remember a picture of a necklace spread out on an Indian blanket. I could see how it was made and decorated. I liked it so I made one. It took lots of my quills."

"Was there anything written about it?" Golly asked.

"I think it said something like: *Apache ceremonial necklace, southern Arizona, late 1800s.*"

"Why did you think it was used to find things?" asked Veronica.

"I don't know."

"Did you just make that part up?"

"No," Needlenose said.

"Then where did the idea come from?" asked Flossie.

"Wait a minute," said Needlenose, "I remember now; there *was* another picture later in the book. It showed Indians sitting in a circle before they went hunting. One of them was wearing a necklace like this. I thought it was a ceremony or part of their tradition or something, and that maybe the necklace helped them find food."

"But their food wasn't lost," Flossie said in frustration. "They were just going hunting!"

"I guess you could see it that way," said Needlenose.

"But that's what *we're* doing," said Turner. "We're hunting for Columbine. Let's sit in a circle."

They formed a circle in the center of the room.

"What now?" said Ssam.

"Maybe we should join hands," said Turner.

"I don't have any."

"That's okay," said Veronica, "Someone can hold your head and someone else can hold your tail." They joined hands, paws, hoofs, wings, head, and tail. A few moments passed.

"Nothing's happening," said Manford.

"Let's close our eyes," said Flossie. "Maybe that will help." They closed their eyes and were silent.

"Still nothing happening," Manford said after a time.

"Think about Columbine," said Turner. "Maybe you can see her in your mind."

They thought about Columbine. Their thoughts seemed to pass from one to another around the circle and the necklace began to glow.

"I see something," Manford said excitedly.

"Tell us," said Flossie. Their eyes were still closed.

"It's Columbine. She's...she's on the ground near a big rock.

She's moving, but just barely. She can't fly."

"Where is she?" asked Golly. "Describe the place around her."

"There are two large rocks about as tall as Turner," said Manford. "They're leaning against each other. A smaller rock is balanced on top. Columbine is on the ground in front of them."

"What direction from here, and how far?"

"She's on the opposite side from the trail. I can't tell how far."

"Can you see anything else?" asked Flossie.

"No, all I see is rocks."

"Let's go, then," said Veronica. They opened their eyes. Manford's necklace was glowing brightly but they paid it no attention.

Golly and Flossie went to look for the place Manford had described. They flew back and forth in close formation, scanning the ground from side to side. But rocks looked different from the air; what might have been distinctive from the ground looked like just another rock from above. They flew outward from The Place With No Trees, looking and looking, until they reached where the mountain sloped off the other side. They found nothing.

"We'll fly lower, as close to the ground as we can," said Golly as they rested. They started again in the opposite direction, flying almost at the tops of the rocks.

The others set out on foot. Manford walked to the left, Ssam peering out of the pack. Turner walked in the middle. Veronica took the right, Needlenose on her shoulder. Each checked the area ahead and from side to side.

Golly and Flossie banked for another turn. They were flying to Manford's left and had nearly come back to where the others were searching.

"There's a balanced rock over there," said Golly. Flossie followed him in the direction he headed. She saw nothing likely at first then they found two large stones separate from the others. The stones leaned close together; another stone was balanced on top in the space between. Flossie landed and found Columbine motionless on the ground. "Go tell the others," she said. "I'll stay with her." Golly took off.

"Princess, can you hear me?" There was no answer. "Princess..."

Columbine moved one wing slightly. Flossie bent closer to listen.

"Can't fly," said a weak voice. "Need flowers."

Golly returned and the others could be heard running close behind.

"How is she?" Golly asked.

"Still alive, thank goodness," said Flossie. "She's very weak."

"Did you find her?" asked Manford, out of breath from his run through the rocks.

"Where is she?" Veronica asked, bounding around the other side of the two tall stones.

"She's here," Flossie told them, "but she can't fly and she said something about needing flowers."

"She wants something sweet to drink," said Turner. "She's had no flowers to sip from since yesterday coming up the mountain."

"But there aren't any flowers here," said Needlenose.

"I have water," said Turner. "That might help."

"Blueberries," said Veronica. "Squash some blueberries for her and give her that to drink. There are still some left."

"I'll get them," said Golly, and he was in the air, soaring with great sweeps of his powerful wings toward where they'd camped. He returned a few minutes later.

Turner mashed a small handful of blueberries in a cup and poured juice into a spoon. He held it down for Columbine to sip. She took no note of it at first then she must have smelled it. She turned her head slightly and began to drink. A shudder shook her briefly as she continued drinking, drinking, drinking.

She stood upright, flexed her stiff wings, and drank more. She fluttered her wings then began to beat them swiftly, still sipping from the spoon. She rose slowly off the ground until she was ten feet in the air, beating her wings faster and faster until they were just a blur.

"Powerful stuff," said Needlenose.

"She thinks she's a hummingbird," said Ssam.

Columbine darted from rock to rock with amazing speed, flew high in the air then circled the group 'round and 'round like a tiny airplane on a string. She went from one to the other of her rescuers, landed on their beaks and noses, and kissed them.

"Thank you," she said. "I thought I was finished. You are all so gallant."

"We're glad you're okay, dear," said Flossie.

"And whatever you gave me to drink, I'd like more of it. It's wonderful!"

They returned to The Place With No Trees. The sun was bright. The wind was still. It was early morning yet so they had much of the day to explore the mountaintop before heading home. But there were questions to answer first.

"What happened to you, Columbine?" said Veronica. "How did you get so far away?"

"I was dreaming," the Royal Princess replied. "I dreamed I saw a big, white flower out on the mountain, and I was so thirsty. I think I started flying in my sleep."

"I've done that," Flossie said. "Got lost every time."

"When I woke up the wind had caught me. The more I fought against it, the weaker I got. I was pushed back and forth, this way and that, and finally crashed against the rock where you found me. After that, I was too weak to fly. How did you ever find me?"

"Manford used his necklace," said Needlenose.

"Everyone else helped, too," Manford said. "We sat in a circle and thought about you. In my head, I saw you lying next to those rocks. Then we went looking for the rocks."

"Manford," said Veronica, "when we were sitting in the circle thinking about Columbine, the necklace started glowing. Did you know that?"

"Uh huh," said Manford.

"I also thought I heard you talking in the night. Did something happen?"

Manford paused, unsure of what to say. He didn't know if they'd believe the story about the Mountain Spirit, yet they *were* his friends, and he *had* found Columbine.

"Yes," he said finally, "something did happen. I didn't know if I should say anything. I was dreaming about a white cloud that moved over the mountain. Maybe it was the same white thing Columbine saw. I dreamed it came into the room, circled around in it, then stopped right above me. I woke up from the dream and the cloud was still there.

"What was it?" asked Ssam.

"It talked to me. It said it was the Spirit of MorningGlory Mountain. It wanted to see the necklace. When I put it on, the spirit touched it and made it glow and told me how powerful it is."

"Why didn't you wake us?" asked Needlenose.

"I wanted to but the spirit said no," Manford said.

"There's a legend of such a spirit," Golly said, "a spirit that has lived in this mountain for thousands of years, maybe always. It has been seen only a few times, and then in dreams or under doubtful circumstances. I never believed it but it must be true, especially if Columbine saw something, too."

"I asked about this room, The Place With No Trees," Manford said. "The spirit built it long ago, it said. I guess it likes being here."

"That answers that question, anyway," said Turner.

"It will be a special place for us now, too," Veronica said. "We'll have to come back."

"The spirit said we should visit it again," Manford said.

They romped about the mountaintop for several hours. They climbed up large rocks and wriggled through narrow openings between them. They played follow-the-leader, hide-and-seek, and king-of-the-hill. They looked from all sides of Morning-Glory Mountain at the country around them. Surrounding peaks looked small in the distance. Clouds drifted below them and the sunny green valleys they'd left three days before were so far down the mountain they were just patches of color.

"Quite a view from here, isn't it?" said Turner.

"Yes," said Golly. "The trees and rocks in the valley are so small I can hardly make them out."

"Trees and rocks?" said Veronica. "I don't see anything like trees and rocks. It's just fuzzy green to me."

"I can see trees down there," said Flossie. "Can you, Manford?"

"No, it's only a blur," Manford said.

"Some animals have better eyesight than others," said Turner. "Those who don't see well can usually hear or smell or sense things better."

"Well, if Golly can see trees and rocks down there," said Veronica, "I want to, also."

"I guess you'll have to get glasses then, my friend."

"My mom has glasses," Manford said. "She's been saying I would need them, too."

"If you had some, you could really enjoy the view. Ask her about them when you get home."

They ate lunch from their supplies in the sandy-floored room as a bright sun shone directly overhead.

"Will you hike down the mountain with us, Mr. Turner?" Manford asked.

"No, this trail goes on over the other side of the mountain. I thought I'd see what's there. Thanks for inviting me, though."

"I'll always remember that you rescued me," said Flossie. "I hope we see you again."

"Maybe you will," Turner answered, "and maybe I'll see Millie someday, too."

They didn't want to leave, but finally said goodbye to Turner, goodbye to the Mountain Spirit, and started back down the trail. The Place With No Trees grew smaller behind them. Soon it was not visible at all. And inside that special place a white cloud was moving, shifting the sand, covering the footprints, smoothing the floor once again.

They spent the entire afternoon climbing down the mountain. What had been steep and difficult going up was just as hard going down. Veronica led, Manford followed, each carrying their usual passengers. Golly and Flossie flew as before but their burdens were much lighter; the berry basket was empty, the pie was gone, and Needlenose had done serious work on the potato chips.

They camped in the clearing where they'd met Turner and awoke the next morning to rain. The rain lasted most of the day but stopped when the adventurers made their final camp. They walked the last day in sunshine, stopping for lunch at MorningGlory Crossing. Ssam slept right through it. When they departed, they took him along.

They stopped to see again the sights and pretty things they'd noted on the way up. Everything looked just as lovely now and promised still to be so the next time they came. Soon they were back in the meadow saying their goodbyes and see-you-tomorrows.

"We should do this again," Manford said.

"Not real soon, I hope," said Flossie.

"Well, maybe not, but the spirit said something that makes me wonder."

"Said what?" asked Needlenose.

"It was about using the necklace to find something that was hidden, maybe something of great value. Do you suppose there's something like that on MorningGlory Mountain?"

"There's nothing in the legend about it," said Golly, "but I wouldn't be surprised."

Veronica headed for Misty Falls and Flossie flew off to her pond. Needlenose offered Ssam the other spare room at Haystack Hollow. Ssam accepted easily.

Manford went directly home and burst in the front door.

"I'm back, Mom," he said. "Oh, we had *such* a great time!"

"You must tell me about it, dear," Manford's mother said, and Manford did, in great detail, to which his mother listened patiently.

"Were you worried about me?" he asked.

"Not at all," Mary Moose replied. "Little moose are *supposed* to have adventures and learn about the world. But I'm glad you're safely home."

"Well, if I'm supposed to have adventures and learn about the world, I'm going to need glasses. . ."

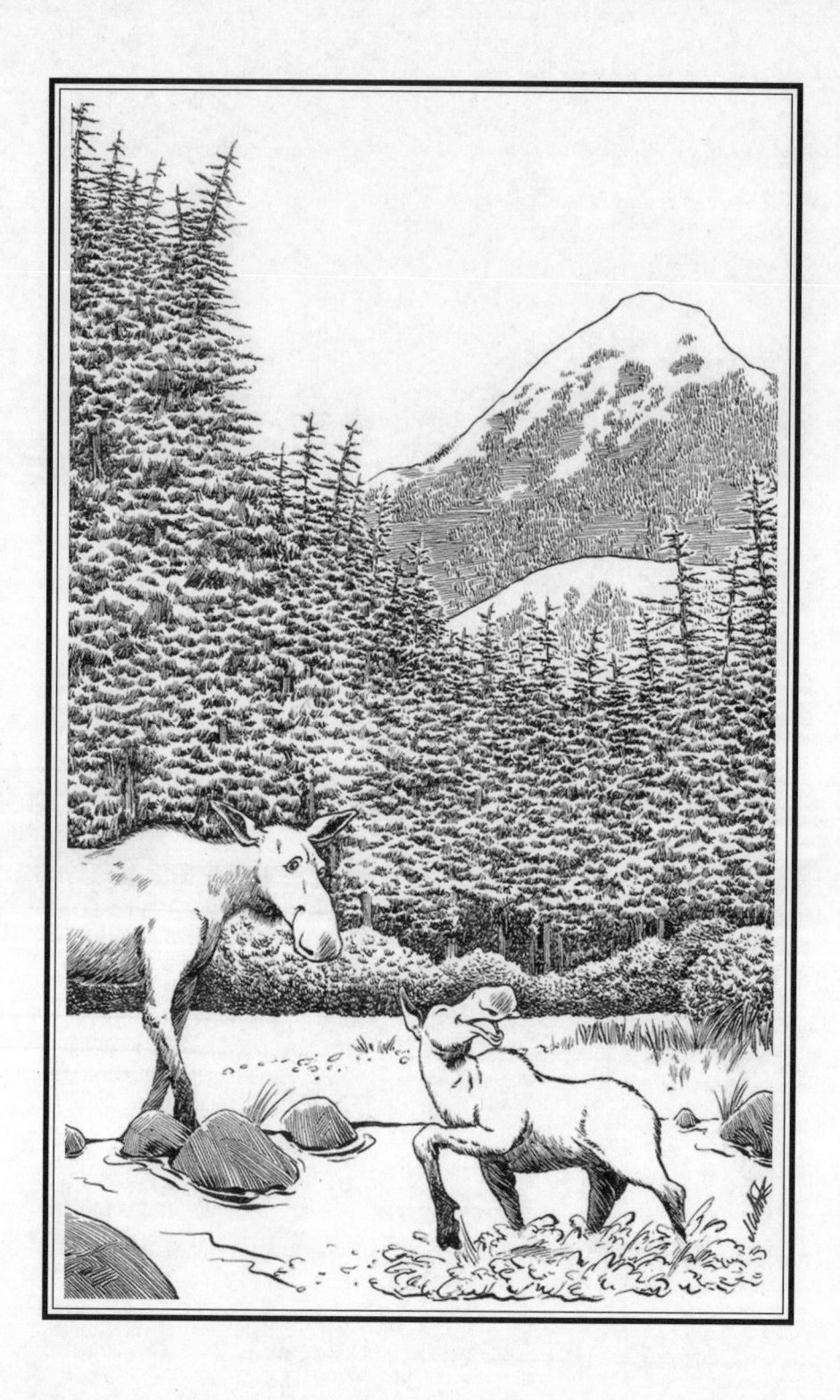

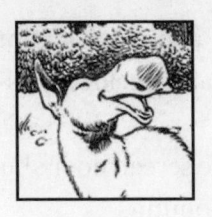

7

Happy To Be Me
In which Mary Moose tells her story

Manford wondered what to do. It was early. He'd eaten breakfast as usual. He'd said good morning to his mother as usual. He'd looked outside as usual, discovering blue sky and sun sparkling on the dew. It was a day to be outdoors, the morning told him. Yet here he was, still puttering about the house, still deciding about absolutely the best thing to do.

'I'll visit my friends,' he was thinking. *Uh huh, but it's early yet.*

'I'll find fresh willow leaves to nibble. Good idea, but I've just finished breakfast.

'I'll walk up Lookout Hill to see MorningGlory Mountain. Okay, but that's a sunrise, sunset sort of thing to do.

'I'll go wading in the pond,' he thought. *'The pond. . .yes, that's it. Moose are fond of doing that, especially in early morning with the water smooth as glass.'*

Manford skipped out the front door to head down the path; the path, in case you haven't been there lately, that led through the woods and across MorningGlory Creek, through WhiteFlower Meadow and past the big tree, over Lookout Hill and down and around and across another creek to the pond that Flossie had found and decided was hers. That's just where he decided to go.

But he stopped as the screen door shut behind him; all around him the roses were blooming.

Pale lavender blossoms covered rows of tall bushes along the front of the house on each side of the door.

Single rows of shorter rosebushes grew in front of those, bright pink flowers bursting from the centers of the rows, pale, whitish pink roses gracing the ends.

Low hedges of roses crossed the yard in front of those, came together at the path, then turned to line it on either side with clusters of deep lavender, almost violet roses, their petals tinged with ruby.

The rose hedges led on to the far end of Moostery Manor's yard. There, tall bushes marked the entrance with showy blossoms of deep pink.

Manford stood on the step on this lovely May day smelling roses, looking at roses, thinking about roses, and almost forgot where he was going. And there he found his mother standing in the yard, humming to herself, deftly pruning roses with her teeth.

"Do those taste good?" he asked.

"I'm not eating them," said Mary, "I'm pruning them."

"Pruning?"

"It means cutting dead parts off the bush so the rest of it can grow. No one has lived here for a while and these roses haven't been tended."

"There sure are a lot of them."

"That's one of the reasons I wanted to live here."

"They're very pretty," said Manford, "but why would you grow so many roses instead of something else?"

"Roses come in more sizes, shapes, and colors than any other flower," Mary replied. "You can always find one you like. They grow in nearly any kind of soil and climate, they survive hot summers and harsh winters, and they bloom from spring to fall. Those are good reasons, don't you think?"

"I guess so."

"They also smell nice and they're easy to grow."

"There must be lots of different kinds," Manford said.

"More than thirteen thousand recorded varieties."

"How many kinds are growing here?"

"Five."

"How do you know that?"

"They still have tags on them."

Manford looked down and saw a printed tag looped around one branch of the hedge.

"*Angel Face*," he read. "Is that a kind of rose?"

"Yes."

"I thought plants had scientific names."

"They have those, too," Mary said. "If you're really interested, I'll tell you a few things about roses."

"Okay."

"The rose belongs to a family of plants that includes many different classes of roses, plus other plants like strawberries, raspberries, peaches, apples, and apricots."

"A strawberry is a rose?"

"No, but it belongs to the same family."

"Can I eat roses on my cereal in the morning?"

"I suppose," said Mary, "but they are much nicer to look at and smell. Now, where was I?"

"You were talking about classes of roses."

"Yes, there are four main ones. The first is called hybrid tea."

"What does that mean?"

"When you cross two different kinds of plants, the result is a new plant called a hybrid. Long ago, someone crossed a tea rose with another kind of rose and called the new one hybrid tea."

"Do you make tea from them?"

"You could, but they're called that because some smell like tea. Nearly all roses sold by florists and three-fourths the roses grown in gardens are hybrid teas. That's what all the roses here are except the hedge."

"What kind is that?" asked Manford.

"It's a floribunda, which means 'abundance of flowers'," Mary said. "It grows close to the ground and has big clusters of flowers. It makes a good border or hedge."

"What are the other two classes?"

"Grandiflora, or 'grand flowers' is one. It grows taller and makes bigger blossoms than the ones I just mentioned. The other class is called climbers. They grow long branches. If you tie them to fences or walls, they look like they're climbing."

"How do they get names like *Angel Face*?"

"New kinds of roses are named by whoever first grows them. The name someone chooses may have to do with the rose's color, or they may name it after a famous person or place, or it might remind them of something beautiful or fun."

"What are the rest of yours called?"

"The lavender roses on the tall bushes next to the house are called *Lady X*. Their color is pale with touches of pink.

"In front of those, the bright pink roses on the center bushes are called *First Prize*. They've won many prizes at rose shows. The pale pink ones either side of them, sort of the color of apple blossoms, are *Royal Highness*.

"*Angel Face*, the deep lavender hedge that runs along the walk, you've already met. It smells sort of spicy.

"The pink roses at the entrance to the yard are *Miss All American Beauty*. They grow as a tall bush and smell strongly like tea. They go kind of nice with the others."

"Everything's lavender and pink," said Manford.

"Whoever planted them must have liked those colors," said Mary. "Some think they don't go well together, but I like them."

"I do, too," Manford said. "They seem kind of special. What other colors are there?"

"There are red roses, of course, plus white, yellow, orange, and coral. Blends have two or more colors, and bi-colors have one color on the front of the petals and another on the back. There are many light and dark shades of each, so you can find almost any color rose you want from white to nearly black, except blue. There are no blue roses."

"Why not?"

"No one has been able to grow one yet."

"Isn't lavender close to blue?"

"Yes, but not close enough. The first yellow rose took twenty-five years to grow. It took that much time to breed out traces of orange, red, and pink and get pure yellow. Lavender still has red and pink in it. It's a long way from pure blue."

"Maybe you could grow a blue rose, Mom."

"I rather like the ones we have," Mary replied.

Manford walked down the path to the end of the yard, then back to the house, smelling each kind of rose as he went. He was quiet and seemed to be thinking.

"Where did roses come from?" he said after a while.

"As near as anyone can tell, wild roses originated in central Asia and gradually spread over the northern hemisphere. Plant fossils found in Colorado show that wild roses were growing here forty million years ago."

"Do wild roses have names, too?"

"No, and in fact, they don't even look like roses. Most of them are red or pink and are simple, five-petaled flowers. Garden roses have big, symmetrical blossoms with dozens of overlapping petals."

"Are they good for anything but looking pretty?"

"That's what they do best. Rose hips, the seedpods that grow when the petals fall, are good for vitamin C. You can make jams, puddings, preserves, candies, and perfume from the petals. Extracts from rose petals were once used in medicines, but it probably just made them taste better."

"I think I'll just smell them and look at them."

"Good idea," Mary said.

"You said there were rose shows. What are they for?"

"Gardeners display arrangements of their most pleasing roses at rose shows and festivals. Judges decide which they like best and award ribbons and prizes."

"What else do you know about roses?"

"Oh, I could tell you how to grow and take care of roses, and how to cross breed them to make new varieties. We could pick some and I could show you how to make arrangements. We could look through rose books in the library and find pictures of hundreds of different kinds. We could learn their histories and figure out how they got their names. But this is enough, don't you think?"

"Uh huh," Manford said. "Thanks, Mom. I like to find out about things." He stood thinking for a moment. "Let's see, I was going somewhere. . .oh, to the pond. Want to come along to the pond?"

"I think so," said Mary. "I've been at this for hours. I can finish after lunch."

It was now mid-morning. The pond, no longer still, rippled gently in the wind and reflected surrounding trees in wavy patterns. Flossie wasn't in sight. Perhaps she was still asleep in Haystack Hollow. Perhaps she was flying somewhere nearby in MorningGlory Forest. She wouldn't be far, Manford knew. She lost her way easily and tried to stay in sight of the pond.

Manford waded into the water to his knees, then to his shoulders. He ducked his head under the surface and opened his eyes. Light shone down through the water and he could see the pebbly bottom. Fish darted out of his path then came back, hanging curiously in the water to watch him.

Mary waded quietly along the pond's edge. She dipped her head in the water at times to pluck and eat plants growing up from the bottom. She waded out farther, allowing cool water to soak into her coat. Then she moved back toward shore and settled down in the shallows to rest. Manford splashed over to her.

"The water feels good," he said.

"Yes," his mother answered, "it's nice and cool."

"Is that why we do this, because the water feels good?"

"Do you need a better reason?"

"I was just wondering."

"The water plants are good to eat sometimes," she continued. "That's a good reason."

"Uh huh."

"Or if it's buggy out, sometimes the breeze on the pond will blow the bugs away."

"I hadn't thought of that," said Manford. "That's a good reason, too. Are there any others?"

"Well," Mary said with a smile, "someone might take your picture and put you in a movie or on a postcard."

"Oh, I'll have to remember that."

"Be sure to pose majestically in front of a mountain."

"Do I need antlers to be majestic?"

"I don't have any," Mary replied. "It never bothered me."

"I'll do my best," Manford said with a laugh.

They were quiet for a time, resting in the rippling water. Birds flew about in the trees around the pond and wind rustled in the branches. There were few other sounds.

"How do you know so much about roses?" Manford asked.

"From reading about them," Mary answered. "When I saw that our new house had roses, I got books about them from the library and studied."

"Is that all there is to it? If I wanted to know about building rocket ships or playing football, would I get books from the library?"

"Well, it helps to understand what you're reading. I learned about plants in school so reading about them now is easy."

"Where did you go to school?"

"In Alaska."

"At a university?"

"No, nothing so fancy. In Alaska, educational television broadcasts classes to remote villages. When I was growing up, I spent winters taking classes on TV."

"What kind of classes?"

"The usual things at first: reading, writing, math, science, history. Then something interesting happened.

"One summer day I was walking in the woods and saw a group of hikers, about a dozen or so. The person in front walked along like he was in his own backyard. The last person in line seemed the same way, but those in between were different. They looked unsure of themselves, like being in the woods was something brand new."

"I've seen hikers like that," Manford said. "Did you follow them?"

"Yes, and I listened as they sat around their campfire and talked. They were city people on a wilderness adventure. They didn't know each other, and they didn't know much about the outdoors, either."

"Did they see you?"

"Oh, sure, and they took my picture," said Mary. "I was part of the 'wildlife.'"

"What did they do on their adventure?"

"They crossed mountains and valleys and forded creeks. They built shelters and fires and cooked. They took sightings with their compasses and charted their direction on a map. And all the while they asked questions—questions about rocks and trees and water and sky and everything else they could think of. The guides knew most of the answers. The thing that bothered me was that I didn't. I'd lived all my life in the woods, yet I'd sometimes wondered about the same things.

"The people became friends during the trip. The guides showed them how to do things. They shared the chores, slowly got better at what they were doing, and when it was over, agreed they'd had a good time. I started thinking it would be interesting to be a guide and help someone through that experience."

"So then you went back to school," said Manford.

"Yes," his mother answered, "and I took subjects that explained how the world works; how plants and trees grow; how rocks were formed; what glaciers do, that sort of thing. I studied Botany, Forestry, Geology, and whatever else sounded interesting. Eventually I got a degree as a naturalist."

"Is that when you got glasses?"

"No, I could see well enough to study. I got glasses to look at things far away, to see what I was reading about."

"And then you became a guide."

"Yes, I figured if people wanted to see the wilderness, who could be better at guiding them than someone who lived there and knew something about it?"

"Was it easy?"

"No, it took a while to get going. I started by following trips other guides were leading, groups like Outward Bound that take people to the woods and teach them wilderness skills."

"Did they ask you to come along?"

"No, I just followed them. They would see me, of course, and would soon start to wonder why a moose was hanging around, especially a moose wearing glasses. Then I'd start talking to them and they'd really get confused. The people on the trips always made a big fuss over this so the guides would let me stay."

"What were the trips like?"

"They lasted five days to two weeks. Every day we'd walk about ten miles to look at scenery and explore the territory. People took pictures, wrote journals, and asked questions about everything they saw all day. Some days they'd go by canoe. Moose don't do well in canoes so I would follow along on the bank. They would go farther on those days but I could always catch up. Moose can move quickly through brush because we have such long legs.

"At first the guides thought I should be a pack animal and carry peoples' gear. I did that a few times, and helped in camp putting up tents and cooking. I learned things from them I couldn't learn on TV. I mean, you can study and read about building a campfire or cooking in the rain all you want but you don't really know it till you do it.

"Before long, they found out I knew the answers to questions people asked. Pretty soon, whenever anyone wanted to know something about the area where we were, about the animals, trees, rocks, mountains, or glaciers, they'd ask me and I'd know. Everyone was amazed. I'd studied the Indian legends, too. Strange rock formations or mountains with unusual shapes almost always have legends behind them. I'd tell those stories when we rested or at night in camp."

"Did the guides invite you back?"

"Yes, after a while. People went home to their cities and jobs and told friends about their Alaskan adventure. Nobody really believed they'd seen a talking moose, but a few signed up for a trip just to find out. When they learned it was true, they told other people, and they told others. The guides got more and more business. Soon all their trips were sold out. And every one wanted me to be on his or her trip so customers wouldn't be disappointed. Each tried to pay me more and more."

"You really must have been busy," Manford said.

"It wasn't long before I could only go a few days on one trip, a few days on another, then a day or so on another. I was running from one place to another the whole summer trying to keep up."

"What did you do?"

"I recruited more moose."

"To be guides like you?"

"That's right."

"How did you find moose who knew what you did?" Manford asked. "Did they go to school, too?"

"Sort of," Mary replied. "The next winter, when moose are pretty bored anyway, I found twelve others that seemed interested in what I was doing. We met every day. They took classes on TV. I helped them with their studies, and taught them other things they needed. Moose know a lot about the woods to begin with, so it wasn't as hard as it sounds.

"In early spring, I took them on trips to teach them the practical things I'd learned from the guides. It's funny now that I think about it. There we were, thirteen moose in the woods setting up tents, building fires, cooking pots of stew. It must have looked odd. But, by the time the trip season started, we were ready. Each of us traveled with one guide for a while then we switched places so we got to go different places and learn different things."

"How did the guides like it?"

"They thought we were great. Their businesses got better and better."

"Did you ever think about running trips of you own?"

"I did. I was going to call my outfit Mary's Mountain Moose Adventures. But then I started thinking. I didn't really want to run a business and do the planning and organizing and paperwork; I wanted to go on trips. We were all enjoying what we were doing and being paid what we needed, so I dropped the idea. Besides, at the end of that summer I was offered a different kind of job and decided to look into that."

"It must have been a good one," observed Manford.

"Yes and no," Mary said. "It was with the Park Service. They heard about my moose guides and me and thought I could help them. But I knew it would be different. Instead of leading five or ten people through the wilderness for a week or two, they wanted me to be a ranger in a small park and give talks to busloads of people, two or three times a day. They figured if I'd done so much for the guides' businesses, I could help them even more."

"Did all of you go?"

"No, the other moose stayed with the guides. I almost stayed myself. I enjoyed being out in the wilderness, going places and seeing things. In the park, I'd have to stay in one place. But it was a chance to learn something new. They gave me a ranger hat and plenty to study about the area and I got busy.

"The park had forest and mountains, scenic drives and hiking trails, and a half-dozen glaciers. Two glaciers flowed into a lake; the rest hung in the mountains. The park was close to a big city so visitors could get there easily by car or bus.

"I studied the area's geology and history. I hiked the trails and identified plants and trees. I researched old records and studied maps of where the glaciers had been the past few hundred years. By the time the first tourists came, I had a ton of new information in my head."

"Then what happened?" Manford asked.

"Well, at first no one believed I was a real moose. They thought I was two people in a costume or some kind of mechanical moose from Disneyland. City people are like that. They don't know that we can talk. In fact, they don't know much about the woods at all.

"But I gave my ranger program, took them on hikes, and answered their questions. Soon, the same thing happened as with the guides. There were two buses a day when I started in the spring and those were barely half full. By summer, we had full buses every hour coming to see the talking moose. I had time to myself only when it rained really hard, and even then some people came."

"So, did you like it?"

"Yes," Mary said, "I guess I did. Most of the people were very nice. They asked endless questions and I enjoyed the chance to help them learn a few things. My second summer there was even busier. So many cars and buses came they had to enlarge the parking lot. People from all over the world wanted to see me and hear my little ranger talk about glaciers and rocks and trees. I felt like a movie star."

"How long did you stay?"

"Three more years. I taught new moose every winter and so did some of the others. Soon every wilderness trip in Alaska had one of my moose guides, and I had moose rangers in all the parks. More people came to visit Alaska during those years than in previous years. Hotels and roadhouses and campgrounds were full all summer long."

"Why did you leave?"

"Working in the park was fun but it wasn't like being in the wilderness. I'd made all the money I'd ever need, so I started thinking about going back to the woods. Then I met your dad."

"Did he come to your school to be a guide?" asked Manford.

"No, he was already a star, dancing ballet in New York. He was in Alaska to do a show. He heard about my moose rangers and guides and arranged a tour to see me. Someone pointed him out in the crowd and told me he was famous. Well, fine, so was I.

"He talked to me afterward and said he was from Alaska, too. He was very nice. That's when I first heard the story Mr. Johnny told at your birthday party. He wrote me letters from New York and other big cities after that and invited me to join him. My guides and rangers were doing fine, so when winter came, I left someone else in charge and spent the next year or so with him on tour."

"Where was I born?"

"The company was in Vancouver, in Canada, in late winter. I'd traveled enough for a while so I found a nice place in the forest to live near there. You were born in the spring. We moved here just about a year later."

"You've done some interesting things, Mom," Manford said. "Don't you miss what you were doing in Alaska?"

"No," Mary replied, "I'm back in the wilderness now and that's where I'm happy. Besides, we still have relatives in Alaska. I can call or visit them if I get lonesome."

"Does it bother you to stay home while Dad's off being a star?"

"Not a bit. I was a star for many years, too. It was fun. I enjoyed it. But now, I like being here, living in the forest and mountains, watching you grow up, tending pink and lavender roses. Here, I can be what I want to be: me. That makes me happy, happy to be me."

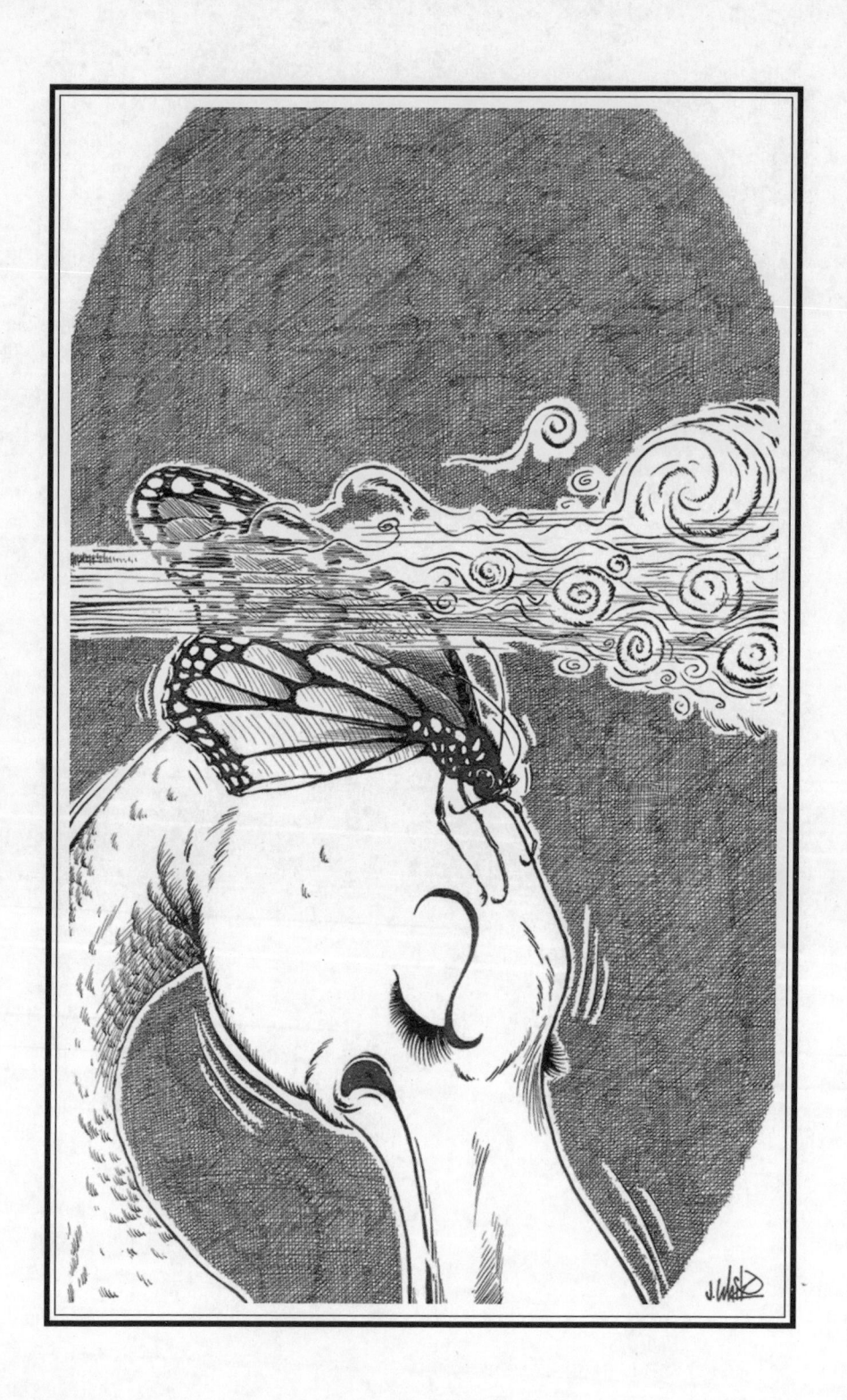

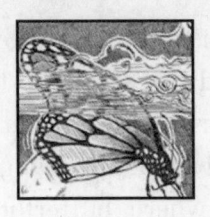

8

A Certain Smelly Something
In which there be dragons

Princess Columbine perched on a bright, yellow daffodil. She flexed her wings slowly, first holding them straight up, nearly touching, so you could barely see her, then stretching them flat to become a bright splash of orange and black against yellow petals. She stuck her head deep inside the flower to sip nectar from its center. It tasted good to her, like honey might taste to a bear. She tasted many flowers each day—daffodils, daisies, poppies—anything as gaily colored as she. Their sweetness gave her energy to fly. Their happy colors made her happy, too.

It was noon. It was June. Columbine began to fly about the meadow. She didn't fly like a bird might, beating wings smoothly and going from here to there in a straight line. No, that was for birds that were fast, and in a hurry. Instead, Columbine fluttered. She flew up. She flew down. She flew from side to side in a zigzag pattern that was really not a pattern at all. It was just fluttering. No one had taught her to fly this way, and she never thought about why she did it; she just did it. It was the way butterflies were.

There was a reason Columbine moved the way she did, as she might have learned had she gone to the library to look it up. Birds chased butterflies and sometimes ate them. But, by flying suddenly up, and suddenly down, and suddenly here and there and who knows where, butterflies weren't always quite where the birds expected them to be. That was how butterflies got away. Everything happens for a reason, you see.

Columbine found Needlenose in the tree in the meadow, sound asleep on a branch. She landed on his head but he didn't wake up. She walked all along him, down his neck and out to the tip of his bushy quill tail and back again. Needlenose kept snoring peacefully and never felt a thing. Columbine didn't want to disturb him, so she flew off to see who else she could find.

Flossie was standing on one leg at the far end of the pond. The Royal Butterfly Princess landed on her head. Flossie didn't stir. Columbine tiptoed down between Flossie's eyes and looked in. Flossie's eyes were closed; she was sleeping, too. Columbine stayed a moment, walking her six-legged walk back and forth, but Flossie didn't move. Butterflies don't wear shoes, of course, and weigh hardly anything at all. A hundred butterflies could land on you while you were sleeping and you'd never feel it, unless you were ticklish. Flossie certainly didn't, so once again, Columbine flew away.

She passed over Needlenose's burrow. Ssam was there, curled up on top in a sunny spot in the grass. She could tell even without landing that he was snoozing, too.

'What a bunch of sleepyheads,' she thought, and she fluttered on through the forest.

She landed on flowers, on leaves, on tree branches, then on a tall blade of grass near the edge of the pond. She looked at everything around her. It was quiet. No wind in the trees, no ripples in the pond—just quiet.

'No wonder everyone is sleeping,' Columbine thought. 'Maybe I should catch a few winks, too.'

She heard a distant buzzing sound. It grew louder and she saw something flying low over the pond. It moved swiftly along the water's edge, its wings just a blur.

'Maybe it's another butterfly,' the Princess thought. *'Maybe it will see me and come say hello.'*

It turned and flew in her direction; the sound of its buzzing grew louder as it approached. Columbine expected it to circle and land, but it didn't. It flew directly at her, looking like it meant to knock her from her perch.

It bore in on her, closer and closer, louder and louder. She wanted to fly and get out of its way but somehow seemed rooted to the spot. She closed her eyes and folded her wings tightly to make herself as small as she could. The buzzing thing zoomed past, swerving away at the very last moment. The draft from its wings set Columbine and the grass blade she clung to bobbing back and forth.

Princess opened her eyes. She saw the creature turning to come at her again. Its wings made a raspy sound that echoed in her tiny ears. Again it flew straight for her, closer, closer, and then pulled away as she scrunched her wings and body to their tiniest size. Columbine was frightened; this was no friendly butterfly. Whatever this was, it was angry. She tried to call for help but couldn't, and besides, her friends were asleep.

Again and again, the buzzing creature dive bombed Columbine, passing as close as it could and sending her bobbing dizzily back and forth. In terror, she clung fast to the blade of grass, too confused and afraid to take off and fly away.

Then it was gone. The sound of its wings grew faint as it flew across the pond. Columbine was shaking. She took a moment to gather her wits then flew unsteadily to where Flossie still stood sleeping.

"Flossie! Oh, Flossie," Princess Columbine cried, sobbing as she landed again on the pink bird's head. Flossie opened one eye.

"Columbine, is that you? Of course it is. Who else would land on top of my head?"

"Oh, the most terrible thing just happened," Columbine said. Tiny tears dripped onto Flossie's feathers and lay there like glistening beads.

"Gracious, Lovely Princess, tell me about it."

"I was sitting in the grass near the pond when a terrible buzzing thing flew at me and tried to knock me over."

"That's awful, Princess. Are you okay?"

"Yes, but it frightened me."

"I can see that," said Flossie. "What was it?"

"I thought it was a butterfly at first, sort of like me but a different kind, but now I'm not sure."

"What did it look like?"

"It had a long body and its eyes were like big jewels," said Columbine. "Its wings went so fast I couldn't see them, and they made an awful sound."

"Did it say anything?"

"No, it was flying very fast. It was scary. I was glad when it went away."

"Where did it go?"

"Across the pond. I hope it never comes back."

"Well, that's a fine thing," Flossie said. "I thought the creatures here were friendly. This one doesn't sound nice at all. Do you remember anything else?"

"It smelled bad."

"How bad?"

"Like garlic!" said Columbine. "A smelly cloud of it wrapped around me every time the thing flew past. I thought I'd faint just breathing."

"This is a puzzle," said Flossie. "I don't know much about the critters here, but it doesn't sound like a butterfly to me. I wonder what it is?"

"I hope we don't have to find out."

The two stayed together through the afternoon. They moved from the water to the shade as the day grew warm, and had long stopped talking about Columbine's experience when she suddenly heard the buzzing sound again.

"There it is," Columbine said, fear in her voice.

"I hear it," said Flossie.

The creature came toward them, apparently unconcerned that Flossie was fifty times its size. It flew closer and closer until Flossie ducked, then it turned to come at them again.

"Peee-ew!" Flossie said. "You're right, Princess, that thing does smell bad. I wonder what it had for lunch."

Again, it attacked.

"Just a minute, buster," Flossie said as it bore in on her again. "What do you think you're doing?"

It didn't answer. It flew straight at Flossie, moving very fast.

"Go away, stinky thing," said Columbine.

Still, the creature buzzed them again and again, saying nothing. Then it flew off, just as before, across the water to the far side of the pond. Flossie and Columbine were left in a cloud of garlicky fumes.

"What's his problem?" asked Columbine.

"Beats me, Princess," answered Flossie, "but the air's a bit thick here just now. Let's find a new spot." She flapped her great wings and flew to a nearby tree.

They descended again when they'd heard nothing more from the creature for several hours. The sinking sun shone brightly by then, reflecting off ripples in the water, backlighting trees on the west edge of the pond, turning MorningGlory Mountain shadowy red and orange.

Before they had a chance to settle, here came the buzzing again.

"Oh, no!" said Columbine. Indeed, the creature was flying noisily toward them once more.

"Hang on, Royal Butterfly," said Flossie. "Let's try a little action of our own." Flossie took off, flying low across the water and picking up speed. The creature pursued. Flossie circled the edge of the pond, moving faster and faster. Columbine held on tightly, looking back now and then to see how they were doing.

It gained on them steadily, following effortlessly and never showing signs of slowing down. Flossie turned in mid-air. Fliers large and small now headed straight toward each other.

"Pilot to navigator, bogie dead ahead," Flossie said to Columbine. *"Prepare to clean windshield."*

Inches away from impact, the small creature veered suddenly into a looping spiral, changing directions and flying around and around Flossie as she sped along.

"Show-off," Flossie said. She turned away but her pursuer was too quick and too good a flier. Everywhere Flossie went, it was there: ahead, behind, on either side. Flossie landed at water's edge. To her surprise, the creature landed on a bush nearby. A strong smell of garlic came to them almost at once.

"What's a rusty bucket of bolts like you doing here?" the insect said insolently. "You fly like you're made of lead." He spoke with an accent of rolling r's.

Flossie looked sourly at their visitor. Its eyes were almost half as big as its head and glowed with rainbow colors of reflected light. Its shiny, twig-like body had six legs at the very front and two matched pairs of transparent wings. After all its acrobatic flying, it wasn't even breathing hard.

"I live here, buzz bomb," Flossie answered, "and so does my friend. What and who are you?"

"I'll ask the questions," the creature went on. "What do you mean you live here?"

"It seemed pretty clear to me. I live here. This is my pond."

"Wrong, Pinky," the creature said. "This pond is mine, and I want both of you out."

"You can't throw us out," said Columbine. "We've been here since Chapter 1."

"Right," said Flossie, "and if you don't watch your mouth, I'll have you for lunch, though you don't look very tasty."

"You couldn't catch me, grandma. I can fly circles around you and you saw me do it."

"I think we need a new approach here," Flossie said thoughtfully. "Shall we begin again?

"Sir Whatever-You-Are, I'm Flossie, the Flamingo. The lovely creature on my head is Princess Columbine, our Royal Monarch Butterfly. We might be pleased to meet you if you could be a little nicer."

"Nice? Why should I be nice? You've taken over my pond and I don't like it. The quicker you leave the better."

"What a bully," said Columbine.

"Why do you think it's your pond?" asked Flossie. "How long have you been here?"

"Longer than you, that's for sure—several years, at least, and my ancestors were here centuries ago."

"It seems odd we haven't seen you around."

"I lived in the water nearly all that time. A week ago I crawled out onto a log, split open my shell, and changed into what I am today."

"Which brings us to my original question," said Flossie. "What are you?"

"I," the creature said, drawing itself up proudly on all six legs and fanning its wings, "am a dragonfly."

"Do you have a name?" asked Columbine.

"I do. I am Dragone Respira-Fuoco. My friends call me FireDragon." He rolled his r's with great drama.

"You have friends?" said Columbine.

"Now who's not being nice," said FireDragon.

"Be polite, dear," Flossie said to Columbine.

Columbine said "Yes'm" to Flossie, and a tiny tee-hee to herself.

"Dra-GO-ne. . .Res-PIR-a. . .Fu-O-co," repeated Flossie,

trying to say it properly. "That sounds important. Does it mean something?"

"It does," replied FireDragon, gesturing expansively with at least four of his legs. "It's the Italian for Dragon with Breath of Fire. But this is getting a bit chummy to suit me. Let's stick to business. This is my pond. Be out of here by sundown. Goodbye." With that, the dragonfly beat his wings and was gone.

"A fire breathing dragonfly," said Columbine. "Well, that explains the garlic, anyway."

"He smells so bad, I wonder how he can stand himself," said Flossie.

"We're not going to leave, are we?"

"Of course not, Princess, we're staying right here. And when Dragon Breath comes back, we'll see what he thinks of that."

Light filtered softly through the trees next morning as the sun rose over MorningGlory Forest. A faint mist drifted across the water. As promised, and after a restful night's sleep, Flossie and Columbine were again at the pond, but this time they stood well away from the edge in the farthest reach of the shallow water. There FireDragon would have no place to land, Flossie figured, and would eventually grow tired and leave them alone.

But Flossie had much to learn about dragonflies. When FireDragon returned, he simply hovered in front of her just out of reach, his wings buzzing with, seemingly, energy enough to last a lifetime.

"Nice try, Feather Brain," he taunted in a threatening voice, "but I can keep this up all day. You can't get away from me. I said sundown, remember? You're packed and leaving soon, I presume."

"Look, Sir Dragoney Baloney," Flossie said loudly, "we're

not leaving. You can pester us all you want but it won't do any good. We're staying. Get used to it. Now before you get too excited, I have a question."

"What?" said FireDragon, who still hung effortlessly in mid-air.

"What do you eat?"

The dragonfly seemed puzzled.

"Mosquitoes," he said. "What's it to you?"

"I wanted to know why you smell like a pound of raw garlic all the time. Whew! It's enough to knock us over."

"What are you talking about?" said FireDragon. "What does smell mean?"

Now Flossie was puzzled.

"Don't you know?" she said. "It's one of the senses we're all supposed to have. You see things, don't you?"

"I certainly do," FireDragon said defensively. "My compound eyes have more than a thousand lenses."

"You obviously hear things."

"Yes, and if you're talking about sense, you're not making much of it."

"Do you feel things; hot and cold, wet and dry?"

"Of course."

"You taste things, don't you?" Flossie went on. "How do mosquitoes taste?"

"Boring," said FireDragon, "but what does this have to do with anything?"

"Those are four of the five senses: see, hear, touch, taste. Smell is the fifth one. It's what noses are for."

"I don't know anything about smelling. What's it good for?"

"It's another way to find out about things," said Flossie. "Flowers smell sweet; pickles smell sour."

"How does garlic smell?" FireDragon asked.

"Strong," said Columbine.

"Isn't that good?"

"Not exactly. It's like you had an invisible cloud of smoke and fire all around you."

"That's how it's supposed to be," FireDragon replied. "I'm a dragon, remember? To make mosquitos taste better, I eat onions, garlic, and chili peppers with them sometimes. Those things taste hot and make me feel like I'm breathing fire, just like a dragon."

"They make you smell like it, too," said Columbine.

"I still don't know what you mean."

"What she means," Flossie said, "is that onions and chili peppers smell strong and hot and fiery, too, just like they taste."

"This is interesting," said FireDragon. "Can you tell me more?"

"If you stop trying to chase us away, we will," said Columbine.

"Oh, I suppose," he said with a sigh. "I wasn't having much luck anyway."

"Then let's go ashore," said Flossie. "Having you buzzing those wings in front of my face makes me jittery."

They settled down on shore and tried to explain. Flossie described the smell of fish. Columbine told about the smell of daffodils. They talked about the smell of spring rain and chocolate cake. But try as they might, he didn't understand. It was like describing color to someone who had never seen, or music to someone who had never heard, to explain the ideas of sweet and sour or fresh and stale to someone who had never smelled. FireDragon grew impatient with their efforts. Flossie saw they needed to do something before he became a problem again.

"Let's go to the library," she said.

"What's that?" FireDragon asked.

"A place with lots of books," said Columbine. "We can look up smell in the dictionary or the encyclopedia and learn about it that way."

"Could you find dragonfly, too?"

"Sure," said Flossie, "let's go."

They flew at once to the library. Needlenose was there, seated at a table, looking through art books and books of Indian crafts. He often did this to gather ideas.

"Needlenose, I'd like you to meet Dragone Respira-Fuoco," Flossie said with a flourish. "His friends call him FireDragon."

"Howdy," said Needlenose. FireDragon, perched on one of the books, nodded.

"We came to read about dragonflies," Columbine said. "He wants to find out why he can't smell anything."

"I know just the book," Needlenose said. "It's one with lots of pictures." He shuffled across to a shelf, returned with an encyclopedia, and began to page through it. "Here you are," he said shortly, pointing to a drawing that looked much like FireDragon. They all crowded round. "Dragonflies are graceful, swift flying insects," Flossie read, "found mostly around ponds and streams."

"That's true," FireDragon said, trying his best to look important.

"It goes on about how you look," Flossie continued, "big eyes, body with shiny, metallic colors, six legs, and four wings; yup, that's you."

"Here's the part about living in the water," said Columbine, walking about on the page. "You spent about four years there before turning into a dragonfly."

"That's just what I told you," said FireDragon. "That book knows a lot about dragonflies."

"It says you're swift and agile in flight, and a skillful dodger," Flossie went on. "That's certainly true. Wow, listen to this: you can sometimes fly all day without landing! Almost the perfect flying machine, it says. That's impressive!"

"That's me," said FireDragon, fanning his wings and buzzing loudly about the library.

"Did you say you couldn't smell anything?" asked Needlenose when FireDragon returned.

"I guess that's true," said the dragonfly, "though I don't know exactly what that means."

"Well, here's your problem," Needlenose went on. "Insects smell with their antennae. According to this, you don't have any. You only have little bristles which apparently don't do the job."

"Does that mean no dragonfly can smell anything?" FireDragon asked, sounding a little sad.

"That's what I read here," said Needlenose.

"That doesn't help me find out what it means. Maybe I'll never find out."

"We could look up other things, like smell, and nose, and antennae," said Columbine. "Maybe that would help."

"Okay," said the dragonfly. His brazen, arrogant manner was gone now and he grew quiet.

They leafed through books for the next hour, reading and talking and explaining. Nothing seemed to make a difference, which isn't surprising, because if you've never smelled a flower or the breeze from a spring rain, you can't really understand what it's like.

"I have an idea," said Needlenose.

"What's that?" asked FireDragon.

"The only way you'll be able to understand smelling is to experience it. But you can't; you don't have antennae. So, why don't we try to make you some? If you wore something like antennae on your head, maybe you would smell things."

"How do we do that?" asked Flossie.

"I don't know," said Needlenose, "but if we go to my place, I'll bet we can figure something out."

They spent the rest of the afternoon upstairs at Haystack Hollow in Needlenose's craft room. The powerful odor from FireDragon made them dizzy at first, but Needlenose picked flowers and brought them inside to help freshen the air. They looked through books and tried ideas one after another.

"I know," Needlenose finally said, "let's make it like a TV antenna."

"Good thinking," said Flossie.

He fastened two pieces of thin, silver wire to a tiny square of wire mesh. He covered the mesh with soft cloth, shaped it to fit FireDragon's head, then added a bit of string to tie under his chin.

"Here, try this on," Needlenose said. "The idea is to get what's left of your real antennae, those little bristles, to stick through the cloth into the grid of wires. Maybe the two long wires will work like antennae and pick up smelles, then pass them down to the grid and on to you. It's worth a try, anyway."

Columbine helped FireDragon wiggle his head into the device, then fastened the string under his chin.

"Aaaaaarghhh," FireDragon gasped, choking and sputtering, "what's that?"

"What's what?" said Columbine.

"I don't know, but I can hardly breathe. It's like fire and smoke suddenly, all around my head."

"Garlic," Flossie and Columbine said at the same time. "See what we told you?"

"Let's continue this experiment outside," said Needlenose. They left the burrow to find the sun going down and long shadows creeping across the grass.

"Much better," said FireDragon, catching his breath. "Whew! So that's what a strong smell is like. But what's this?" He had flown and landed in a patch of clover. "It's like honey being poured on my head. Mmmm, this is nice."

"That's what a sweet smell is like," Columbine said. "Now

do you understand what we were telling you?"

"Oh, yes, this is wonderful," FireDragon said, and he plunged into a frenzy of discovery, flying from place to place and reporting his new sensations.

"The grass smells good," he said, "not sweet like the flowers, but sort of heavy and nice. The tree bark has a smell; kind of sharp, I think; and the moss growing on it has a different smell. Amazing! The green leaves have a smell, and the evening air has one, too. I bet everything has its own smell. Gee, this is really something!"

"Listen to our bully-boy now," Flossie said to Columbine. "Nothing but a marshmallow inside, don't you think?"

"Tee-hee," she replied. "He's just a snapdragon, after all."

They followed him around till well after dark, then off and on through the next several days. Each time they met him he was still reeling from exciting smells his antennae were bringing to him.

"This is super," he said one afternoon. "I never knew what I was missing."

"Do you still want us to leave your pond?" Flossie said.

"Oh, no," he said, "I want you to stay. You were nice to me even when I wasn't very nice to you. I want to be friends. In fact, I've been thinking that you and the Lovely Princess should have your own burrow like Needlenose. I'm sure there are plenty of places for one around here. Or maybe you'd like a nest in one of these trees. Why don't you think it over? You'd be very good neighbors."

"We wouldn't be intruding?"

"Not at all," said FireDragon. "The pond is big enough for all of us."

"Will you stop eating onions and garlic and chili peppers now that you know how they smell?" Columbine asked.

"No, I won't stop that. I'm still the Dragon with Breath of Fire, you know. The smell's not so bad a little at a time. I might even get to like it."

"Nobody's perfect, I suppose," the Princess sighed.

"Your antennae are still working well, I gather," said Needlenose.

"They are," the dragonfly said, "and they're going to make my life wonderful. Thank you for making them."

"You're welcome. I've never made anything quite like that before."

"You came up with just the right idea," FireDragon said, "but there is something slightly odd about them. Whenever I sit a certain way or in a certain place, I not only get smells, but I hear sounds, too."

"What kind of sounds?" Needlenose asked, puzzled.

"Music sounds, mostly, but talking sounds sometimes, too. Nothing I've ever heard before. Wait, I'm hearing some right now. . .do the words 'bases loaded and bottom of the ninth' mean something?"

"Oh, for goodness sake," Flossie said. "You built him a radio. He's picking up a baseball game."

"What's baseball?" asked FireDragon.

"Well, folks, back to the library," said Flossie. "This boy's education has just begun."

"You'll probably like baseball," said Needlenose.

"Why do you think that?"

"Well, the encyclopedia said you're a 'skillful dodger'."

"That's terrible, NeedleKnothead," squawked Flossie, "terrible, terrible, terrible!" and she chased him along the path, swatting him with her feathers as he laughed and laughed.

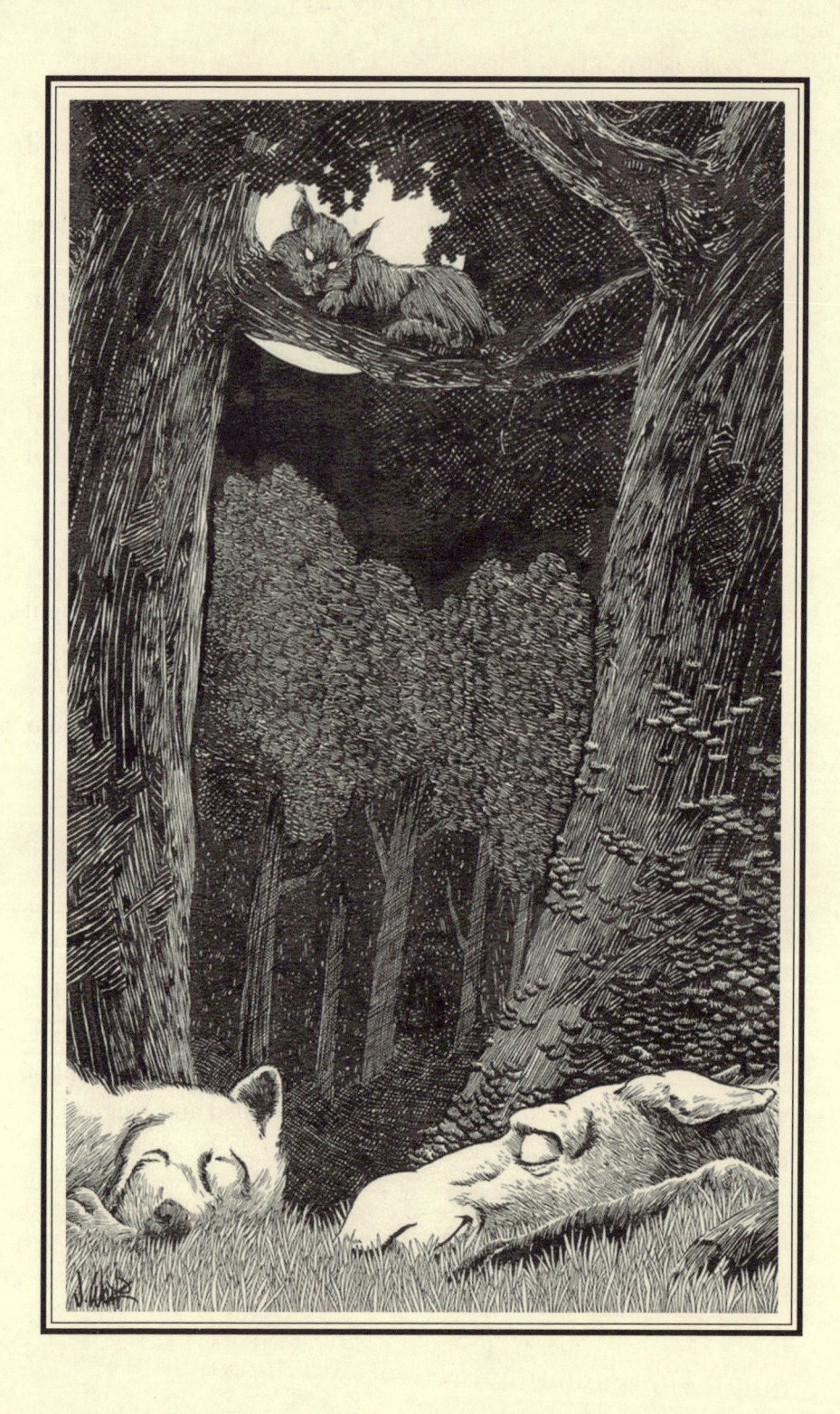

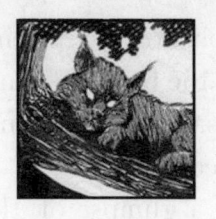

9

Eyes in the Forest
In which Manford and Veronica are followed

"Our garden is growing," said Veronica. "You can see it's going to make a picture."

"Yes," Manford said, "the sky looks blue, the clouds are turning white, and the mountains are already brown and red. Some of Golly's wildflowers are coming up, too."

They were standing where the trail to MorningGlory Mountain crossed the creek that flowed from Flossie's Pond. Flowers now grew where they'd planted them in bare dirt a month before—pansies, petunias, columbines, and morning glories, too.

"Your strawberries have blossoms," said Manford.

"Ooh, they'll be so good when they're ripe!" Veronica replied. "And my lettuce is coming along. The picture will be pretty when everything grows; maybe too pretty to eat!"

"I'd like to see it from up high like Golly does. It's too bad bears don't have wings."

"Or rotating antlers like my dad."

"A bear with helicopter antlers would be cool, or maybe jet engines. *Fooooom!* I could fly right over."

"You should probably stick to dancing."

"Maybe we can see the picture from Lookout Hill."

"Maybe," Manford said. "Let's go find out." They walked to the meadow and climbed Lookout Hill. Looking back through the trees, they caught a glimpse of the garden. "It's upside down," Veronica said. "MorningGlory Mountain is standing on its head."

"But you can tell what it is even from here. I think it's going to look nice."

"Me, too."

They stood on the hilltop and looked at everything around them. It was a pleasant morning in the middle of June, a morning that looked much like the picture in the garden soon would. The sky was bright blue. White clouds drifted past the mountains. Trees in the forest were now fully leafed out.

"What should we do?" Veronica asked.

"Let's go exploring," replied Manford.

"Exploring where? In the forest? In the mountains? Along the creeks?"

"Somewhere we haven't been. That's what exploring is, isn't it, going where you haven't been?"

"Uh huh," said Veronica.

"Where haven't we been?"

"Look around and see. We've been to MorningGlory and the mountains over there (Veronica pointed east), and to the meadow and pond near here (she pointed to the area around them). We've gone that way (Veronica pointed west) to Misty Falls and up to where Golly lives. There are plenty of other places we could go. Should we look at the map at the beginning of the book and see what they are?"

"Okay."

"Here we are on Lookout Hill," said Veronica, pointing to the map with a stick. "See where the trail comes up from the meadow?"

"Uh huh."

"And here's the trail past the garden that goes to MorningGlory Mountain."

"It sure doesn't look very far," Manford said. "It took us days to get there and back."

"It's a small map," said Veronica.

"What about this trail that says, 'To Mexico'? We haven't been on that."

"The sign at MorningGlory Crossing said it's 2,490 miles to Mexico, Manford. That's a little too much exploring for today, don't you think?"

"We wouldn't do all of it," Manford replied.

"No, I suppose not, but we could go the other way, 'To Canada.' That's only 148 miles."

"Okay, I'll tell my mom we'll be gone a few days and we can start right away."

"Wait a minute, wait a minute that was just an idea. Let's keep looking at the map; there might be something else."

"Like what?"

"Well, look. See what you see."

"There's Misty Falls where you live," said Manford, "and there's the trail down to my house. But Haystack Hollow isn't on here, and it doesn't say Flossie's Pond on the pond. Why is that?"

"This is the far away view. Those things are on the close-up on the next page."

"Oh."

"I have an idea," said Veronica. "See where the creek flows out of Flossie's Pond and down to another pond?"

"Yes, it goes to a road from there, my mom said."

"I think she's right. We don't want to explore roads, but we could follow the creek the other way. We've never done that."

"We've been to the store," said Manford.

"Sure, but the creek goes much farther than that," said

Veronica. "See, it goes right off the map."

"What do you suppose is up there?" Manford asked.

"I don't know, but we could find out. That's what exploring is—isn't that what you said?"

"Uh huh, but let's not just go for today; let's stay out till tomorrow."

"Okay," said Veronica, "and if we can, let's come back through the forest to Golly's place. That would be something new."

"Sounds great."

"Then get your things and tell your mom and we'll go."

"Should we ask the others to come along?" asked Manford.

"Not this time. Let's just the two of us go on this adventure."

Manford went home for his backpack and supplies and they were on their way a while later. They followed the creek north from where the path from Lookout Hill crossed it. They walked in the water or beside it on one bank or the other. They passed the store and the library—they could see them through the trees—then continued north through the forest. They were exploring, going where they had never been before.

The creek twisted and turned. The bank was level at times, other times it rose up as the land became hilly. They followed along it, sometimes climbing high into the woods above the water, then making their way back down.

"Does this creek have a name?" Manford asked.

"I've never heard of one," said Veronica, "and the map didn't say anything about it."

"Maybe we could give it one."

"Flossie probably should; it comes out of her pond."

"She hasn't even named that yet," said Manford. "We just call it Flossie's Pond."

"Oh, she'll get around to it."

The trees grew tall and close together. Sunlight brightened the tops of them but only reached the ground in streaks or patches. Manford and Veronica walked quietly. If you'd been following, sometimes you could see or hear them and others, they'd blend into the forest and disappear. Even the pink feather on Manford's hat would sometimes be hard to spot.

They entered a canyon after they'd gone about a mile and a half. The creek narrowed. The water ran deeper and faster. The creek banks rose sharply beside them, becoming too steep to walk along. They saw rocky cliffs overhead on either side.

"Looks like we go swimming," said Manford, and he charged into the stream. His feet touched bottom for a while as he forged against the current, then he had to paddle. Veronica came right behind, easily making her way through the swift water. They paddled and thrashed through the narrow passage, then waded ashore to a rocky beach. Veronica shook like a dog, sending water flying everywhere.

"Look," Manford said, pointing across the creek to the canyon wall a hundred feet above them, "there's something up there."

"You mean above that rock slide, that dark place?"

"Uh huh," Manford said, "I can't see it very well but I'll bet it's a cave. Let's go up there."

"Okay."

They crossed to the east side of the creek and began climbing. The way was steep and led over boulders and loose rock that shifted and slid. They climbed carefully, zigzagging through rocks and brush to find the best way.

Details of the cave became clear as they approached. The opening was large but the cave was not deep. Rock had apparently broken out of the canyon wall and smashed into pieces as it fell down the mountain, leaving behind a huge hole. It was nearing noon and much of the cave was still in shade. Veronica and Manford continued upward over the jumbled rocks and soon reached the entrance. They climbed up inside.

The floor slanted steeply uphill in a series of broken ledges. In places it was bare rock; in places shallow sand. Water dripped from the overhanging roof to make puddles and stains. The cave had never been lived in or even recently visited. There were no footprints except those of birds. The explorers looked about.

"No drawings on the walls," Veronica said.

"No old tools or pots," said Manford.

"No lost civilization here, I guess; just a cave."

They looked back the way they'd come. The creek flowed silently through the valley below, blue where it reflected the sky, white where it rushed over rocks, shining and glittery where struck by the sun. The canyon they were following stretched north and south into the distance, much farther than either of them could see.

Soon they climbed down the rocky slope and again headed up the creek, lunching along the bank as they went. Their course led them deeper into the canyon and to higher ground. The creek narrowed and widened, flowing swiftly and slowly accordingly. It rounded bends to the left and right. They followed through the twisting canyon wherever the water led.

"Have you noticed anything unusual?" said Veronica as they stopped to drink from a shallow pool.

"What kind of unusual?" asked Manford.

"Well, I don't exactly know, but I've had the strangest feeling for about the last hour that something is watching us."

"I haven't felt anything like that. What's it like?"

"Strange and creepy, like if you turned around quickly there would be something behind you or something looking at you from behind a tree or rock."

"Have you seen anything?"

"No, I haven't," said Veronica, "but I've looked a couple of times. It's probably nothing, but it really feels weird."

They went on and soon heard rushing water ahead where the canyon narrowed once again. Rounding a bend, they saw where the creek raced toward them down a long, rocky cascade. Water frothed and churned. The way grew steeper and they had to make their way carefully along the bank. The canyon walls closed in ahead of them and the creek became a waterfall of many levels. Water flowed through a cut a hundred feet above, fell noisily to a pool, then ran down a steep, rocky course and fell again. They stopped at the base of the falls.

"That's lovely," Manford said. "I like to watch water fall and splash and run down the rocks and then come all together and make a creek again at the bottom. It always seems to know where it's going."

"Just like us," said Veronica. "We know where we're going."

"Where?"

"Exploring."

"Right," said Manford. "So what do we do now?"

"We have to get to the top to keep following the creek."

"Then let's go back and find a way up. We surely can't climb here."

"Goodbye, waterfall," said Veronica. "Thanks for the show."

They backtracked to a place where the canyon was wider and not so straight up and down. Veronica led the way up the slope through a thick stand of trees. Manford followed, picking his way easily through the brush and rocks with his long legs. They climbed to a rocky cliff, crossed a ridge from there to a low spot in the canyon wall, then went on up to the crest. They walked atop the canyon wall, stopping and looking, taking in fuzzy, out-of-focus views of the cave they'd visited across the canyon and of MorningGlory Mountain rising far beyond.

Soon, they were at the top of the falls. Manford pushed leaves into the stream and watched them race off with the current and fall down, down, down till he lost sight of them in the rush of water below. Then they walked on, following the creek north once again. It was mid-afternoon.

The land around them became more hilly and forested. They walked through a jumble of humps, steep banks, and rocky knobs. They passed among large boulders and through areas of deep grass and tall flowers. Always, the creek led them deeper and deeper into the woods.

"Will we find this creek's source?" Manford asked.

"It's hard to say," said Veronica. "We might find the beginning, but it might go on for miles and miles."

Manford suddenly looked behind him.

"What's the matter?" asked Veronica.

"I thought I heard something," Manford said. "Did you hear anything?"

"No, what was it?"

"Footsteps crunching in the leaves, but only one or two."

"Maybe there *is* something back there," said Veronica.

"I'm starting to think so, too. It's real strange."

"I don't know why it has to hide. We're friendly. We wouldn't hurt anything."

"Let's keep looking and listening," Manford said. "Maybe we'll spot it."

They came to a fork in the creek a while later. Two smaller streams flowed together there, giving a choice of going left or right.

"Which way?" asked Manford.

"Left," said Veronica. "That will take us toward Morning-Glory Creek."

The left-branching stream led along the base of a tall peak. Soon it turned and led them into a narrow valley. The stream became narrower, shallower, slower moving. Leaves drifted lazily down it instead of rushing as they had farther back. The water was clear; the bottom was muddy.

The valley sloped gently uphill between peaks to either side. They followed along it. The creek became smaller and smaller. Then, as the land rose suddenly before them, they saw where the creek began—a small trickle of water bubbling out of the ground.

"Wow," said Manford, "this little dribble turns into Flossie's Pond? That's really something!"

"This one and others like it," said Veronica.

"Well, now we've explored to the source of the creek without a name, at least one source, anyway."

"You'll have to write about this in your journal."

"I plan to; I brought it along in my pack."

"It will be dark in a little while," Veronica said. "Let's go on around this hill and find a place to stop on the other side."

"Okay," said Manford.

"Tomorrow, we'll walk south through the forest. We'll find GloryView and go back home from there."

They climbed past the bubbling spring and continued their walk around the mountain. It was bigger than it first appeared, which is how things usually go when you're exploring, and it took them till early evening to find a pass around the far side to lead them south. The forest was thick and dark. Though the evening sky was still light, less and less light filtered through the dense leaves overhead. Manford and Veronica walked on in deepening shadows looking for a place to stop.

The light had nearly gone before they found a small, grassy opening in the trees. They chose places to sleep and settled down. Deep woods surrounded them and soon they could see nothing but the dim shapes of trees on all sides. The sky was black. The forest was black. They would rest until morning.

"What a great day!" Manford said. "We found a cave and looked around in it; we found a waterfall and climbed to the top of it; and we explored to a source of the creek. That's the kind of things I like to do."

"Me, too," said Veronica. "I'm not so sure I want be a dancing bear in the circus after all. I think I'd rather be an adventuring bear. Exploring is fun. Seeing what there is to see is fun. Maybe I'll keep doing that."

"Do you want to be my partner?" Manford asked. "Should we be explorers together and go see what we can see?"

"Oh, yes," said Veronica. "Friends and companions and adventurers together always; that's us."

They talked a while longer then gradually quieted down. The forest made night sounds around them; wind rustled in the trees; insects chirped and hummed and buzzed. It was too dark for Manford to write in his journal so he soon fell asleep. Veronica lay awake. There in the dark and the quiet she was having strange feelings again, feelings that they weren't alone.

"Manford," she whispered.

"Wha. . .what?" he said, waking up.

"There's something *watching* us; *I just know it.*"

Manford looked around but saw nothing in the dark.

"I feel it, too," he said. "I wonder what it is."

"I thought I heard footsteps in the leaves," Veronica said. "Maybe it was just a squirrel, but I don't think so."

"Should we take turns staying awake to watch?"

"No, I don't think it's anything that will hurt us. I'd just like to know what it is and why it's being so sneaky."

They watched a while longer then settled back down. Soon, Veronica was breathing evenly and snoring. Manford kept looking here, looking there, then finally laid down his head and closed his eyes. Almost instantly, they shot open again. He'd heard a noise, leaves faintly crunching in the woods somewhere to his left. He looked in that direction.

He saw eyes. Two yellow, unblinking eyes were watching him from the dark.

"Veronica," he whispered, *"Veronica, wake up!"*

"What is it?" she said, waking at once.

"*I saw it!* I saw it out there. There were eyes watching us—big eyes, far apart eyes—not some little chipmunk or squirrel."

"Where?"

"Over there," and Manford pointed but the eyes were gone.

"It must be moving around us," said Veronica. They looked around them but saw nothing.

"I know it was there," Manford said. "I wonder why it doesn't just say hello."

"WE KNOW YOU'RE WATCHING US, WHOEVER YOU ARE OUT THERE," Veronica said loudly. "EITHER GO AWAY OR COME OUT SO WE CAN SEE YOU."

There was no answer.

"WE WON'T HURT YOU," Veronica went on, "AND YOU CAN'T HURT US, EITHER. IT'S A MOOSE AND A BEAR YOU'RE DEALING WITH HERE. IT WOULD BE BETTER IF YOU JUST CAME OUT."

Still, they heard nothing. They watched the dark woods. They listened for sounds in the night. They waited for something more to happen, but nothing did. In time, they grew tired and fell asleep.

And the yellow eyes watched them. From a tree high above where Veronica and Manford slept, the yellow eyes watched, unblinking, through the night.

It was long past dawn when they awoke. They looked immediately into the woods on all sides but saw no sign that anything had been there. They started walking.

"How do we know we're going the right way?" asked Manford.

"We don't, really. We're just going this way because last night we came from that way."

"I guess if we're exploring and going where we've never been, then anywhere we haven't been is the right way."

"And anywhere we've already been is the wrong way," added Veronica.

"That sounds right," said Manford. And thus they walked on through the forest, following no trail or creek or map, but definitely going the right way because they'd never seen any of it before.

Now, if you really must know where they actually are, if you're the type who worries about these things, they're walking south through the woods between MorningGlory Creek and the creek where they began. Each creek flows through a canyon, so it'll be pretty hard for them to get lost. If they stray too far from side to side they'll eventually run into one creek or canyon or another, so don't be too concerned about it.

"I'm getting tired of this," Veronica said suddenly.

"Tired of what?" asked Manford.

"Whatever is following us; it's back there again."

"Then let's find out what it is."

"How?" asked Veronica.

"I have an idea. I'll show you when we come to the right spot."

They were walking in a forested valley between two hills. In time, they turned right and passed into a stand of dense trees that blocked the view from behind.

"Quick," Manford said, "hide in the trees and stay very still. I'll keep going. Maybe what's following us will pass you by." Veronica vanished in the trees. Manford kept walking and talking as if his partner were still close by.

Veronica waited as quietly as she could. Nothing happened for a long while. Then she heard a sound: cautious footsteps in the leaves. She looked back the way they'd come. There was something. . .something crouched behind a tree. It moved quickly to another tree, then another, making soft footsteps as it went. It came closer, closer, then passed near where Veronica lay hidden.

It was a cat, a large cat with gray and white fur, tufted ears, and huge paws. The tip of its tail was black. It continued in the direction Manford had gone. Veronica waited till it was almost out of sight, then followed.

Cat followed moose; bear followed cat. Manford made as much noise as he could and stayed where he might always be seen. The cat crept along, intent on what lay ahead. Veronica followed quietly, keeping the cat in sight, getting nearer and nearer.

Manford climbed to the top of a ridge and disappeared down the other side. The cat sped ahead, then suddenly stopped and looked around. It froze; Veronica was fifty feet behind.

"Hello," Veronica said. "Now, I'm following you."

The cat seemed about to spring and run when Manford appeared again at the top of the ridge.

"Hello," said Manford, and he and Veronica walked toward the cat from opposite directions. Soon, the three of them stood together. The cat looked at the ground and seemed very nervous and shy.

"What's your name?" asked Veronica in a friendly way. There was no answer for a while then the cat slowly lifted its head.

"Aurora," it said.

"You look like a cat," said Manford. "Are you?"

"I'm a lynx," it said.

"He's a lynx, Veronica. Is that a kind of cat?"

"She," said Aurora. "I'm a she, and yes, a lynx is a kind of cat. We're called bobcats sometimes."

"Why have you been following us?" asked Veronica.

"I wanted to see where you were going."

"We're exploring," said Manford.

"Yes, I heard you talking about it."

"I saw your eyes in the dark last night. Why didn't you come out when Veronica called?"

"I didn't want to," Aurora said. "I just wanted to watch. I'm not very sociable."

"Where do you live?" asked Veronica.

"Anywhere; I just go from place to place."

"Do you have any friends?"

"What's a friend?"

"Someone to be with and have fun with and go places with," said Manford.

"Someone to do things with and talk with about things," said Veronica. "Manford and I are friends, and we have lots of other friends in MorningGlory Forest."

"No, I don't know anybody like that. I'm just me. That's all there is."

"We could be your friends," said Manford.

"You could?"

"Uh huh."

"Why?"

"Because friends are nice to have," said Veronica.

"What other friends do you have?" asked Aurora.

"Oh, lots," said Manford. "Right now, we're going to Golly's house; he's our friend. He's an eagle."

"And there's Needlenose, the porcupine," said Veronica, "and a monarch butterfly named Princess Columbine."

"Butterflies are pretty," said Aurora.

"She'd like to hear you say that," said Manford. "We also have Flossie for a friend. She's a pink flamingo."

"What's that?"

"A big pink bird."

"I've never seen one of those."

"Don't forget Ssam," said Veronica. "He's a garter snake."

"I don't like snakes."

"Everybody says that, but I'm sure you'd like Ssam. He's very smart."

"We live where there's a pond and a meadow," said Manford,

"and lots of forest and a really big mountain."

"That sounds nice," Aurora said.

"And we have a garden," said Veronica.

"What's that?"

"A place where you grow flowers or things to eat," Manford said. "Ours will make a picture when it grows."

"Of what?"

"Of where we live," said Veronica.

"I think I'd like to see that."

"Why don't you come back with us?" said Manford. "You could see where we live and meet our friends."

"I don't know if I could," said Aurora.

"Why not?"

"I told you; I'm not very sociable. I wouldn't know what to say."

"No problem," said Veronica. "With seven of us talking, you'll hardly need to say anything. But if it doesn't work out, you can come back here. We'll let you be."

"You promise?"

"Yes, we promise," said Manford, "and friends always keep promises."

They walked south through the forest all morning and afternoon. Aurora said little but kept pace as they passed through wooded valleys, along sloping ridges, across grassy clearings. They strayed west from their course and came to MorningGlory Creek. After walking along it for a time, they followed a ridge back to where they thought GloryView to be.

"What are we looking for?" asked Aurora.

"A house in a tree," said Veronica. "It'll be hard to spot until we're almost upon it because of these woods."

"I'll take a look," Aurora said, and she climbed to the top of a tree.

"Is that how you watched us last night?" Manford asked. "I saw you once on the ground but never thought to look up in the trees."

"Yes," said Aurora, "I stayed watching almost till morning. Climbing is easy for me."

"What do you see?" asked Veronica.

"There are trees out here, but I don't see any with houses."

"It's down in the branches. You probably still won't be able to see it."

"Way over there (Aurora pointed southeast) I see some kind of box in the top of a tree. Is that what we're looking for?"

"It's Golly's lookout," said Manford. "His house is nearby."

"Looks like we're almost there," said Veronica. "Are you ready to meet our Golly eagle?"

Aurora was quiet for some time. She seemed to be thinking, perhaps wondering if she really wanted to go on.

"I guess so," she finally said. "I guess I'd like to see what having friends is all about."

So Manford and Veronica headed southeast toward GloryView, toward Misty Falls, Flossie's Pond, and MorningGlory Mountain. Their shy new friend followed quietly behind.

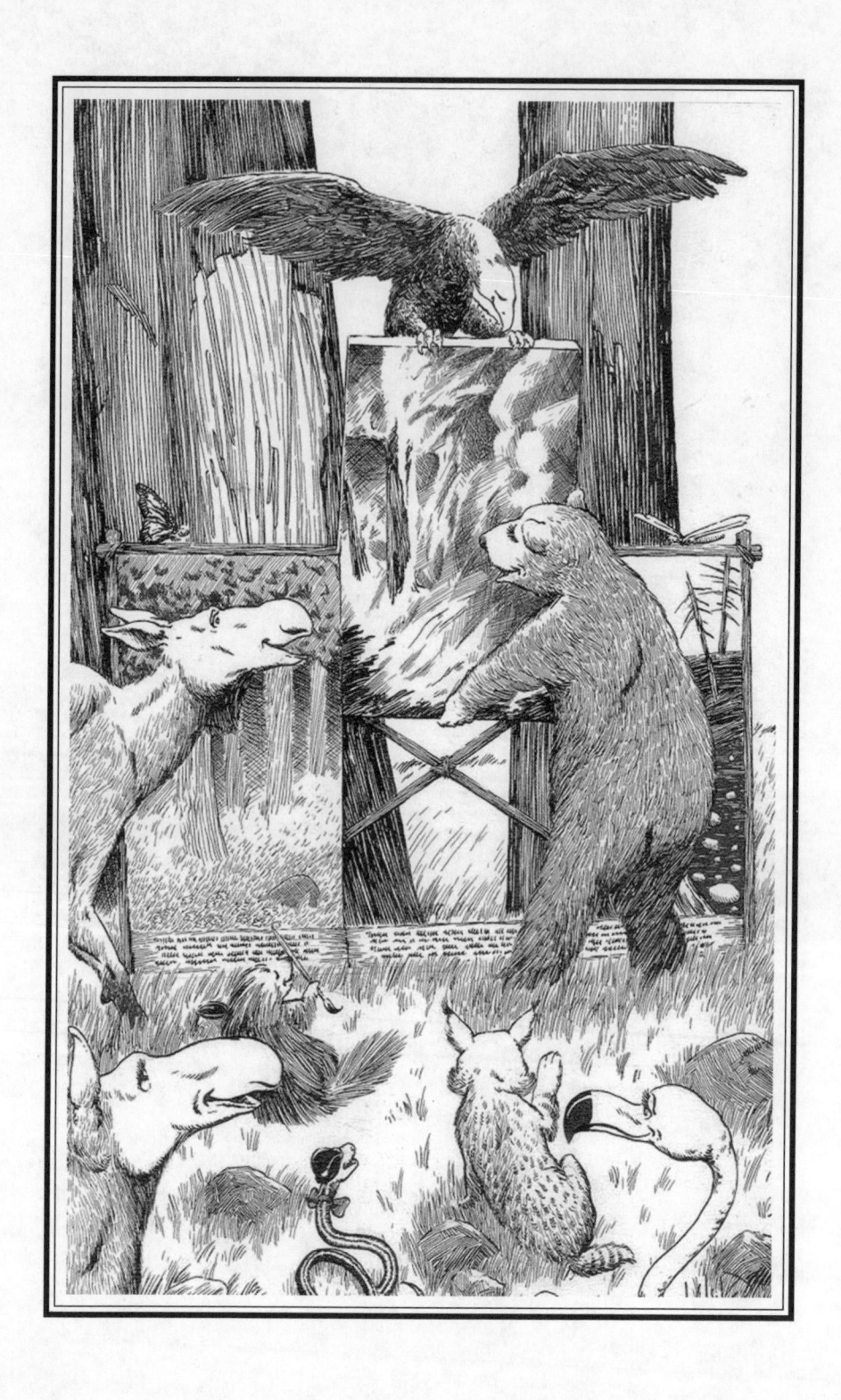

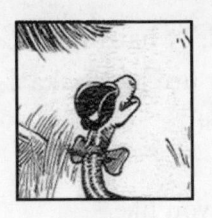

10

Good Neighbors, Unite!
In which Needlenose brings life to art

Manford watched the rain from his bedroom window. Straight down it fell, pattering quietly on the roof, making soft, overlapping circles in puddles in the yard. It had been doing this for hours.

He'd gone walking in it, ambling through the forest and along the creeks, feeling water fall gently on his head and run down his back, letting it drip from his nose. He'd gotten soaked, as wet as if he'd been swimming in the pond. Manford enjoyed the rain. He walked in it often. He thought it felt good.

Now it was evening and he was dry once again. Still, he watched and listened as the sky grew dark. Rain was such a magical thing, helping the forest grow, washing dust off the leaves, keeping the creeks and ponds full. Manford liked to watch it do its work.

"Manford." That was his mother calling. She was probably in the living room reading the Sunday paper. He went to see.

"What, Mom?"

"Did you see this story about the fire?" Mary Moose was settled on the floor with the paper spread before her.

"No," said Manford, "what fire?"

"There was a forest fire in Alaska a couple weeks ago. This is the first I've heard of it."

"What happened?"

"You can read it if you like."

"Oh, read it to me," Manford said. "I like it when you do that."

"Okay," said Mary. She adjusted her glasses and began to read:

FOREST QUIET AFTER FIRE

TETLIN JUNCTION, Alaska - Two weeks ago these hills were burning. Flames a hundred feet high roared through this forest, reducing dry stands of spruce to blackened stumps. Pushed by high winds, fire raced down one hillside and up the next, burning with such heat that trees exploded into flame before it.

Columns of gray and white smoke rose thousands of feet in the air. Flames burned in bright yellows, fierce oranges and reds, and through swirling smoke, sometimes seemed edged in green. The fire jumped creeks and roads and raced through a campground, devouring heavy picnic tables like kindling. It snapped and crackled angrily as it raged through the woods with a rumbling roar. People and animals alike fled before it.

Firefighters pumped water from ponds and streams, dropped water and retardants from helicopters and planes. They cleared wide firebreaks with shovels and bulldozers and lit backfires to stop advancing flames. A hundred and fifty square miles of forest burned in a matter of days. And the fire continued, shifting one way then another in the path of the wind.

Then it rained—soft, gentle, soaking rain. The fire slowed, then stopped. Smoke hung over the area for days like a blanket hiding the damage done.

It is quiet here now. What once was thick, shady forest now is open meadow. The smell of charred grass and wood is ever-present. But the smoke has cleared; the sun is shining.

The fire didn't leave total ruin. There are hopscotch patterns in the grass where flames suddenly turned or skipped ahead, leaving patches still growing. Some clumps of trees were missed completely or only lightly singed and are still green.

Life is already returning. Shoots of green among the blackened stubble are an inch high. Mice and squirrels dash about. Birds land in the skeletal branches of trees still standing. Fireweed will grow by August and spread throughout the area next summer. Always first after a fire, the tall, showy flowers will turn these burned woods reddish-violet.

Ashes will enrich the soil. Unburned tree roots will send up new shoots. Willows and aspen will soon grow, bringing moose to browse where they found nothing to eat before. Cones from some conifers release seeds only in a fire. Winds and birds will scatter them and the forest will grow once again.

Fire destroys. Fire brings life. The cycle has repeated for millions of years.

"Lots of fancy words," said Manford.
"Newspapers can be a little grand at times," Mary said.
"What's a backfire?"
"Firefighters light a new fire and keep it burning toward the main fire. When the two come together, there's nothing to burn on either side so the fire goes out."
"I see," Manford said, "and a conifer, what's that?"
"A tree that grows cones like a pine or hemlock."
"And the cones have seeds in them to grow new trees."
"That's right," said Mary.
"What did the story mean about fire destroying and fire bringing life?"
"When trees are tall and close together, they're the only thing that grows. They use up all the moisture and not much

sunlight reaches the ground through their branches. When fire destroys the trees, the forest becomes a meadow. Sun shines on it. Rain falls on it. Soon, life returns. Grass, small plants, and trees grow again. Before long, animals can hunt and graze where there was nothing much to eat before."

"So fire isn't a bad thing?" Manford asked.

"Fires set through carelessness are always unfortunate," Mary said. "They cause much needless destruction. But fire itself isn't good or bad. It's part of what happens, like day and night, winter and summer."

"But it's not good when fire hurts animals or people."

"No, it isn't, just like it isn't good to be cold in the winter or lost on a dark, rainy night. But rain happens, and winter happens, and forest fires happen. When they do, some things end and new things begin. It's the way the world works."

"I see," Manford said, "spring starts over after winter, and the forest starts over after a fire."

"That's exactly right," Mary said.

"What about our relatives and friends in Alaska? Do you suppose they're okay?"

"I was just thinking about them," Mary went on. "I'd better call them right away."

Manford listened to his mother's part of several conversations and tried to fill in the missing lines. After *"Oh, that's too bad,"* and *"Was anyone hurt?"* and *"I'm sorry to hear that,"* about three times each, he was getting worried.

"What's going on, Mom?" he asked when she finally put down the phone. "Who have you been talking to?"

"I called my friends, the moose guides, at least those I could find. Most of them were out on trips. The fire burned a big area, they said, but only came near a few moose we know; three of the guides, one of my older brothers, and two of your dad's sisters.

"Are they okay?"

"They escaped the fire but the places they lived were burned. They'll have to go somewhere else."

"Did they live in houses like us?"

"Bucky's sisters did," said Mary. "He found a nice place for them but it's gone now."

"Oh, that's sad."

"Yes, and they're getting rather old and set in their ways. Going to a strange area will be hard for them."

"Is someone helping them?" Manford asked.

"Of course. We always help each other when it's needed, don't we? But the fire isn't their only problem, it turns out. Alaska had a hard winter this year. Snow was deep and temperatures were extremely cold. Moose and other winter animals had trouble getting food. My guides organized help for those who were doing poorly but by spring, reserves were low. The fire made things even worse. They'll need a good summer guiding tourists just to get everyone back on their feet."

"We should help, too," said Manford.

"We should," his mother replied, "but I'm not sure what to do."

"You could send them money."

"Yes, I could. We have plenty to help family and friends."

"So, why don't you?"

"I will, but I don't think that's enough. I'd also like to do something that helps in a different way."

"How?"

"I don't know," Mary said.

"We could go there ourselves and help out."

"I thought of that, but it isn't the answer. My guides are smart enough to handle things."

"You said they were busy," observed Manford.

"That's true, but we're still better off staying here."

"Doing what?"

"Something to call attention to the problem and get others

to help. If we get a hundred others involved, that's better than if we worked alone."

"Uh huh, but how do we do that?"

"I don't know," Mary said.

"Neither do I," said Manford. They were silent for a time as they thought about what to do but had no great ideas.

"Keep working on it," Mary said. "Maybe we'll find a way to be really useful."

Manford lay in his bed that night thinking. *'Maybe we should invite them here. There's plenty of room in MorningGlory Forest. They'd surely be happy.'* He thought about it some more. *'Hmmm... it would be a long trip for moose that are getting old. Maybe not. What else?*

'I could tell their story for the newspaper. Headline: Moose Homeless After Fire. *That might get others to help. But...what is their story? I would have to find out. I would have to talk to them or go there and see. That would be fun. I wonder...'*

Manford's thoughts drifted. *'Fire in MorningGlory Forest... miles of lovely woodland, all gone up in smoke. That would be sad— Golly's house, Haystack Hollow, Moostery Manor—gone. How awful!'* Manford frowned. *'I should think about something else,'* he decided. Soon he fell asleep.

Not much later, the light snapped on in the hall and Manford's mother came into his room.

"Manford, I've got it," she said excitedly. "I've figured it out."

"Mmmm," Manford said, waking up. "Wh-what? Figured what out?"

"How to help up north."

"How?"

"There's an art contest."

"A what?" Manford asked. He looked puzzled.

"I read about it in the paper after you'd gone to bed," Mary said. "It's a contest with categories for different kinds of crafts. We could enter it."

"Um. . .I don't get it," said Manford.

"If we made something that told about the fire, perhaps we could draw attention to it and get help."

"Are we artists?"

"Well, no, but we could give it a try."

"Uh huh."

"We might even win prizes," Mary said.

"Maybe so, Mom," said Manford.

"You don't sound convinced."

"I think I'm just sleepy."

"That's okay, dear. I'm sorry I woke you. We'll talk about it more in the morning."

But Mary was already gone in the morning, off to visit the neighborhood. Manford found his breakfast on the table. Alongside it was a printed note that said: Come to the meadow.

Finding no one in WhiteFlower Meadow, he settled down to wait under the tree. Soon his friends began arriving—Flossie, Columbine, Needlenose and Ssam, then Golly and Veronica, too. Mary got there last.

"I asked Aurora to come," she said, "but she thought she'd stay in the woods today."

"She's very shy," said Manford.

"Why did you want to see us?" Princess Columbine asked.

"I want to tell you about a problem, and about an idea I have to help solve it. I'm hoping you'll want to help, too. First, listen to this." Mary held up the article from the paper and read it to them.

"I saw that story," Golly said when she'd finished. "I wondered if you might have family or friends there."

"We do," Mary said, "and I called some of them. No one got hurt, they tell me."

"That's good to know," Golly said.

"But some lost their homes," Mary went on. "They'll have to find something new and I'd like us to help them."

"How do we do that?" asked Needlenose.

"I think she's going to tell us," said Veronica.

"Yes, I am," Mary said. "I read about an art contest in the paper. It has many categories and, of course, prizes. Each of us could create an art work and enter it."

"I still don't get it, Mom," Manford said.

"Our art would tell a story about forest fire, about its causes and results, like what was said in the article. We'd tell about our friends' situation as part of it and perhaps draw attention to their problem. We might get others to help them, and we could win some prizes."

"It's a plausible idea," said Golly.

"I see what you mean now," Manford said.

"Excuse me, Mary," said Flossie. "You're thinking big here, which is fine, but I'm confused. How will a bunch of animals who don't know the first thing about art suddenly create something so wonderful it wins prizes?"

"Now just a minute," said Needlenose. "I happen to know quite a bit about art and I'd like to enter."

"He made Manford's necklace, remember?" said Ssam.

"He also drew the picture we planted in the garden," said Manford.

"A thousand pardons, good sir," Flossie said with a penitent bow and a sweep of her wing. "I'll begin again; we have one artist, and an excellent one, to be sure. What are the rest of us going to do?"

"I wouldn't know where to start," said Veronica, "unless there's a category for dancing."

"No, there isn't," said Mary. "That's a performing art."

They heard a raspy buzzing just then and FireDragon, their dragonfly friend, circled 'round and 'round and landed on Flossie's head.

"What's this, a secret meeting?" he asked.

"No, join us," said Mary.

"I thought you never left the pond," said Columbine.

"I do when there's something interesting going on. So what's going on?"

Mary explained what they'd been talking about. By the time she finished, FireDragon was sputtering and fanning his wings.

"You're going to do art works about fire," he said, "and you didn't invite me? Fire isn't just my middle name, it's my whole name. It's what I'm all about! I want to be in this, too."

"Don't be so touchy," said Flossie, "or I'll start calling you Dragon Breath again."

"Sorry, Ms. Flossie," FireDragon said, trying to be nice, "but I want to be part of this, if it's okay."

"Certainly," Mary said with a smile, "you can be part of whatever we do."

"So, what are we going to do?" asked Veronica.

"I suppose we should talk about that," answered Mary.

"I could write a story," said Manford.

"Let's see," Mary looked through the contest information. "Hmmm, there's no category for stories," she said.

"Writing isn't art?"

"Writing is *literature*, Manford," Golly said.

"Picky, picky."

"Since Needlenose is our artist, maybe he has an idea of what to do," said Columbine.

"Possibly," said Needlenose. "If we want to attract attention, it seems to me we should make something big. To make something big, we should all work on one thing rather than each doing something on his or her own." The others nodded.

"Okay," Mary said, "that sounds good."

"What kind of thing?" asked Golly.

"I'm not that far yet," Needlenose replied.

"How about a rug or wall hanging," suggested Flossie. "I've

seen some with pictures woven into them that tell stories."

"That might work," Mary said. "Do you know how to do that?"

"No."

"I do," said Needlenose. "It's not terribly difficult. . . ." He suddenly left off talking. His mind was thinking, churning, whirring. His eyes began to brighten. He seemed to be watching something far away. When he spoke again, it was to nobody in particular.

"We could work on it together," he said. "We'd make it fifteen feet long, maybe four feet high." He paused. "It would be a weaving showing a forest of green trees on the left side, fire burning and smoking in the center, and a meadow on the right—black and burned near the fire, slowly turning to grass, flowers, and small trees on the far edge. It would hang on a wall or a frame."

"Yes, I see it," Mary said. "It sounds right."

"I like it, too," said Ssam. "What parts will each of us do?"

"I'm still thinking," said Needlenose.

"While you're thinking, here's another idea," said Columbine. "You want to tell a story about animals as much as fire, don't you?"

"Yes," said Mary.

"Well, we're the animals. If we're part of the story, we should be part of the art. If I landed in the meadow on this weaving, I'd look like a butterfly on a flower. But I'd be real and moving. I'd give your art life.

"I'm also orange and black, sort of like fire. If I landed on that part and moved my wings, I'd make the fire look like it was burning."

"Splendid idea," Mary said.

"I can be in it, too," said FireDragon. "Put a pond in the picture and I'll be its dragonfly."

"Since you're such a great flier," said Veronica, "why don't you be a helicopter dropping water on the fire?"

"We fire-breathing dragons start fires, we don't put them out."

"Force yourself," said Flossie. "You're working on a new image, remember?"

"I was just kidding," FireDragon said. "Sure, I'll be the helicopter."

"This is really coming together," said Mary.

"You still need a story to explain things," Manford said. "Maybe something short that's lettered at the bottom of each part of the picture."

"I agree," said Ssam, "and having a narrator would be good, too. I'll trade my bowler and bow tie for a ranger hat and green neckerchief and be part of the art, too. I'll tell the story to everyone who comes by. We'll be living, talking art."

"That sounds wonderful," said Mary.

"Veronica, what will you do?" asked Columbine.

"I just figured that out. Needlenose said this could hang on a frame, didn't he? Well, I can build that. I'll get poles and tie them together; it shouldn't be hard."

"I think we have it," Mary said. "But Golly, we haven't heard anything from you."

"It's an excellent plan," Golly said, "but I suggest we do this weaving in three pieces instead of one. The left panel will be the forest, four feet high and five feet wide as Needlenose said. Flossie can do that one. I'll do the middle panel that shows the forest on fire. Needlenose, if you do the panel on the right, Flossie and I can learn what to do by watching you."

"It's a deal," said Needlenose. "We'll start by drawing pictures to work from so the panels match when we put them together."

"What can I do?" said a new voice. They looked around and saw Aurora sitting quietly in the grass. They'd been so intent on their project, they hadn't heard her approach.

"Hello, Aurora," said Manford. "Gee, what can she do, folks?"

"Rocks," said Veronica, "she can find rocks."

"What for?" Aurora asked.

"When we hang this work of art upright on the frame, the bottom six inches or so will have to lay flat on some kind of shelf. That's where Ssam will be, moving back and forth to tell the story. Since the flat piece will still be part of the picture, Aurora can find rocks to blend in with it. Rocks for a stream or the pond, maybe; rocks that might be boulders in the forest."

"Oh, this is going to be fabulous," said Mary. "You sure can be a creative bunch when you get ideas going."

"What are you going to do, Mom?" Manford asked.

"Make arrangements, buy materials, and work out problems. Are there any that come to mind?"

"When does this have to be finished?" asked Flossie.

"In less than two weeks," Mary said. "We should probably get moving."

Later at Haystack Hollow, Flossie and Golly perched near the studio table as Needlenose drew. He sketched quickly with colored chalk and soon the picture he'd imagined began to emerge. He'd completed all three drawings by evening and the next day drew them again, full size, for the scenes that would be woven on four-by-five foot backing sheets.

He demonstrated weaving for Flossie and Golly. It wasn't like making flat cloth, he said. They had to bunch up the fabric so it stood out to give the picture texture and depth. Golly nodded that he understood. Flossie wanted to work with Needlenose in case she needed help.

Mary shopped. Armed with lists, she scoured local stores and had basketloads of supplies delivered to Moostery Manor where they would build their creation. No other indoor place was big enough.

Veronica roamed the woods looking for downed trees the proper size. As she found each one, she stripped off its branches and added it to a growing pile. Aurora tagged along picking small rocks out of streams. She gathered a colorful collection in the course of a few days.

Flossie and Needlenose started work on their weavings in Manford's living room. They sorted materials by color, laid out their backing sheets, and began. Needlenose made swift progress, the picture of what he wanted still vivid in his mind. Flossie watched, partly in fascination, partly hoping she would soon see the picture, too.

Manford sat in the kitchen trying to write. He'd saved the newspaper story and had read it again and again. Anything he wrote sounded just like it. Soon he found himself staring at the kitchen wall, writing nothing.

"This is hard," he said to his mother.

"Go to the library," she said. "There are lots more materials there to help you." Manford did, glad for a change of scene.

For some reason, Golly preferred to work at home. There was enough room there, he said, and he liked being alone to think. He carried his drawing and supplies to GloryView and stayed. Asked how he was doing the few times others saw him, he always replied, "Just fine."

Work continued for a week. Flossie finally began her own weaving and stuck to it most of each day, doing small parts, then ripping them out and starting over.

"They don't look like trees," she kept saying. "This is supposed to be a forest. It looks like a bunch of bushes on stilts."

"It's getting better," Columbine said to encourage her. "It's starting to look really good."

Needlenose, meanwhile, was nearly finished. His weaving of the blackened area slowly turning green and sprouting new grass and trees was lovely. He'd added colored beads for new flowers and some of his quills as downed trees. If the other two pieces turned out as good as his, the whole work would be a winner.

"I wonder how Golly's doing," Flossie said one day.

"He has the drawing and the material we selected," Needlenose said. "He should be doing fine."

"He didn't ask many questions. I hope he gets it right and not backwards or something."

"He's too smart a bird for that," said Needlenose.

"You're right, I suppose," said Flossie.

"Do you really worry about things like that, Flossie?" Mary asked. "It never crossed my mind."

"Maybe I'm bothered that we haven't heard from him. It just seems odd. Where do we have to take this when it's finished, by the way?"

"To an art gallery on the coast," Mary said.

"How do we do that?"

"I've arranged for a truck to pick it up down the trail at the road crossing."

"That should be interesting," said Needlenose.

Manford was back at the kitchen table. He'd looked through books at the library and found more material. He'd made notes on cards, sorted them into order, and again was trying to write. But he was still staring at the kitchen wall. Writing something that sounded right just wasn't that easy. The wastebasket overflowed with crumpled paper. Wanting to be useful, Ssam offered to help.

Needlenose made a silver outfit for FireDragon, stenciling black numbers on it so he'd look like a helicopter. He added a dangling line with a bucket whose bottom could be opened. FireDragon would trail it behind him to put out the fire.

Veronica built the frame in the front yard, lashing poles at the junctions with strips of bark. She hung Needlenose's finished piece from it, patted the bottom six inches of it flat on the shelf she'd installed, then adjusted everything to fit. A third of the work was complete.

The deadline approached. Manford and Ssam finished two of the descriptions they were writing and started working on the last. Flossie finally got the drift of what she was doing and made good progress. She'd be finished in a day, it appeared, just when the work had to be carried to the road.

No one had seen Golly in days. He was at home, they knew that, and he was busy, too. Flossie had flown by to check. How he was doing on his weaving, nobody knew. He kept news of it entirely to himself. Flossie finally flew to his door and knocked.

"We have to take everything to the truck tomorrow," she told him when he answered.

"I'll be there," he said.

"You're sure."

"Don't worry, I'll be ready."

They assembled their creation in the yard the next morning. The day was cloudy, one that would surely bring rain by afternoon.

Flossie admired her finished panel hanging on the frame. Dark tree trunks rose into bursts of rich, textured leaves that seemed ready to enfold the viewer. It was a forest that looked deep and mysterious, like you could walk into it and disappear. Flossie was pleased.

"At last, it looks like woods," she said.

"What are you going to call this great work?" asked Columbine.

"I think it should be Forest Fire Trilogy," Needlenose said.

"That's not very exciting," said Veronica.

"I know, but you have to understate these things. Calling it Rising From Its Ashes or some such thing would be overdoing it."

Manford and Ssam finished their compositions then Needlenose lettered them carefully on three narrow boards. He nailed the first to the front of the flat shelf under Flossie's weaving of the forest, then stood back to read it:

> This forest took hundreds of years to grow. It offers shade and protection for animals, and homes for birds. Its leafy canopy renews the air. Fires caused by lightning or carelessness can destroy it in a matter of hours.

He nailed the second board next to it where Golly's weaving of the fire would go.

> Where there are no breaks in the forest to stop fire, such as rivers or roads, firefighters dig them. They pump water from ponds, drop chemicals and water from the air. The most effective firefighting tool is rain.

Needlenose's work, already in place, had a creek running through the blackened meadow into a pond. Aurora put stones from her collection in place; real rocks for the stream to flow through, and real boulders to lie among the trees. Needlenose nailed the third lettered board below it.

> The forest is gone but its charred ruins are not dead. Sun shines here now and rain falls. Grass will grow soon, then flowers, then trees once again. Animals will come to feed. In time, the forest will return.

"Your descriptions are great," said Needlenose. "They don't sound like they were hard to write."

"Ssam made it seem so easy," said Manford.

They finished everything by noon. Everything except for the four-by-five foot hole in the center where, they fervently hoped, Golly's part would fit. The work would be meaningless without it. Golly knew what he was doing, they kept telling themselves, but it would be nice to know for sure.

FireDragon was the first to see him.

"There he is," he said, and he buzzed into the sky toward the eagle circling carefully overhead. Golly was carrying something wrapped in brown paper. He circled low and settled it slowly to the ground, leaning it against the wooden frame.

"Welcome," Mary said, "you're just in time."

"Do we get to unwrap it?" asked Flossie.

"Of course," said Golly with a confident smile. "Mary, this was your project, why don't you do it?"

"All right," she said. Mary pried the paper loose at a corner then tore it away. She caught her breath and stepped back.

It wasn't a weaving at all.

It was a brilliant watercolor painting.

Flames of angry reds, oranges, and yellows leaped from the forest as if the painting itself were on fire. White and gray smoke clouds swirled along the ground and rose to tower in the sky. Trees in the path of the fire seemed to cower and wither before it. Some of them already blazed like torches. The colors were lustrous and intense, dazzling and alive, as if one were watching the actual scene.

"Totally awesome," said Needlenose, looking on in obvious wonder.

"Magnificent," said Flossie.

"It's fantastic," Mary said. They set it between the left and right panels. "Golly, it's absolutely beautiful, and it fits perfectly with the others. You never told us you were a painter."

"Yes," Golly replied, "I guess I've been keeping a little secret."

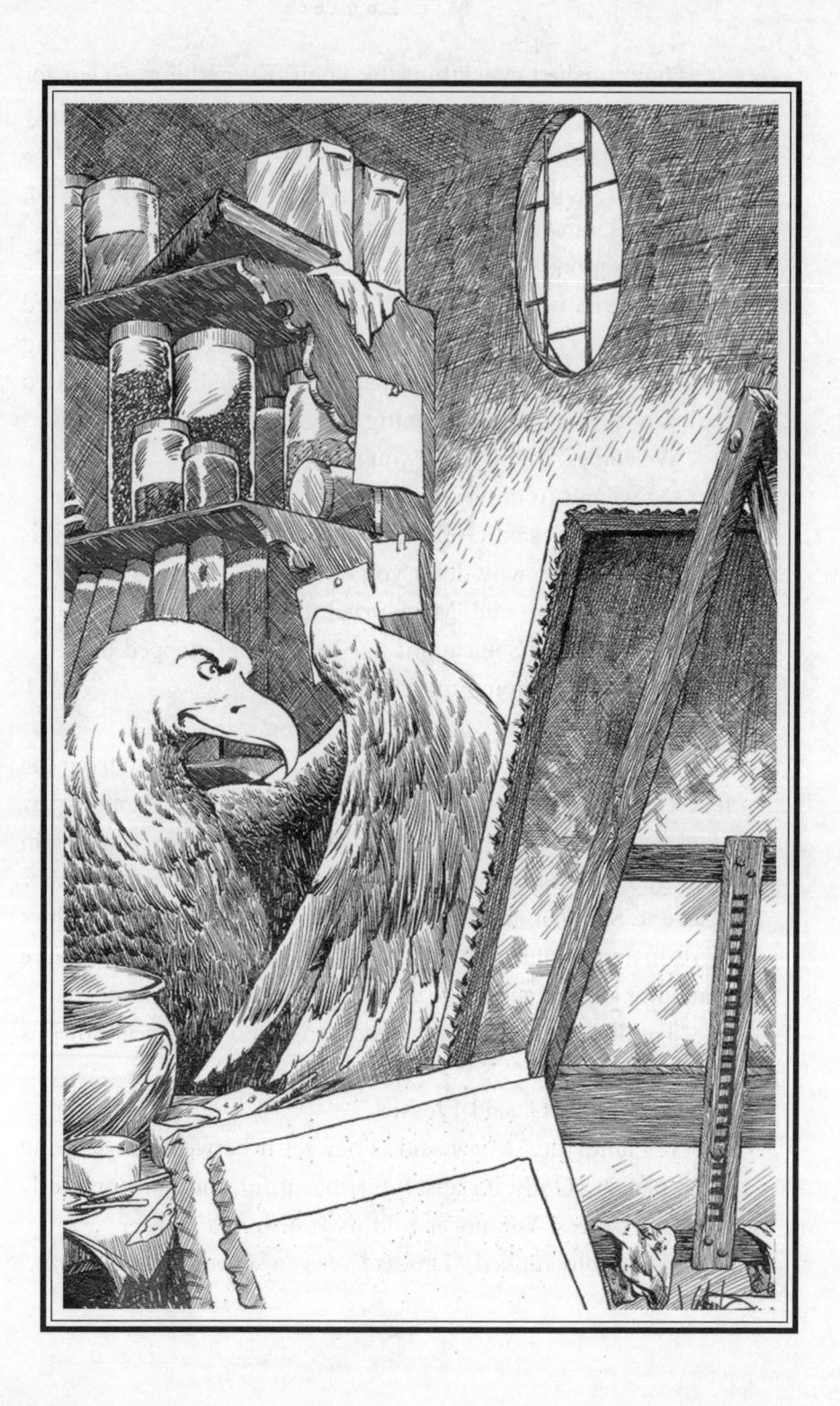

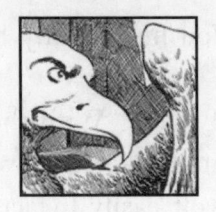

11

Secrets Revealed
In which we find something unexpected in Golly's closet

"How long have you been painting?" asked Needlenose.

"Years," replied Golly. "I have quite a collection."

"And you never mentioned it?"

"No."

"Why not?" asked Columbine.

"It's just for my own enjoyment. I didn't want to make a big fuss."

"But this is so good, and so professional," Mary said. "Didn't you want to hear others say so?"

"I'm pleased that you like it," Golly said, "but since it was just for me, I didn't need to show it. I guess I've enjoyed keeping it a secret."

"GloryView isn't that big," said Ssam. "You must have art from floor to ceiling *everywhere* if you've been painting so long."

"No, I burned the old ones. I have thirty or so of my better works hanging up or stored in the study."

"How do you paint?" asked Needlenose. "These don't look like regular brush strokes."

"I use my wing feathers. It's very convenient."

Flossie laughed. "You must really be a sight sometimes," she said.

"You're right," Golly said. "With the tip of each feather a different color, I look rather like a lady who's been painting her fingernails. But it comes off easily. In fact, when it rains, I simply sit outside and spread my wings to wash the paint off."

"Do you paint only watercolors?" asked Mary.

"I do only this style," Golly said, "but it isn't exactly watercolor."

"What is it?" Veronica asked.

"It's more like a dye. I make the paints from plants, you see."

"You make them?" said Columbine.

"Yes, very much like the Indians do. Different plants make different colors."

"What plants do you use?"

"Oh, dozens. Remember back in Chapter 3 when I planted wildflowers in our garden?"

"Yes," Manford said.

"Well, I didn't pick them just because they looked nice. There was a reason I didn't mention at the time why I chose each one I planted."

"Wasn't one of them scarlet bugler?" asked Flossie.

"Yes," said Golly, "I get pink dye from that."

"But its flowers are red."

"True, but when you boil them, the dye comes out pink."

"Did you use pink in this painting?" asked Ssam, arching his head high and scanning the angry flames.

"Only to lighten the red. Red comes from Indian paintbrush. Since it's very dark, I had to mix it."

"What other plants did you use in this painting?" asked FireDragon, hovering before it.

"I made green for trees in the path of the fire from red onion skin. That's actually purple but it makes a green dye. The dark, grayish brown for the tree trunks came from juniper berries, and the patches of light brown came from Brigham tea."

"How did you get such color in the flames?" asked Ssam.

"There are many colors there," Golly continued. "I told you about the red; the orange came from wood lichen. That's green when you gather it but it makes orange dye. The yellows came from several plants: the dark shades from Navajo tea and wild buckwheat, the light yellows from wild sunflowers and goldenrod. A plant from our garden makes a light yellow, too. Can you guess which one?"

"Butter-and-eggs?" guessed Manford. "You planted that, I remember."

"That's correct. I used white onionskin to make an off-white dye for the smoke rising from the fire. And the bluish, greenish, and dark shades of gray in the smoke came from blue flower lupine, wild walnut leaves, and juniper mistletoe. Black came from combining sumac leaves, pinon pitch and ocher."

"You planted globemallows in the garden, too," Manford said. "Those flowers are orange. What color comes from them?"

"Light purple," Golly said. "The blossoms turn that color when they dry. Dark purple comes from wild blackberries. I didn't use either in the painting, except to mix with other colors to make different shades."

"How do you make the dyes?" asked Columbine.

"I gather plants in the summer when their colors are brightest. I pick as many as I think I'm going to need for the year all at once, then preserve them by pressing them between boards. To make a certain color dye, I boil the plants I need in water until I get the right color. Some vegetable plants have to be fried first and others, like cactus, which doesn't grow around here, first have to be left to rot and turn mushy."

"Does a particular plant always make the same color dye?" asked Needlenose, clearly interested in this new idea.

"No, colors always vary. What I get depends on when the

plants were picked, what the weather was like before I picked them, how long they were pressed, and the length of time they're boiled. Sometimes I boil different plants together to get new colors, but it's better not to. To produce its best colors, each plant must be boiled a different length of time."

"You learned this from the Indians?" asked Veronica.

"I read about how Pueblo and Navajo weavers have made their dyes for more than two hundred years. I was curious, so I tried it. I kept trying until I got it to work. Of course, when the Indians do this, they shear sheep, clean the wool and hand spin it into yarn then soak it in dyes for several days. After drying, they have different colored yarns to make patterns in their blankets and rugs. What I'm doing is somewhat the same; I'm just painting with the colors instead."

"This is fascinating," Mary said. "I'd like to hear more and see the rest of your work."

"That can be arranged, I suppose," said Golly, "but at the moment, we have an art work to carry to the road crossing, and it looks like it'll be raining soon."

Flossie and Golly flew the art panels to the road. Manford and Veronica carried the frame to the meadow then down a trail that ran beside the creek which flowed from Flossie's Pond to the spot where it met a dirt road. Columbine and FireDragon flew ahead; Mary Moose followed with Needlenose and Ssam riding along. Aurora was gone again, likely to the woods to spend the day alone.

The truck, a large, enclosed van with its pull-down rear door standing open, was waiting on the road.

"I don't see anyone around," said Manford.

"That was the agreement," Mary said. "I asked that the driver park the truck here, leave the back door open, then take a walk for a couple hours. When he returns, he's to drive whatever's in the truck back to the gallery."

"Didn't they think that was an odd request?" asked Flossie.

"Yes, but I told them the artist was a recluse and didn't want anyone to know where he or she lived."

"Well, that's true enough," Flossie said.

"I hope the driver has a raincoat," said Manford. "We're going to get wet pretty soon."

They loaded the frame into the truck, then hung their art pieces on it and fastened them in position. They tied the finished work to the inside of the truck to keep it from shifting during the ride.

"It looks wonderful," said Mary. "It's sure to cause comment."

"Is the rest of the art ready?" asked Golly.

"I think so," said Ssam.

"Get on board, then. It's time to shut the door."

Columbine and FireDragon flew into the truck; Veronica lifted Ssam aboard. Each found a place to hide to avoid discovery.

"Goodbye," Golly said. "Good luck at the show."

"Thanks," they heard FireDragon say. "This sure is going to be different."

Veronica shut the door, then returned with the others the way they'd come. Rain began a few minutes later. The driver soon returned and saw the truck door closed, so he started the engine and headed slowly back down the dirt road. That was part of his instructions, too: drive carefully to avoid damage to the art.

The truck followed the dirt road to a highway then continued west, driving down out of the Cascade Mountains about forty miles to the Washington coast. On the outskirts of a large town sometime in late afternoon, the driver pulled into a parking lot and backed to the entrance of an art gallery. He opened the truck's rear door and looked inside. A helper from the gallery joined him.

"What is it?" the helper asked.

"Beats me," the driver said. "First I've seen it."

"Get a look at the artist?"

"Nope. Went walking like I was supposed to. Saw a bear and a couple moose on the way back, but nobody that looked like any reclusive artist. Grab an end of this, will ya?"

They undid the tie-downs and carried the cargo into the gallery. There was no one there. The exhibition was scheduled to open the next afternoon; the building would be closed till then. They set the fifteen-foot piece where they thought it should go then turned out the lights and departed.

Soon the building was quiet. Patches of light from scattered windows began to fade. Ssam poked his head out from his hiding place under Needlenose's weaving.

"Are you okay, Columbine?" he said.

"Yes, I perched in the middle of the flames and no one saw me."

"How about you Mr. Dragonfly?"

"I'm hanging onto the back of Flossie's forest."

"I guess we can come out now," Ssam went on. "The show starts tomorrow. What shall we do till then?"

"If this is an art gallery," said FireDragon, "I suppose we should go see the art."

"That's what I was thinking," said Columbine.

"I've never seen art before. I hope you can explain it to me."

"Ssam and I will try," Princess said.

"And while we're looking," said Ssam, "maybe we'll find something to eat."

"Mosquitoes with chili peppers would be tasty," said FireDragon. Soon, the three were slithering, fluttering, and buzzing through the gallery in search of whatever they might find.

They were in their places when the first people arrived next morning. There was much to do. Ssam heard the people say they had entries to put into categories, works of all kinds to hang and arrange, cookies and wine to set out. There were nearly two hundred entries, they said.

"I counted two hundred and six," whispered Ssam.

"I got up to eighty-seven," FireDragon whispered back, "then I found that open bottle of Tabasco sauce on the counter. Whoa, do I feel like a dragon today!"

"Be careful where you breathe," said Columbine. "Don't burn a hole in the art."

The gallery people bustled about the rooms, walking past the entry from MorningGlory Forest, pausing to talk to each other about it, even moving it to a new spot a time or two. Its residents stayed motionless. If the people ever noticed them, they must have figured, and correctly so, that they were part of the art.

The show opened at 3 p.m. Only one or two visitors came at first, but toward evening a crowd began to gather. People wandered through the rooms, some looking at the art, some talking together, others seemingly more interested in the food.

Ssam, Columbine, and FireDragon waited patiently. Then, with seventy people gathered, fifteen of them in front of Forest Fire Trilogy, Ssam raised his head and spoke in a loud, commanding voice:

"LADIES AND GENTLEMEN, GOOD EVENING."

Heads turned.

Talking quieted.

Puzzled looks crept across faces.

"MY NAME IS SSAM—SSAM WITH TWO Ss—ONE BIG AND ONE SMALL. THE SMALL S IS SILENT." Ssam paused and looked around to make sure everyone was listening.

"You are looking at a story of destruction and renewal," he went on in a regular tone. "This brilliant work's news is bad and yet, is good, or perhaps it is neither. Follow me from left to right as I explain." Ssam moved along his crawlway to the forest panel on the left.

"Here, the artist has captured mature, old growth forest. Trees are tall and sturdy. They've been here a hundred years, quite likely more. Their leaves renew the air. Birds live in their branches and animals make homes among them. But nothing grows on the forest floor. Sunlight rarely reaches it and rainfall and groundwater go to give life to the trees. . ."

As you can tell, Ssam is elaborating on a story we've already heard. But is anyone hearing him? A few are, but others are whispering.

"Is that a snake?" said one. "I can't stand snakes."

"Can't be," said another.

"Must be something mechanical," offered a third, "especially with a voice like that."

"It's a good job, whatever it is."

"Let's see how it handles questions," said a young man in a dark suit and bright yellow tie.

"Shhh," said the woman with him.

"Pardon me, Mr. Ssam," the man went on, ignoring her. "How do leaves renew the air?"

"Leaves absorb carbon dioxide from the air and give back oxygen," Ssam replied. "When people and animals breathe, they turn oxygen into carbon dioxide. It's a sort of balance, you see. Plants need something from us; we need something from them. There are lots of people and animals, so we need lots of plants and trees to keep the air breathable. That's part of the bad news in the story told here. With the forest gone, some part of the work isn't being done. Nice tie, by the way."

"How did it do that?" the woman beside the questioner whispered.

"Must be someone watching us with a microphone," he answered. "There's a speaker in that thing, I'll bet." A man on the edge of the crowd took out a cellular telephone, punched out a number, and talked quietly.

Ssam moved to the center panel now. He began relating the story told in Golly's painting of the fire, about how swiftly a fire moves and what firefighters do to stop it. Columbine, perched in a matching orange section of the painting, flexed her wings and moved from side to side.

"It's moving, almost like it was burning," someone said, pointing. "That's clever." The crowd had grown to fifty people watching now, squeezing close together to see. FireDragon took off, buzzing loudly and trailing an orange bucket on a string. Hovering above the painted flames, he dumped a load of cayenne pepper. The falling orange powder looked like chemical fire retardant. Columbine closed her eyes and stopped moving. One or two people in the audience sneezed.

"This is getting realistic," someone said.

Ssam talked on. The dragonfly helicopter returned to reload then buzzed back across the painting dropping a bucketload of salt that looked like water as it fell. Flying low over the flames, he passed our Fire Wing Princess.

"Salt on your tail, Columbine, tee-hee," he said.

Ssam moved on to panel three. Contest judges gathered with the crowd as Ssam explained the process of regrowth after a fire. Columbine fluttered across, shook salt and pepper from her wings, and landed on a flower Needlenose had represented with a bright yellow bead. FireDragon flew behind the wooden frame, wiggled out of his helicopter costume, then buzzed around the right side to land on the pond. Ssam reached the end of his story and began to tell about the homeless moose in Alaska.

"Thank you for your attention, everyone. You might like to know that this work is based on an actual fire..."

A TV camera crew bursting through the door cut Ssam short. The man with the phone had called them. They worked their way to the front of the crowd.

"We heard about a show going on," said one of the crew.

"You just missed it," someone said.

"Not a problem," said Ssam, seeing Channel 12 News lettered on the camera. "We'll start over from the beginning." He slipped quickly back to the first panel, Columbine returned to her perch in the flames, and FireDragon flew behind the frame to get into his helicopter suit.

The camera crew set up their gear and handed a microphone to the man with the phone. He would be the announcer, it appeared. He made introductory comments as the cameras rolled, then turned to Ssam.

"Go ahead; you're on."

Ssam told his story once again, in a clear voice, left to right, with helicopters and butterflies and dragons.

Everyone in the gallery was now watching. The moving figures weren't mechanical, that much was clear—the second show was different from the first. This was the real thing, they realized, and they strained to see and hear everything.

The judges assembled hastily in the corner of the room. They compared notes then quickly toured the rest of the exhibit, pointing, conferring, and eventually agreeing. The chief judge whispered something to one of the crew. When Ssam finished, the announcer returned and invited the judge to step before the camera.

"This is such a surprising work," the judge said, "so excellently done with such a variety of materials and effects, we are awarding it this special blue ribbon as the most creative and educational piece in the show." He pinned the ribbon above a flower growing in the blackened meadow. Columbine fluttered to it and landed as the camera focused on the ribbon's gold-lettered words. The crowd applauded.

"You'll be on tomorrow with the six o'clock news," the announcer said as the crew packed to leave. "Thanks for the show."

"May I use your phone before you go?" asked Ssam.

"Sure thing," the man said. He pulled out the antenna and set the phone down where Ssam could reach it. Ssam punched out Mary's number with his nose. He listened to it ring three times, then heard Mary's voice, "Hello, this is Moostery Manor. We're not in just now. Please leave a moosage at the tone. . . ." Beep.

"This is Ssam," said Ssam. "We've won a blue ribbon and we'll be on Channel 12 News tomorrow at six. Don't miss us. This show stays open for a week, by the way. We'll have to do this every night. Bye."

Back at GloryView, meanwhile, Golly was selecting paintings for his own exhibition. With his secret out, his friends had eagerly asked if they could see his other work. He was flattered and, he had to admit, pleased that they were interested.

Mary had suggested he pick the paintings he liked best and bring them to Moostery Manor. He could hang them throughout the house and leave them up until everyone had seen them. He'd readily agreed. Now, while the final visitors were leaving the gallery and Ssam, Columbine, and FireDragon were settling down for another night, Golly paced about his rooms, picking items from the walls and from those stacked in closets in the study.

A one-eagle show, he was thinking; this is really special. I'll have to choose very special works. Through the late evening hours he picked one, then another, then another. By midnight he'd chosen twenty he could show with pride. He smiled. This will do, he thought. This will do nicely.

He flew his paintings one at a time to Moostery Manor the next morning. Flossie, Veronica, and Needlenose joined Manford to hang them wherever Mary specified. They marveled and exclaimed over each painting. Golly explained what each was and told how he'd obtained the more exotic colors. One painting captured Mary's eye.

"I know what this is," she said. "It's lovely."

"I was hoping you'd like it," Golly answered. "It's an Alaska scene, though you can see this spectacle other places, too."

"Those are northern lights," Mary said. The painting showed a black night sky crossed by folding curtains of shimmering brightness in red, white, and green. A dark landscape of frosted trees reflected their glow.

"Yes," Golly said, "you see them mostly in the winter, so I've shown the ground as tundra covered with snow. It's called 'Fire and Ice'."

"You should have entered it in the show," Mary said, "and some of these others, too. They're wonderful."

"I didn't want to compete with what we did enter," Golly said. "Besides, I've decided to give this one to you. I'd be honored if you'd hang it in Moostery Manor to remind you of your original home."

"I'd love to," Mary said. "Thank you very much. Let's see, we'll hang it. . .there," she decided, pointing to a spot between two windows.

"What's this one?" asked Veronica. She was looking at a small painting still in the stack to be hung.

"I painted that a few weeks ago," said Golly. "I was thinking about Needlenose that day. Perhaps it would fit in Haystack Hollow."

The painting showed a forest clearing with a large mound to the left, identified by a sign as Haystack Hollow. Puffy, yellow clouds filled the sky, from which fell a blizzard of golden potato chips that covered the ground, and the burrow, and piled up on branches of trees. A bushy figure stood knee-deep atop the burrow lifting his head and front paws to the sky. "Yes!" it seemed to say.

"A potato chip snowstorm," Flossie said. "What a concept."

"Gorgeous yellows," Needlenose said. "Absolutely my favorite shade. Thank you, Golly."

"You're welcome. It's called 'Let the Chips Fall'."

"I'll put it in my pantry."

"Right above your lifetime potato chip supply, no doubt," said Flossie.

"Oh, there's hardly enough there for a month," Needlenose replied.

"There's also one in the stack for Misty Falls, Veronica," Golly said.

"It's this one, I'll bet," Veronica said. She held up a circus scene. Clowns darted about in little cars, riders stood on galloping horses, gymnasts vaulted atop one another to form a human tower. The audience cheered and waved. Behind the center ring, a twenty-piece orchestra in striped blazers played fast music. In the ring, with top hat and cane, danced a happy, smiling bear.

"What's it called?" Manford asked.

"'Millie'," Golly said. "That seemed to be enough."

"It looks like her, too," said Veronica. "Thank you. I like it, and so will Mom."

"Do you ever do portraits?" asked Flossie.

"I painted my reflection in the mirror once."

"Did you call it 'Double Eagle'?" asked Needlenose.

"Actually, I did," said Golly, "but then I burned it."

"Why?"

"When the title is better than the art, one or the other needs to go."

"Maybe you should get Mary to sit for a portrait," said Flossie. "You could call it the 'Moosa Lisa'."

Mary laughed.

"That's not that bad an idea," said Golly.

"Time for the news," Manford said. "Ssam said they'd be on at six." He turned on the TV and they all gathered round it. The feature opened with an announcer standing outside the gallery.

"It was just a simple art contest," he began. "An announcement in the paper invited local artists to bring paintings, weavings, sculptures, and other crafts."

The camera switched to the inside of the gallery to show paintings hanging neatly on the walls, and carvings, pottery, beadwork, and a dozen other types of art displayed about the rooms.

"These are the works they entered," the announcer said. "Truly lovely and interesting pieces, as anything usually is when someone clever does something for the joy of it."

They saw their forest fire scene.

"But this work is different. Its two outer panels are weavings; the center is a watercolor painting. It tells a story, a story about forest fire—not just in paint and fabric and printed words, but it tells you, listen."

The camera singled out Ssam, ranger hat on his head, green neckerchief where he usually wore his bow tie. Ssam was telling the story they had crafted into Forest Fire Trilogy. They saw Columbine flexing her wings, and FireDragon buzzing overhead dropping orange powder on the fire.

"The storyteller here is a garter snake, friends," the announcer went on. "He said his name is Ssam—Ssam with two s's. We don't know how this is being done, but maybe we don't need to. Ssam has a story, and a message. Let's listen once again." The camera had followed Ssam to the third panel where he was just finishing:

"...trees will grow, and one day the forest will return. Thank you for listening, ladies and gentlemen. We've told you this story, my friends and I, so you would understand a little more of how nature works.

"You might also be interested to know that this work is based on a real forest fire that happened in Alaska just a month ago. The people there are safe but many animals, particularly moose, are homeless. After a difficult winter, their prospects are bleak. Perhaps you'd like to help us help our friends in the fire. I'm hoping you will."

"Amazing things are happening here," the announcer said in conclusion. "Not only is this work amazing, and its special effects amazing, but even before this broadcast is aired, we have begun getting dozens of calls at the studio. People are asking how they can help. People are sending money.

"Channel 12 has established a 'Give a Moose a Home' fund and we'll be sending whatever comes in to assist wildlife relief efforts in Alaska."

The camera again showed the outside of the art gallery with a long line of people waiting at its doors.

"The show will be open the rest of the week," the announcer said. "See it for yourselves. Adam Hill, Channel 12 News."

The living room at Moostery Manor was quiet as those gathered there looked at each other in wonder.

"It worked, Mom," Manford finally said. "Your idea worked!"

"I can hardly believe it," said Mary. "This is really too amazing."

"I guess it shows you the power of art," said Golly.

"Pardon me for being too practical," Flossie said, "but where are we going to put that thing when this is over?"

"Don't worry," Mary said. "With all this publicity, even after Golly brings Ssam, Columbine, and FireDragon home, someone will want to buy Forest Fire Trilogy. We'll have enough money to build homes for half the moose in Alaska."

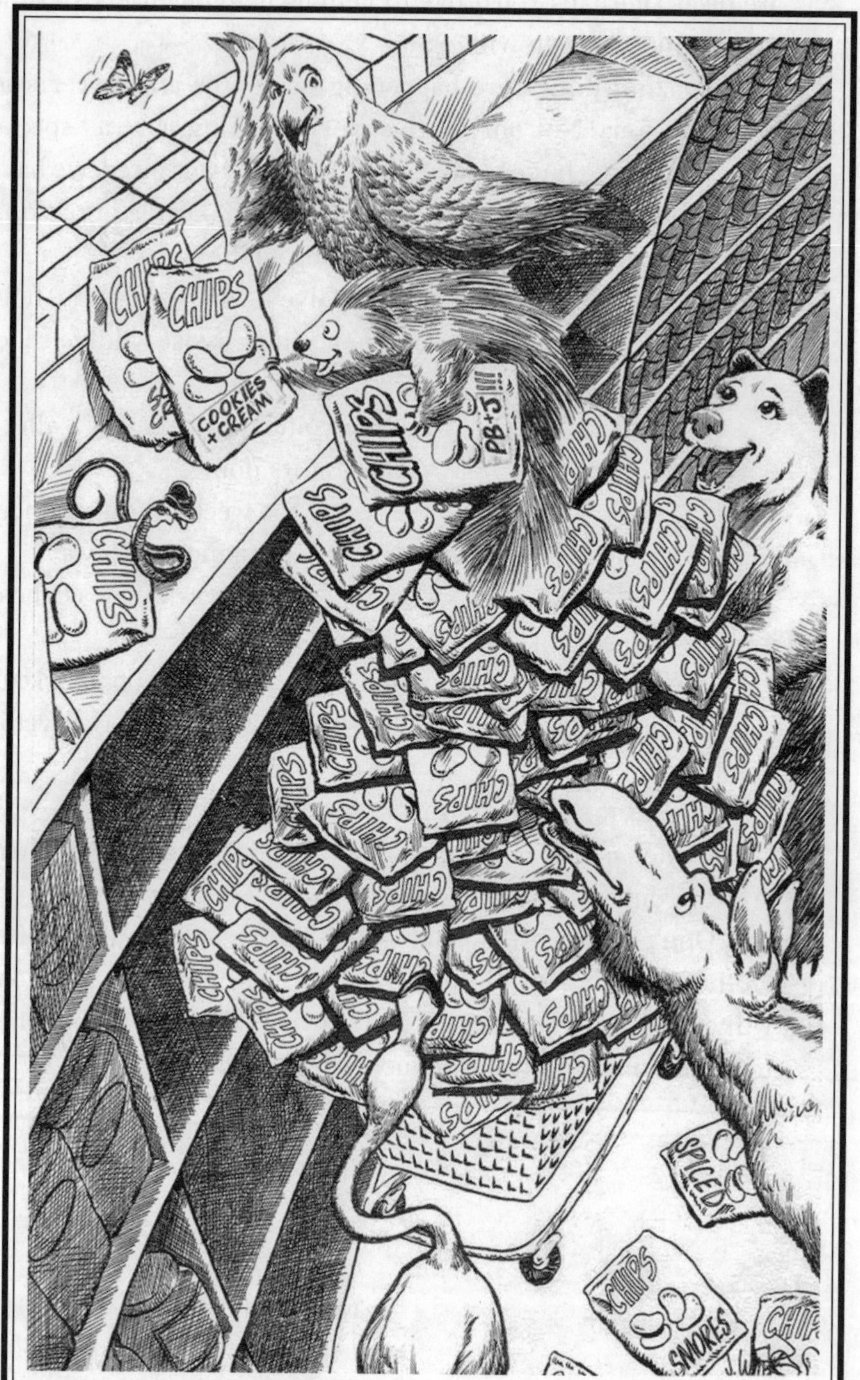
CHIPS
CHIPS
COOKIES + CREAM
CHIPS
PB+J!!!
CHIPS
SPICED
CHIPS
SMORES
CHIPS

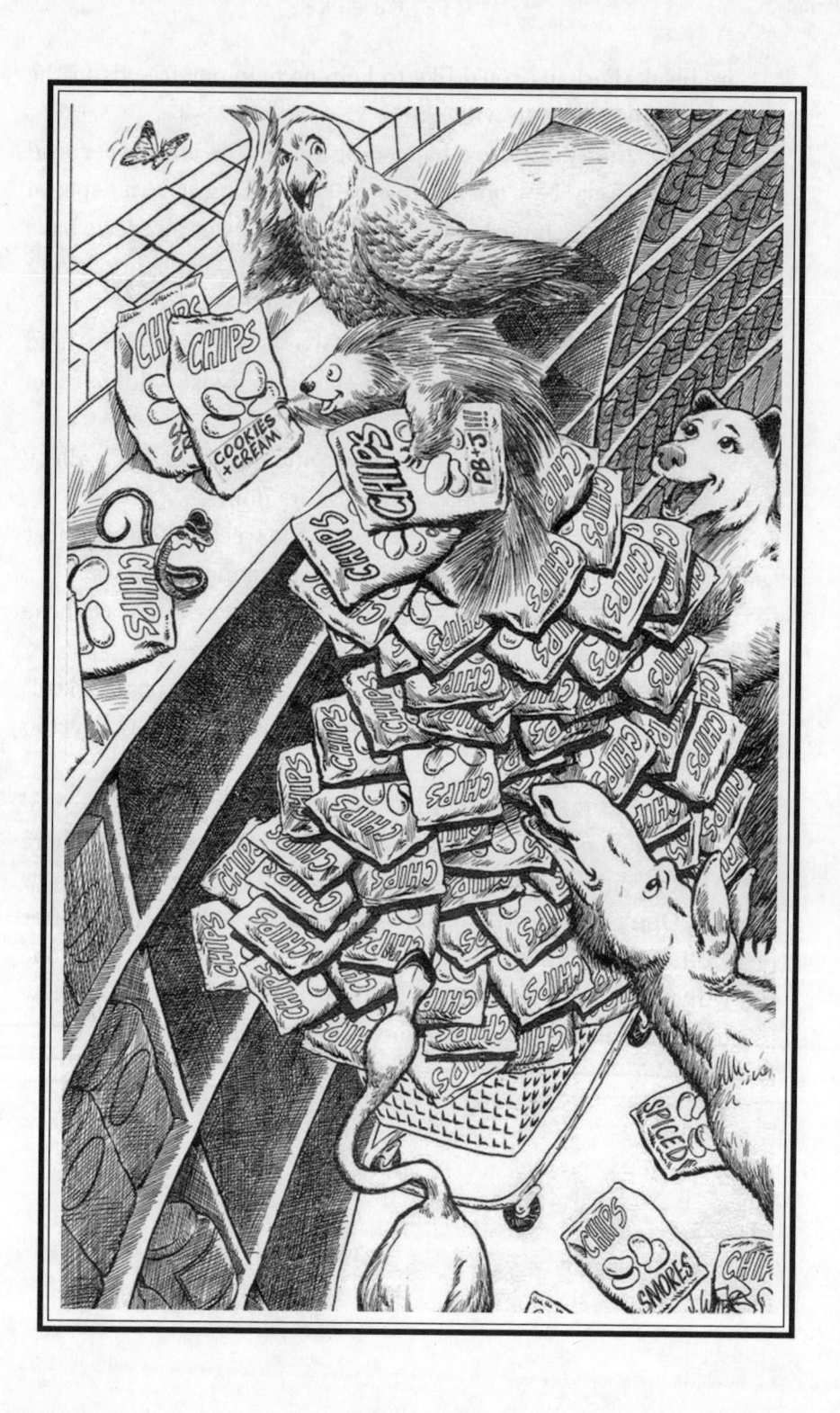

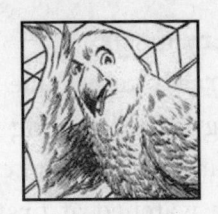

12

Improving the View

In which Manford, Veronica, and Ssam get glasses

Aurora had moved into Moostery Manor. There was plenty of room, Mary said. She'd outfitted a spare room in pleasing colors and had welcomed her to stay as long as she liked. This was something new for Aurora. Living alone in the quiet woods, she'd never known about houses, cooked meals, or a room of one's own. She had to admit it was kind of nice.

There were other new things as well.

Books were amazing. Pages of words and pictures about things she never knew existed—she started learning to read right away.

Movies were like magic. Stories of far off places, especially big cities, were wonders she'd never imagined.

Machines were incredible, too. Devices to heat the house and make toast, to stir things and light things and talk to friends in other houses—life chasing mice for dinner and sleeping in trees was never like this.

But she learned quickly. She asked questions and watched how things were done. She practiced reading and writing with Manford, making her letters round. Soon she felt at home, which pleased Mary very much.

What caught Aurora's interest like nothing else, however, was the kitchen. Peeling things, mixing things, cooking things, baking things, rolling and cutting and chopping had a strange fascination for her. She watched at first as Mary made meals and treats. Soon she wanted to help and would leaf through cookbooks pointing out things that looked good.

"Can we make a pie?" she asked Mary one evening.

"What kind?" Mary asked.

"Like the brown one in this picture. Pumpkin, is that how you say it?"

"That's right, but we'd have to get a pumpkin."

"What's that?"

"It's a fruit. It's big and round and orange and grows on a vine along the ground. You scoop the seeds out of the inside, peel the skin off the outside, and use what's left for cooking. It makes excellent pie if you add plenty of spices."

"Can we get one?"

"We won't find pumpkins in the store until fall," Mary said, "but we'll get canned pumpkin. Tomorrow's Saturday and we're going out anyway; I'll put it on the list."

"Oh, good," said Aurora.

Next morning at ten, Manford, Veronica, and Ssam were to visit the optometrist. Several chapters ago, you'll remember Mr. Turner telling them how much better they'd be able to see wearing eyeglasses. They saw things clearly up close, but the world far away was a fuzzy, colored blur. Mary had phoned for their appointment and added other errands to make it a full day's outing.

They started out after breakfast on the path to the meadow, met Veronica there, then crossed Lookout Hill and descended toward Flossie's Pond. Ssam would be waiting where the path turned north toward the store. It was a cloudy day and looked like it would rain by afternoon.

"GOOD MORNING, FRIENDS," Ssam's voice boomed before they even reached the bottom of the hill.

"Good morning," Mary said, when they'd come closer. "If you see so poorly, Ssam, how did you know we were coming?"

"I pick up scents in the air with my tongue. I know what moose and bear smell like, so I figured it was you. I wasn't sure about Aurora. She has such a dainty smell, it'll take me a while to recognize her." Aurora didn't know what to think about this, but smiled.

Needlenose and Flossie had come along with Ssam, as had Princess Columbine, perched on Flossie's head. Each said their good mornings in turn.

"Want a ride, Ssam?" Manford asked.

"Sure," he said. Veronica lifted him so he could crawl into Manford's pack, then the party moved on toward the store.

"We're happy to have you home from the art show," Mary said to Columbine and Ssam. "I presume FireDragon is busy buzzing around the pond this morning?"

"No," said Columbine, "he didn't come back."

"He didn't?" said Manford. "Why not?"

"The art gallery was on the coast," Ssam said. "The sight and sound and smell of all that water overwhelmed him. It was the biggest pond he'd ever seen. He decided to stay and explore it."

"That will keep him busy," said Needlenose.

"The Italian restaurant he found also might have had something to do with it," added Columbine.

"He asked us to say goodbye to everyone and thanks for being nice to him," said Ssam.

"And we were just getting to like him," said Flossie.

In MorningGlory Forest, whenever anyone ran short of something or needed something new, they went to the store. Bears still gathered berries in the woods, of course, and moose still ate willow leaves off trees, but for such civilized characters to live as they did in houses and furnished caves there had to be a store.

The store was many stores, really, eight buildings large and small clustered on either side of the path about a mile north of Flossie's Pond. Nearly anything a forest creature wanted could be found at one or another.

"Where are we going first, Mom?" Manford asked.

"To the furniture store," Mary said. "If Aurora's going to help in the kitchen, she needs a tall stool to sit where she can see."

The path soon opened into a wide clearing. The florist and movie theater stood on their right, the post office and library on their left. They entered the furniture store just beyond the library.

"Be careful where you sit," Mary said. She was like mothers everywhere, you see, reminding you of the obvious just in case you didn't think of it yourself.

The showroom was large. One part had dozens of couches and chairs with big pillows and footstools, all pushed close together. Wood or glass topped tables stood in front of things or beside them holding lamps, picture books, or centerpieces of small bowls and candles.

Manford and Veronica followed, weaving pathways in and out. They sat up straight in straight chairs, rocked back and forth in rocking chairs, then settled into huge reclining chairs and made weary sounds like they badly needed rest. Needlenose turned lamps on and off, some just by touching them, and talked about someday wiring his burrow for electric lights. Ssam disappeared into a long and many sectioned couch.

"Found a quarter," he said, popping up between the cushions about halfway along.

That display led to one of dining rooms. Like the couches and chairs, items here came in many styles and sizes for different kinds of animals. Some pieces, nearly as small as doll furniture, were arranged on shelves. Columbine found one such setting done in mahogany and red velvet. It was so elegant and plush it seemed fit for a queen. She perched in the tiny chair at the head of the tiny table and flexed her royal wings regally.

Finding the beds next, Veronica plopped in the middle of one and rolled onto her back.

"Whoa, it's a waterbed," she said as it surged and rippled beneath her.

"I had one once," said Needlenose. "Bad idea! My quills poked it full of holes and it turned into a fountain."

Ssam found the others looking through kitchens.

"Finding anything?" he asked, spiraling up the leg of a tall wooden stool.

"There are wonderful ideas here," Flossie said. "I'd have a great time outfitting a place of my own."

"Try that stool, Aurora," Mary said. "See if you like it." Aurora climbed atop it with Ssam.

"Seems fine to me," she said.

"Okay, I'll have it delivered home. Ssam, where's Columbine, and what are the others doing?"

"Our Monarch is in the royal dining room just now," said Ssam. "The others are sitting or snoozing."

"Round them up, will you? It's time for their appointment, and yours, too."

"TIME TO GO, EVERYBODY," Ssam thundered, vibrating mirrors on the walls and silverware on the tables.

"That wasn't exactly what I had in mind," Mary said with a patient smile.

The optometrist was upstairs in the last building on the right. The waiting room was decorated in soft colors and, like the furniture store, had many sizes of chairs for its visitors.

Magazines were stacked neatly on tables. Pictures on the walls showed drawings of the workings of the eye. A gray, clouded light came in the windows. The arriving party sat down to wait.

"What's he going to do to us?" Manford asked.

"What is she going to do, you mean," Mary replied. "The doctor is Miss Melinda, according to her diplomas on the wall."

"What's a diploma?" asked Aurora.

"It's a certificate you earn for going to school. It means you've completed the necessary studies and are qualified to do what you do."

"Oh," Aurora said, "do you have one?"

"I studied forestry and botany and learned to be a naturalist. I have a diploma for that."

"Oh," Aurora said again.

"What is she going to do to us?" Manford persisted. The office door opened then and the doctor appeared. Miss Melinda had a soft, pretty face and big, sparkling, brown eyes. She wore a white jacket and held papers in a clipboard.

"Good morning," she said in a gentle voice. "Manford, Veronica, and Ssam, would you like to do this together?"

"Sure," they replied.

"Follow me," she said, leading the way to the examination room.

She sat them at a long counter. Veronica lifted Ssam from the pack so he could move about. The doctor opened a book and showed them a circle filled with green dots, with a number made of orange dots in its center.

"Do you see a number here?" she asked.

"Twelve," Manford said.

"How about here?" She turned to another picture with different colors, the number less clear this time.

"Twenty-nine," said Veronica.

"And here?"

"Seventy-four," said Ssam.

They answered in turn for several more pages, the numbers becoming harder to see each time.

"What was that for?" Manford asked.

"It tells how well you see colors," Melinda replied. "Some don't see green or red very well. To others, the colors are confused: reds, greens, yellows, oranges all look alike. A few don't see blues, and some see only black and white. If you had your colors mixed up, you couldn't see some of the numbers."

"That's interesting," said Veronica. "What happens next?"

"Come over to this instrument and rest your chin on the bar." The doctor adjusted knobs to line up a camera with Veronica's right eye.

"Watch the red dot inside the lens. . .ready. . ." Flash, went a very bright light.

"Oooh," Veronica said. She clamped her eyes shut but still saw a white disc that seemed to grow and grow, then slowly turn pale.

"Don't worry; what you're seeing will fade in a minute. Ssam, your turn."

Photographing Manford was a problem. The instrument didn't have room for his long nose. The doctor raised and lowered and extended as far as things went but the lens was still too far away.

"Turn sideways," she finally said. She made adjustments again. "Hold still now. . ." Flash.

"Oooh, it's like seeing the sun," Manford said. "Do you have to do our left eyes, too?"

"I'm afraid so. Back to you, Veronica."

"What do the pictures show?" asked Ssam.

"The inside of your eyes," the doctor said. "I can tell if they're normal or damaged in some way. I can see if your lenses are clear or cloudy. I can see whether veins and arteries are the right size or if they're too fat, too thin, or twisted. And I keep the pictures for next time to see if anything has changed."

She next put glasses with Polaroid lenses on Veronica and showed her a sheet of nine diagrams.

"These pictures each have four circles," the doctor said. "For each one, tell me which circle seems lifted up."

The first was easy. Veronica pointed to one circle of the four that looked to be an inch off the page. The second was harder and by the time she reached number nine, the circles all seemed flat to the page.

"What are we doing now?" Manford asked.

"A stereopsis test, it tells how you see depth. If you can't see depth, the world looks flat like a picture."

The patients passed this exam and went on to another instrument. Ssam positioned himself in front of it, watching while Melinda adjusted a small nozzle.

"Keep your eye open," she said, "I'm going to squirt a puff of air at it." Ssam blinked when she did so, and then held still to test the other eye.

"This measures pressure," the doctor said. "A disease called glaucoma increases pressure in the eye and ruins your vision. If you have your eyes checked regularly, this test will tell me in time to help you."

"Are we okay?" Veronica asked when they'd finished.

"Normal as can be," the doctor said.

The next instrument peered into their eyes, clicked, purred, and shifted back and forth, then calculated the lens prescriptions each would need to see normally. The doctor took this information and led them to another room. She sat Manford in a padded chair and swung a device in front of him with eyeholes to look through.

"This is a phoropter," she said. "I start by setting it to the prescription we just calculated. While you look through the eyeholes, I'll change lenses one at a time. Tell me which ones help you see better." She turned on a projector to show a chart of letters on the wall twenty feet away. The chart's left half was red, the right green.

"Which side looks clearer?" the doctor said.

"Red," Manford answered.

"Now which one?" she said, changing a lens.

"Still red." She continued until the two sides looked the same to Manford, then the green side looked clearer.

Next she showed a white chart with four rows of black letters. She reset the lenses again.

"Tell me which lens makes the letters look clearer—this, or this?"

"The second one is better," Manford answered.

"Try this now—number one, or number two?"

"Two is still better."

The doctor changed lenses until Manford said both choices looked the same. Then she placed a chart sixteen inches in front of Manford's eyes, showing paragraphs in type of decreasing size.

"We've checked your distance vision; now we'll see how well you do up close. Does the tiny paragraph at the bottom look clear?"

"Uh huh," Manford said.

"I thought it would. Most youngsters can see close up and far away with the same lenses, but now and then I find one who doesn't."

"Do you need two sets of glasses then?"

"No, you get bifocals. But you won't need those."

Manford's final test involved crossed lines.

"This tests your ability to focus," the doctor said. "Which lines seem darker—vertical or horizontal?"

"Does vertical mean up and down?" Manford asked.

"It does."

"That's what looks darker." The doctor changed lenses until all lines looked the same, then the horizontal seemed darker.

"This is really something," Manford said. "I can see through those lenses. I can read things far away. It's wonderful. But you tried many lenses; which is best?"

"Several will work," Melinda explained. "I started each of your tests with a lens that wasn't strong enough, and then gave you stronger and stronger lenses until they were too strong. I'll pick one from the middle to get the best for you. By testing you several different ways, I can be sure to choose the right one." She wrote numbers and symbols on Manford's chart.

"The world will sure look different when I get these," he said.

Veronica and Ssam then went through the same tests. Their prescriptions were even stronger than Manford's.

"That's it," the doctor said. "I'll be giving you all contact lenses. Once I show you how to wear them, you'll be seeing more of what's around you than ever before. You'll be discovering the world all over again."

"I like that idea," said Manford. The doctor escorted them back to the waiting room.

"I'm going to see, Mom!"

"It's going to be great!" said Ssam.

"They've been excellent patients, Mrs. Moose," Melinda said. "I'll order their glasses and you can pick them up in a few days."

"They asked a million questions, I'll bet," Mary said.

"They did," the doctor replied with a smile, "and good ones, too. Goodbye, and thanks for coming to me."

"Where to next, Mom?" Manford asked.

"To the library first, then I thought we'd see a movie."

"What do you need at the library?" Veronica asked.

"Aurora was asking about school while we were waiting," said Flossie. "Since Miss Melinda has a diploma from eye doctor school, and Mary has one from naturalist school, Aurora wants to know if there are diplomas for cooking."

"Let's find out," Manford said, and they headed downstairs and back along the path.

The librarian, a large spotted owl, nodded at their request and took them to a row of reference books. He pointed out guides to colleges and universities then pulled out one for trade schools. He flipped through the pages for a moment.

"Schools are listed by state," he said. "Let's try the index." He turned to the back of the book. "Cooking, you wanted?"

"Yes," Aurora said.

"Cooking; let's look under Food. Yes, here are some listed under Food Service. Just a minute. . .yes, there are more under Restaurant Management and there might be some others as well." The librarian showed Aurora the categories in the index.

"Many states have schools, it appears," he went on. "Find their names in the index, then read about them in the front of the book."

Aurora sat at a table and paged through the book with Mary and Flossie. They found a dozen schools in as many states that looked promising. Mary wrote out the names and addresses.

"Do you want this for some special reason?" asked Columbine.

"Maybe," Aurora said, sounding a bit mysterious.

They walked across the path to the theater. Golly, who'd been circling lazily above, drifted down to join them. "It's a Roy Rogers double feature today," he said.

"I suppose you could read that from way up in the sky," said Ssam.

"I could, indeed."

"Pretty soon we'll be seeing things far away, too," said Veronica.

"You'll like that," Golly said. "May I join you at the movie?"

"Sure," said Needlenose.

Old westerns were featured on Saturday afternoon and already there was a long line. Rabbits, beavers, birds, even a few woodchucks and coyotes stood waiting and moving slowly forward.

Inside, the usher seated everyone by height: rabbits down in front, moose and bears in the back, others in the middle by increasing size. Our party of friends took six seats in the back row. Ssam watched from Manford's hat; Needlenose sat on Veronica's shoulder; Columbine perched on Flossie; and Aurora sat on all fours in the seat. The screen was a bit far away for them all to see clearly but they enjoyed being there nonetheless.

The theater was nearly full. Creatures chattered at each other and went back and forth to the refreshment stand. The audience cheered when the theater lights dimmed, then continued to talk loudly and crinkle candy wrappers while cartoons starring Mickey Mouse played.

"Aren't we supposed to be quiet?" Aurora asked.

"Yes," Mary answered, "this is disgraceful."

"I'll fix that," Ssam said. "Hold your ears." He took a deep breath. "SILENCE," he roared. "EVERYONE PLEASE BE QUIET."

Everyone in the audience slapped paws, wings, or hooves to their ears then turned around to see who had made such a sound. The theater fell silent at once and soon the movies began.

"Thank you, Ssam," whispered Mary.

"No problem," he replied.

The films played out basic themes. Bad guys plotted to take things that didn't belong to them—gold, some cattle, a ranch—and Roy, our hero, used sixty-seven minutes of black and white film to stop them. There were ambushes, horse chases, fist fights, runaway stagecoaches, and fair ladies who could ride, and rope, and shoot right along with the men. The audience, led by Ssam, booed the villains, cheered Roy and his crew, and applauded when all turned out well. By the time the double feature ended, it was four in the afternoon. Rain hadn't yet fallen from the cloud filled sky but it would very soon.

"That was fun," Manford said.

"Yes," said Golly, "I'm glad I went along."

"Come to the market with us, if you like," Mary said. "That's where we're going next."

"Okay," said Golly.

The grocery, largest of the eight buildings, was next to the theater. They found it crowded with afternoon shoppers. There was one cart left, with one wheel that wobbled and another that wouldn't turn.

"I want to ride," said Needlenose.

"Okay," Veronica said, carefully lifting him into place. "Fasten the seatbelt."

"Roger," Needlenose replied. Golly perched on the edge of the basket, Princess Columbine rode on his shoulder, and they were off, Veronica pushing. They went first down the produce aisle where fresh fruits, vegetables, and greens caught their eye.

"They have nice willow leaves, Manford," Mary said. "Would you like some for pie?"

"We could just pick some, couldn't we?"

"Of course, but it will be raining soon, and these look very good."

"Okay."

"I don't see any blueberries," Veronica said, sounding disappointed. "In fact, there are no berries here at all."

"It's not the season yet," Mary said.

"Berries must be in season somewhere. I thought sure the store would have some."

Turning the corner, they came to a display of fresh fish on crushed ice. Flossie pointed out a salmon that might have weighed thirty pounds.

"Just think, Golly," she said, "if you and I started at either end of this, it would take days to reach the middle."

"I'd be happy to help," said Veronica.

"Let's try something smaller," Golly said.

"The trout looks good; how about that?" said Flossie. Golly chose a four pounder and had it wrapped.

"Planning a party?" Needlenose asked.

"No, but we could," Flossie said.

"Since we're baking a pie," Mary said, "why don't you all come to Moostery Manor from here and spend the evening?"

"O-kayyy," said Ssam.

"I'd be delighted," said Princess Columbine.

"For a party, we'll have to have blueberries," said Veronica. She was pushing the cart down the aisle of canned fruits and vegetables.

"Here are some canned blueberries," Manford said.

"Oh, come on," Veronica said, "a bear buying blueberries in cans; what kind of story is this?"

"There are frozen berries two aisles over," said Mary.

"Frozen blueberries!" Veronica sounded even more disappointed.

Aurora, following quietly at the back, studied the cans on the shelf as she passed. *'Beets, beans, corn,'* she said slowly to herself, matching the words to the pictures on the cans. *'Plums, cherries, pumpkin. There it is, pumpkin.'*

"Is this what we want?" she said aloud, showing a can to Mary.

"That's it," Mary said, "just put it in the cart."

"Would you like juice, Princess?" Ssam asked. "There are many kinds here: orange, grapefruit, cranberry."

"Daffodil would be nice."

"I don't see any daffodil."

"Do they have something like Mr. Turner gave me on the mountain?" Columbine asked.

"That was blueberry juice, as I remember," Ssam said. "Here's cranberry and blueberry mixed; that should fix you up."

"Sounds wonderful," said Columbine.

"I told you we needed blueberries," said Veronica.

"Hey, grumpy bear," said Needlenose, "how about blueberry ice cream?"

"Now there's an idea," said Veronica, brightening at once. "I'll get some for sure."

Mary had found other items from her list as they went along and the cart was starting to fill. Rounding another corner, Veronica came to the potato chips.

"Company, halt!" barked Needlenose. "Push me closer, will you? I think it's time to stock up. Let's see, are there any kinds here I haven't tried?"

Flossie read from the bags "onion and garlic, sour cream and chives, Hawaiian style, jalapeño and cheddar, Italian pizza, smoky bar-b-q, Cajun spice, salt and vinegar, extra thick ripple crunch. Looks like every kind here but amaretto and cream."

"A party needs one of each," Needlenose said. He unfastened his seatbelt and loaded chips in the cart.

"Let's finish before it starts raining," Mary said. Needlenose buckled up and Veronica resumed pushing.

"Look, Ssam, fresh mice," said Manford, pointing out black and white mice darting about in a cage. "They're imported from Venezuela."

"They look great," said Ssam, "and South American mice are so tasty and spicy. It must be the chili peppers and maraca music."

"Would you like one or two?"

"One, thank you."

Mary found the last items she needed and Veronica pushed the cart through checkout. Outside, it had started to drizzle. They parceled out groceries between them and hurried toward Moostery Manor. The rain increased steadily, but they were protected by trees most of the way and reached home without getting soaked.

While Mary and Flossie made dinner, Aurora followed

cookbook instructions to make a lovely pumpkin pie. The others helped or played games until Mary called them to the table.

"Anyone for pie?" Mary said afterward.

"Yes," a chorus of voices replied.

It was gone in one pass around the table. Aurora was pleased. She saw the looks on their faces as what she had made was served. She listened to their compliments and comments about how tasty each thought it was. It made her feel good. It was as if making this treat was something nice she had done for each of them. Seeing her pie enjoyed and appreciated made her feel happy and warm.

"Manford, will you help me write some letters?" she said.

"Sure," he replied.

"Have you decided something?" Flossie asked.

"I want to go to school," said Aurora. "I want to learn everything I can about this magic in the kitchen. I want to know a hundred ways to make my friends smile and make myself happy, too. I want to have something I can really do well; something I can feel good about all the time."

"When will you leave?" asked Needlenose.

"Soon," Aurora said, "maybe even before we get to Book Two."

"We'll miss you," Mary said quietly, "but we'll write to you, and we know you'll do well."

Aurora smiled. It was nice having friends, she decided. She was glad she'd come to live with them. She would go away and she would return, and she would always have good friends in MorningGlory Forest.

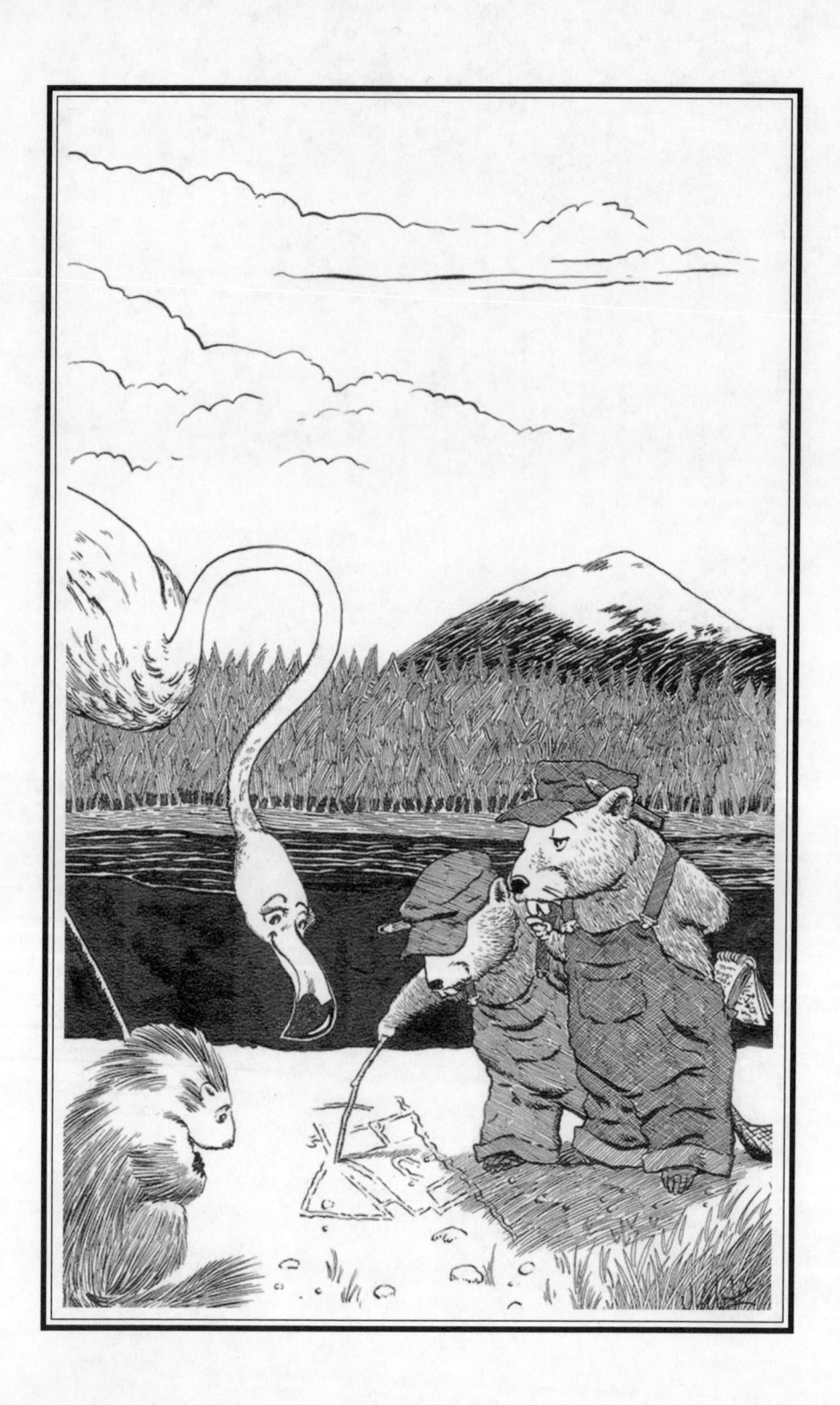

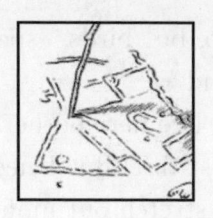

13

Florida-by-the-Pond
In which Flossie builds a castle in the air

Summer had come to MorningGlory Forest. Days were sunny, blue-skied, and warm. Afternoon showers were frequent and refreshing. The animals played in the meadow and woods and talked of going on new adventures soon, but they weren't in any rush. They had plenty to do and plenty of time to do it.

Flossie and Needlenose were having breakfast in the kitchen at Haystack Hollow. Flossie had been thinking things over for several days and had made a decision.

"I'm not going back to Florida," she said. "I'm staying here. This is much better than standing on a beach with ten thousand other look-alike birds that never had an original thought in their lives."

"Sounds fine to me," said Needlenose. "Just keep the room upstairs and consider yourself at home."

"I didn't mean here here, NeedleNoodle," Flossie went on. "I want to stay in MorningGlory Forest with the rest of you, but I want a place of my own."

"Isn't your room here okay?"

"It's fine, dear chap, but birds, especially flamingos, don't usually live underground."

"Does having Ssam live here bother you?"

"No, no, Ssam is just fine. But I need air and water and a view. I need a place to stretch out in, a place to invite you to, and the others as well, at least those that fit."

"What kind of house do you want?" asked Needlenose.

"A Gothic mansion would be nice—gables, peaked roofs, screened-in porches, and fancy woodwork, maybe about forty rooms. It would remind me of Florida, but I suppose that's impractical here."

"A bit."

"Well, I'm definitely not the log-cabin-in-the-woods type."

"A log cabin would be the easiest," said Needlenose, "so, naturally, we wouldn't want to consider it."

"Right," said Flossie, "rule that out from the start."

"What else have you thought about?"

"Something on the pond that has lots of room and is warm through the winter. Beyond that, I have no idea."

"I've always lived in burrows myself," said Needlenose, "so I can't really say what would be best. But I know who to ask."

"Who?"

"Beaver Brothers; they're about a mile downstream. They remodeled my burrow, so I'm sure they could build something for you."

"Do I have to know exactly what I want?"

"No, in fact, it might be better if you don't. Let them come up with the ideas."

"Then lead the way," said Flossie.

They headed down the stream that flowed from Flossie's Pond. Needlenose walked in his pokey, shuffling way. Flossie strutted beside him, picking the way carefully with her long, spindly legs.

"Are you ever going to name your pond?" Needlenose asked. "We've been calling it Flossie's Pond and it even says that on the map. It's getting kind of permanent."

"Sounds like a done deal to me," Flossie said. "Flossie's Pond. . .*Flossie's Pond.* . .it has a nice sound to it, don't you think? That should definitely be its name."

"Okay, but what about this creek? It doesn't have a name."

"Flossie's Creek would work."

"That might be overdoing it."

"Oh, sure. Half the countryside is named MorningGlory this, MorningGlory that, or MorningGlory something else and two Flossie somethings is overdoing it?"

"Yeah, I think so."

"We could name it for our dragonfly friend, I suppose," said Flossie. "He lived here a long time before going off to be Grand Poobah of the Pacific. It would be a nice way to remember him."

"That's a good idea," Needlenose said. "We'll call it Dragonfly Creek."

"Is that all it takes?" Flossie asked. "Two of us walk down a path and decide what to name things? *That's it?*"

"That's it," said Needlenose. "We're in charge here, you know."

"I like this place more all the time."

The stream soon widened into another large pond. Several buildings stood back from the water's edge at the far end of it; one of them was a sawmill. There was a sign over the main entrance:

Beaver Brothers, General Contractors
Never too busy to take time for you

A beaver in heavy bib overalls and a denim cap, with a flat pencil stuck behind his right ear, greeted them as they entered.

"How may I help you today?" he asked, sounding like a whistle as air rushed through his big front teeth.

"I want a house built," said Flossie, "a nice house on a pond and I don't want a log cabin."

"No, you certainly don't," the beaver answered at once, whistling (in the key of D) with certainty. "Too hard to insulate. Can't keep them warm in winter without tending the fire. And the insurance! Oh, my, no! No log cabin for you Miss. . .um, Miss. . ."

"Flossie," said Flossie.

"Thank you, Miss Flossie, a fine name, that. A house on a pond, you say. Nearby, I presume?"

"A mile upstream," said Needlenose.

"Oh, yes, Flossie's Pond, I was just reading about that. Pleasant place, big enough to be a lake, it is. Nice woods around it, too. Where on the shore were you wanting to build?"

"I don't want it on the shore," said Flossie. "I want it in the water."

"In the water, hmmm, yes, extraordinary," said the beaver, taking it all in stride, "a challenge, indeed. The water is high during heavy rains, it even floods sometimes. And, of course, the pond freezes in winter.

"Hmmm, in the water," he continued. "We build lodges in the water. No windows, though, and the entrance is underwater—doesn't seem right for you.

"Hmmm, I'll ask my brother to join us; he might have some ideas. Take a moment to look through this catalog while I find him."

Flossie and Needlenose paged through the catalog, looking at drawings of ranch homes, bungalows, oceanside villas, forest cabins, and even a tree house that looked like Golly's.

"Something for every occasion," said Flossie. "No Gothic

mansions, though."

The beaver soon returned with an identically dressed twin wearing his flat pencil behind his left ear.

"I've been discussing your most interesting idea with my brother, Ms. Flossie," said Right-Ear, the one they'd first met.

"Yes, yes," said Left-Ear, whistling his s's in the same way (though in the key of A-minor), "and we think it would be helpful to visit the site. The area itself may suggest some solutions."

"Follow me," said Needlenose. The party left the office and headed upstream.

Flossie's Pond was no small puddle. It was oval in shape, about a third of a mile long and a quarter-mile across, or half again as big as the meadow. A stream fed the pond at the north end where the trail from the meadow passed. Many small trickles of water flowed in from springs around the edge. Thick woods of aspen and birch surrounded the pond. The shore was flat, sandy beach in places; in other places the bank rose steeply, sometimes many feet high. A stream flowed out from the southern end where water rushed in a splashing cascade down a long slope of rocks.

"Delightful, delightful," said Left-Ear as they walked around the pond. "Many possibilities here, many." The brothers went from woods to water's edge and back again, looking at everything, making notes on pocket pads. The stream flowing from the pond drew their attention. They talked, paced about, pointed, drew in the sand, and looked at each other thoughtfully.

"Are you thinking what I'm thinking?" said Right-Ear in a low voice.

"I'm sure I am," said Left-Ear. "Do you think it might be possible?"

"We'd have to do tests."

"Yes, of course, tests."

"But it might work, don't you think?"

"It might."

"What are you two muttering about?" Flossie asked, stepping up behind them.

"Ms. Flossie," began Left-Ear, "we may be in a position to make you a generous offer."

"Yes, generous," said Right-Ear.

"I'm listening," said Flossie. Needlenose sat with his ears up as well.

"First," said Left-Ear, "tell us why you want the house in the water."

"I'm a *water bird*. I want to swim up to my house, not walk through woods or across rocky beach. I want to sit on the front porch and be in the water, or at least very near it. Water is my natural habitat. I want it all around me."

"Perfectly understandable," said Left-Ear. "You know, of course, that building in the water presents many problems. Water flowing and eroding is one, freezing and thawing, another; each leading to damage and, unfortunately, constant repairs."

"I know what I want," Flossie said.

"To be sure, to be sure," said Right-Ear, "but think about this." He led the group closer to where the stream flowed out of the pond.

"Listen," he said, "what do you hear?"

"Water," said Flossie. Indeed, the stream flowing down its rocky course gave the pleasant sound and feeling of a waterfall.

"Now, look," and Right-Ear pointed to a place a few hundred feet east of the stream. "See how the shoreline drops back over there to form a small bay? Water is rushing out of the stream here, yet is quite still over there. It even has a nice stretch of beach."

"I see that," said Flossie, "but what's that got to do with my house?"

"Everything, Ms. Flossie, everything," said Left-Ear. "Notice the bank is steep here, making a point of land between the stream and the bay. It's twenty feet high, maybe more, before it levels into the woods above."

"Could you get to the point, please?" said Flossie.

"It's quite simply this," said Left-Ear.

"Yes, simply and elegantly this," added Right-Ear.

"We propose," Left-Ear continued, "to build you a house over the water. We'll burrow into the side of the steep bank and build half the house there, underground. We'll extend the other half out over the pond."

"The front of the house will wrap around the bank from the stream to the bay," said Right-Ear. "With windows and porch all around, you'll see the pond straight ahead to the north, the cascading stream to the west, and the bay and beach to the east. Windows in the roof will let in sunlight. Glass floor panels will show the water below."

"The floor of the house will be a few feet above the water, five, maybe six," said Left-Ear. "We'll build a trap door there, giving you an entrance from below as well as those on either side."

Flossie looked interested.

"With the back of the house underground," said Right-Ear, "it will be out of the wind, thus warmer in the winter. You can have guest rooms there for someone like your needled friend here."

Needlenose looked interested.

"Building over the water avoids the problems we mentioned, yet gives you everything you want, maybe more."

"What keeps it up?" asked Flossie.

"Science," said both brothers at once, "balance and counterbalance. It won't fall down. We will stake our reputations on that."

"It does sound attractive," said Flossie, "but how will I ever afford it?" Smiles lit the faces of the look-alike brothers beaver.

"This brings us to the generous part of our offer," said Right-Ear.

"Indeed," said Left-Ear, "we've dreamed of a project like this for years, many years. If you bring a crew of steady workers to help with building, and agree to give a tour now and then for interested parties, we'll be pleased to build your home for the mere cost of its materials."

Flossie pressed for details. The brothers calculated, estimated, and paged through their pocket reference guides. They quoted an amount. Flossie bargained; the brothers wavered. Then they agreed.

"Your offer is generous," Flossie said. "I see only one problem."

"What is that?" they asked.

"I'm just a bird," Flossie said. "I don't have money in the bank, or anywhere. I really don't know how I would pay you."

"That's not a problem," said Right-Ear. "Do what your friend here did when we rebuilt his burrow. Work for us until the bill is paid off. With this wonderful new home, you'll be the perfect one to take over our advertising. Your house will be paid for in no time and we'll have enough business to keep a hundred beavers busy."

"It sounds wonderful," Flossie said, and she accepted their offer. She would have a delightful new home; a magnificent command post hanging just above water at the end of the pond, with views to all the world nearby.

"We're certain you'll be pleased," said Left-Ear. "We'll give Mary Moose a call at once and have her inspect the site."

"Manford's mother?" asked Needlenose.

"Yes, with her background in natural sciences, she's able to tell us which trees and plants are common and which shouldn't be disturbed. She helps us lay out the structure and grounds to take best advantage of the surroundings: the view, the foliage— that sort of thing. She's been most valuable to us. We're engineers, you know; we know about building—materials, construction, stability. Ms. Mary helps make our buildings fit with the land."

"Sounds sensible to me," Flossie said. "Okay, Needlenose, let's go find helpers."

"Who do we need?" he asked.

"Veronica is powerful and can dig. We'll have to ask her."

"Manford is strong, too," said Needlenose. "I'll bet he can lift and pull and do all sorts of jobs."

"Then we'll ask him," Flossie said. "Golly will be useful. In fact, let's ask everyone. There's sure to be something for us all to do."

They met Veronica and Manford at the other end of the pond coming down the path from the store. Ssam was looking out of Manford's pack. He was darting his head about and talking a steady streak.

"Look at those leaves on the trees. Aren't they amazing? And the flowers, so many shapes and colors, I can hardly believe it. What's that in the sky? Are those clouds? So that's what they look like! Wow, this is something. Heads up! Flossie and Needlenose ahead."

"What are you chattering about, Ssam?" Flossie asked.

"I can see, Flossie, I can see! Oh, it's so wonderful, *so unbelievable*."

"We all can see now," said Manford; "we got our new glasses today. Things aren't fuzzy and blurry anymore."

"It must be nice to see the world around you for a change," Flossie said.

"Where are you going now?" Needlenose asked.

"To the top of Lookout Hill," said Veronica, "to look at things far off and see what they're really like."

"Before you go," Flossie said, "In a few days, I'm going to need help. Are you available?"

"Sure," Manford said, "what kind of help?"

"I'm having a house built by Beaver Brothers. I'm supposed to bring workers."

"Sounds like fun," said Veronica. "We'll help."

"Where's your house going to be?" asked Ssam.

"At the end of the pond where the creek flows out."

"Yes, I can see it from here. Lovely spot. Can I help, too?"

"You're all invited, and tell Golly and Princess Columbine. Tell Aurora, too, if she hasn't already left for school."

"She's leaving tomorrow," Manford said. "The cooking academy has more openings in the summer. Even though they thought her application a bit unusual, they accepted her right away."

"You're having a going away party for her, I presume," said Needlenose.

"Of course," Manford said. "It's tonight, and we're expecting all of you."

Work on Flossie's house began a short time later. Flossie arrived early with six helpers. Beaver Brothers brought a crew of twelve, each wearing denim overalls and tool belts, each with a flat pencil in one location or another. The entire beaver crew whistled in a sort of harmony when they talked. The site was staked and marked with orange ribbons to show exactly where the house should go.

Veronica began digging the hole in the bank. Needlenose pushed dirt down a chute the beavers built, sending it into a wagon. Manford pulled the wagon downstream and dumped it in a sunken area of land. Flossie and Golly flew posts and planks to the site, holding on to slings fastened around the ends. The beavers used these to support the walls of the hole Veronica was digging, to keep it from caving in. The hole would extend thirty feet into the bank when completed, and be twelve feet high and twenty feet wide.

Ssam, scholar that he was, offered creative ideas and assisted Left-Ear and Right-Ear with designs, tests, and calculations.

Columbine flew back and forth carrying messages from one worker to another, becoming known as the Royal Princess Express. Mary came every day to help, too, often bringing lunch.

When the opening in the bank was finished, Veronica dug holes eight feet deep in a dozen places inside. These would be filled with concrete to help anchor the house in place. Manford mixed concrete by stomping up and down in a great tub and lifted buckets of it up to Veronica.

To support the house itself, four long, steel beams would be fastened to the concrete anchors once they had dried. Beaver Brothers had the beams in stock. To move them upstream, they made two pulling harnesses and cut short logs to use as rollers underneath. Veronica and Manford pulled the beams slowly along while Flossie and Golly flew roller logs from back to front. The crews lifted an end of each beam into the hole by cable, then pushed, pulled, winched, and dragged until each was bolted in place.

The house then began to take shape. Beavers did the framing while Flossie and crew hauled supplies. Columbine carried messages all the while: requests for more nails, measurements for cutting, orders for snacks.

The underground part of the house was built of concrete block, reinforced with steel, and sealed with tar. Manford and Veronica carried blocks while the beaver crew built walls. Ssam slipped about from place to place, sighting along edges, making sure everything was straight.

Needlenose did the tarring, crawling in the tight space between the dirt wall of the hole and the outside of the house. When he'd finished, the beavers hosed this space full of insulation to support the bank and keep the house warm. Needlenose lost more than a few quills in the process. In fact, he looked like Bre'r Rabbit's tar baby by the end of the day and had to have a bath in turpentine.

The house was planned to extend twenty feet over the water

at its farthest point. The front of it would be a three-quarter circle to give a 270 degree view. The framers left openings for huge windows all around and built a wraparound front porch. From inside the house or on the porch, Flossie could see the stream, the pond, the beach, the woods, and plenty of clouds and sky. She grew more excited as each day passed and more of the house came to be.

They completed the front roof by the end of week two. It was steep and gray shingled and extended from bank to bank around the front of the house. More than one beaver, denim overalls, tool belt and all, slid off it during shingling and splashed into the pond.

The top of the house would be a large sundeck, with the pitched roof around the front edge making a railing about three feet high. The deck would hold, the beavers said, the weight of birds, porcupines, moose, bears and all their friends and relations.

The crews soon moved inside. They built two guest rooms in the back of the house, along with a room for Flossie and a studio for her projects. The front part of the house had no dividing walls. Half the space was given to kitchen and dining areas. A lift, built into the kitchen wall, would allow Flossie to send refreshments to the upstairs deck. The rest of the area would be a large, open parlor. The openness would give Flossie a feeling of freedom and space, the beavers said, especially with windows catching light from all angles during the day.

The time came for Flossie to choose colors.

"Pink and gray," she said. "Those are my colors and that's what I want."

She had the outside of the house painted gray to blend with the surroundings, but inside was a different matter. Here she wanted pink walls and ceilings and gray carpet throughout. By the time woodwork, cabinetry, and windows were installed and the painting finished, every one had grown accustomed to pink and gray. Some even thought it rather nice.

Manford and Veronica kept busy outside. The house was built for a flamingo, not a moose or bear. Even though its outside measurements might have sounded large, the house wasn't big enough for them to fit inside. They hauled materials upstream and down and cleaned up the grounds. Sometimes, they went to the sundeck on the roof to sit. Flossie, Golly, and Needlenose joined them there now and then, until Columbine came fluttering up to them with a message for one or another.

The front part of the house hung six feet above the water. Flossie went there often. She had room underneath to swim and stand on one leg. The water was calm there, but she could swim outward into the current where the pond flowed into the stream.

Furniture Flossie had ordered began to arrive. A truck offloaded several dozen items a mile or so beyond Beaver Brothers where the dirt road crossed the creek on a bridge. Manford hauled them wagonload by wagonload upstream. There were couches, beds, tables, chairs, and lamps, all in pinks and reds and the white and gray shades of driftwood. Beavers carried everything inside through the bottom trap door.

It was special ordered furniture, built to the taste and size of a flamingo. It fit Golly and Flossie comfortably. Needlenose had to jump to reach the chairs. Had Manford and Veronica tried it, they would have splintered everything in which they sat. No worry, Flossie said; the deck would have iron patio furniture. It would support a bear or moose and not blow away in the wind.

The house was finished four weeks after work began. One day, beavers bustled about everywhere to finish small details, the next day they cleared away their tools and scraps and were gone. Flossie was left with her wonderful new house, her favorite old friends, and her non-stop view of the pond.

"I want to thank you for helping me," she said to the group gathered on the deck, "and I think the best way is with a party."

They cheered.

"Give me a few days to plan it, and some time to be alone in this new place then we'll have a grand wing-ding to celebrate."

They shouted hooray.

"Everyone rest up, clean up, and come back here at noon in three days and we'll fill up. It will be the official, grand opening celebration. I'll have things ready for you to have a good time."

They said they wouldn't miss it for the world.

And no one did. The forest friends arrived at Flossie's sundeck promptly at noon three days later. At Mary's suggestion, each brought a house warming gift. Left-Ear, Right-Ear, and several of the beaver crew came, too. Flossie had strung paper streamers along the deck railing and put festive tablecloths and napkins on the tables. The sun shone brightly that lovely summer day and made rippled reflections in the pond. The animals sat under patio table umbrellas to keep from getting too warm.

Flossie offered sodas and punch, sandwiches and salads, and snacks for those with particular needs. She'd filled an entire washtub with potato chips, for example, to make sure Needlenose felt at home. They played games, talked and chattered, and those who wanted to took a dip in the pond.

Flossie led a tour about mid-afternoon. Veronica and Manford watched through the windows as she took the other animals through the house to show off her guest rooms, her parlor, her color-coordinated furniture, and her wonderful, wraparound view. She'd decorated the guest rooms cheerily to make her friends feel at home should they want to stay. Her own room had a pink flamingo painted on the door, wearing a gray top hat, cut-away coat, and a long string of pearls.

Flossie served dessert outside—ice cream, cookies, chocolate cake with heaps of frosting—then opened her presents while the others ate. They'd brought her kitchen things, decorative things, things that would be useful around the house. She thanked each and everyone, assuring them their gifts would be used.

Then it was time for the announcement, time for the christening celebration.

Flossie stood at the very front of the deck. Just beyond her, over the railing, the roof pitched steeply down toward the water.

"It means a lot to me to have good friends," Flossie began, "friends nice enough to make a southern bird want to stay through a northern winter. You've made me feel welcome. I want you to feel welcome here in the house you helped build.

"I was lost when I first arrived. I wanted to go home, back to where I thought I belonged. Living here has been such fun that now I'm here to stay. This is my home—MorningGlory Forest, Flossie's Pond, and this house we've built. Thank you all."

The listeners cheered and dabbed at their eyes with kerchiefs.

Flossie had filled a large balloon with champagne. She threw it high in the air over the steep front roof. As it came down, burst on the roof, and splashed down into the pond, she said, "I christen this place Florida-by-the-Pond. Welcome one and all."

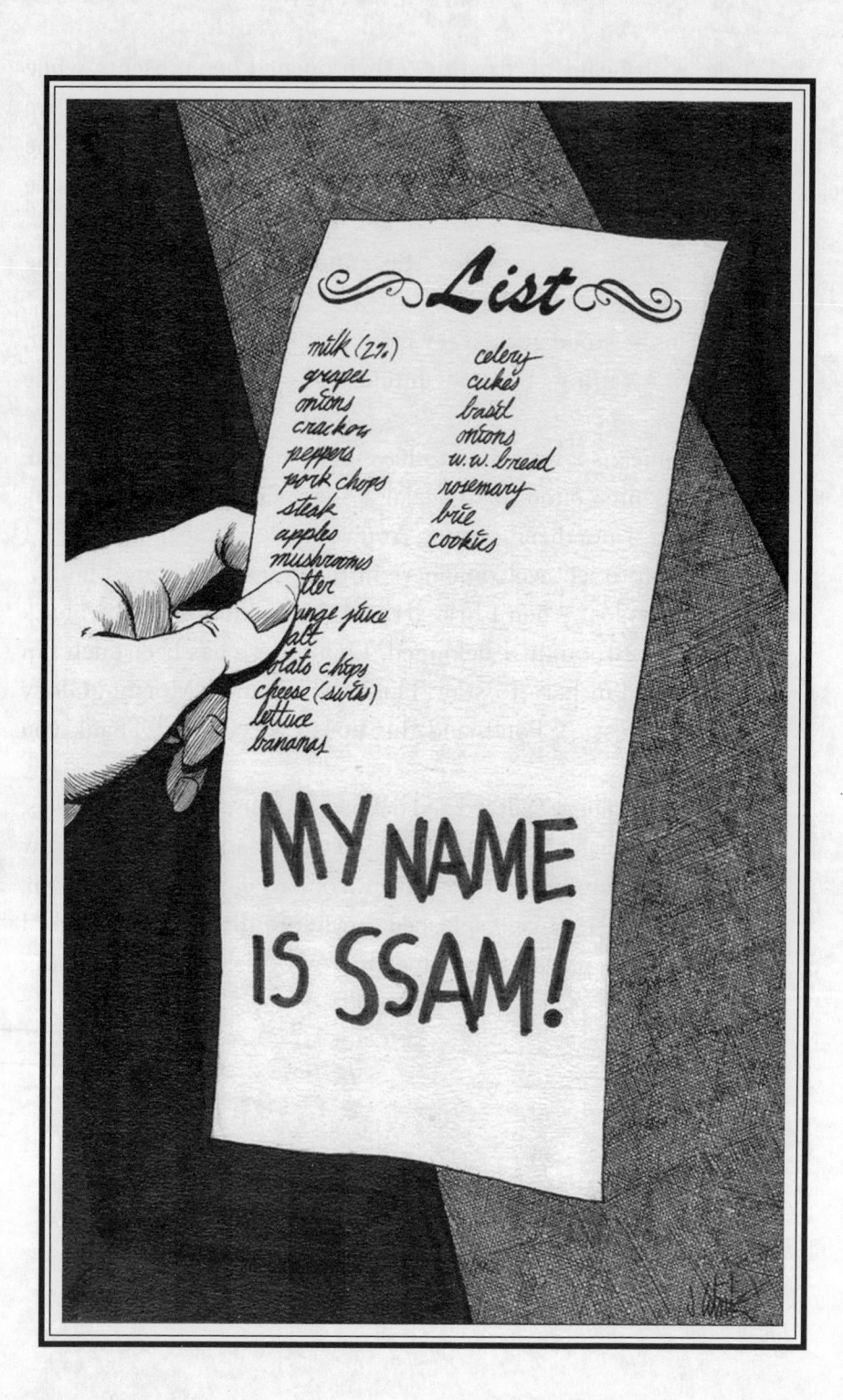
List
milk (2%)
grapes
onions
crackers
peppers
pork chops
steak
apples
mushrooms
lettuce
bananas
celery
cukes
basil
onions
w.w. bread
rosemary
brie
cookies
MY NAME IS SSAM!

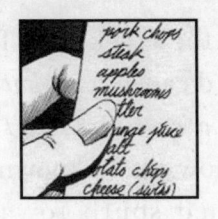

14

Message in the Dust
In which Ssam goes exploring and is taken prisoner

Ssam awoke at noon. He crawled from the pillow where he often slept near the fireplace and scooted up the entranceway to look outside. He saw a pleasant August day. Usually that meant he'd seek the nearest patch of sunshine and spend his time enjoying being warm. Not today. No, today he felt charged and full of energy. This was a day for traveling, for scouting out the neighborhood to see what he could see.

He wrote a note for Needlenose: GONE EXPLORING, BACK SOON. To write, Ssam held the pencil in his mouth and printed carefully in small, block letters. It wasn't easy. He didn't spend time on long explanations.

He went west along the path to the shore of Flossie's Pond. Another path, which he took south, joined it there. This was familiar territory; he'd seen it many times before. He came to Flossie's house as he rounded the end of the pond. He looked it over, remembering how busy they'd been building her this wondrous place to live. So many windows, he thought. It looks like a control tower for directing arriving and departing flocks of birds.

Ssam went on to the creek that flowed from the pond. Dragonfly Creek, they'd called it. *'That's nice,'* he thought. *'And there's a path along it, a route I haven't taken. Good, something new.'* He turned to follow the unknown path.

The way continued south toward Beaver Brothers' lumberyard. Ssam didn't walk, of course; he had no feet or legs. But that didn't matter. Moving back and forth in a constant S or "serpentine" pattern, he would rest on the back part of his body, push the front part forward, then rest on the front of his body and bring the back part up. Over and over he'd do this, so fast and smooth you'd think he had wheels and was zipping along tracks like a model train.

It was a mile downstream to Beaver Brothers' pond. This was beyond where Ssam might usually have gone but today he was exploring. He stopped to look at colorful rocks and mossy trees. He stopped to listen to chattering birds and water flowing in the stream. He stopped to flick his tongue and smell the scent of flowers in the air. It was a lovely way to spend the day.

He stopped at the garden they'd planted months before. He couldn't see it from the trail so he climbed a slender tree to look. The flowers' brilliant colors had made a lovely picture: MorningGlory and its brother-and-sister mountains in red and brown, a sky of blue with clouds of white, Golly's wildflowers making a forest of green, yellow, orange, and red. The animals came to see it often, to watch its progress as the flowers grew. *'Veronica's been eating the strawberries,'* Ssam said to himself. He returned to the trail and moved on.

Things looked different from Ssam's point of view. His head was barely an inch off the ground. Grass looked tall to him. A fallen log looked like a wall. And trees seemed impossibly big, almost like giants standing all around. With his new contact lenses, Ssam saw for the first time how big things really were. It filled him with wonder. He stopped again and again to note things as he passed.

He reached the pond in about an hour. Had he been an early riser and arrived by eight o'clock, he'd have found the water still as glass and reflecting the surrounding scene. Now breezes brushed the pond and pushed ripples gently to the shore. Ssam peered over the edge to look into the water. His reflection bobbed up and down. In places, it came apart. Ssam made a face at his image, then turned and headed round the pond to follow the creek farther south.

The path grew rougher here. Some distance ahead was the back country road where trucks had bumped along to deliver Flossie's furniture. Manford had brought the furniture from there in wagonloads, leaving wheel and hoof tracks where the ground was soft. Ssam followed the creekbank instead of staying with the trail, moving easily through grass and weeds along the water's edge. He covered another mile this way before returning to the path.

Being built close to the ground had advantages. Small openings were like wide doorways to Ssam. He could wiggle through the weeds and barely touch them as he went. And you could hardly see him. With his paint job of camouflage black-and-green, he blended with his surroundings and nearly faded from sight.

Which makes it hard to understand how what's about to happen ever happened. It's true Ssam's mind was drifting. Instead of tuning in to sights and sounds around him as he'd been doing up till now, he was thinking about the road. *'Should I cross it? Is it safe? It should be. It's narrow and dirt and has traffic only now and then.'* Or so Ssam supposed. And that's what he was doing, supposing about something that lay ahead instead of paying attention to what was happening nearby, when he ran into a foot.

Not a bird foot. Not a moose or bear foot, either; nothing like that at all. This particular foot wore a sneaker and belonged to a small boy standing in the trail. Before Ssam had time to think, the boy grabbed him behind the head and lifted him up to look into his eyes. Ssam felt silly to be so taken by surprise. Being small and fast and protectively colored doesn't do much good, you see, if you aren't paying attention.

'This was clever,' thought Ssam, but he wasn't really worried. There were several scary snake things he could do. He flicked his tongue to frighten the boy. It didn't work. The boy stuck his tongue out, too. He wrapped himself around an arm and tried to squeeze. The boy tightened his grip until Ssam began to want for air.

"What's your name?" the boy asked.

Ssam tried to shout it—the boy would surely drop him then—but he was being held too tightly to talk.

"I'm Eddie," said the boy. "Would you like to come home with me?"

'No, I wouldn't,' Ssam was thinking. *'I have a nice home already.'*

"I think I'll call you George," Eddie went on. Still firmly holding Ssam, he walked down the path toward the road.

'He can't be here alone,' Ssam figured. *'He's heading toward a car. Whoever brought him here will make him put me down.'*

Yes, there was a car ahead, a small red one, parked just off the road. A woman looked to be sleeping in the driver's seat—the boy's mother, Ssam presumed.

Creeping quietly to the car, Eddie reached through an open window and carefully pulled his yellow raincoat from the back seat. He stuffed Ssam into a pocket and zipped it shut, then rolled the coat into a ball and returned it to the car.

Ssam was left in the dark. He could breathe but was jammed so tightly in the pocket he could barely move. He heard no sound. Eddie had apparently gone away.

'Things are not improving,' thought Ssam. *'Time for strategy. Should I yell? A deafening voice booming,* "HELP, I'M BEING KIDNAPPED!" *from a rolled up raincoat in the back seat; would*

that work? Hmmm. . .the boy isn't afraid of me, but the lady might be. She might smash me with a shovel. Bad idea; I'll try something else.'

'Can I open the zipper?' Ssam asked himself. He worked his nose around to the inside of the pocket's zipper and tried to push it down. The entire pocket moved. He tried again, this time also wedging his tail above the zipper and pushing. No good; it still wouldn't move.

'Can I bite through the coat?' He tried, but garter snakes don't chew things, they swallow them whole. Their tiny teeth curve inward to hold the things they swallow, and they break off easily. Ssam bit the pocket repeatedly but the material was rubbery to shed the rain and seemed like chewing on a tire.

"EDDD-IE!" Ssam froze. It was the mother calling.

"I'm here," the boy answered, some distance away.

"Let's be going now."

Soon Eddie got in. The car started and moved slowly down the road.

'Bad news,' thought Ssam. He had more problems to deal with now, not only how to escape, but how to find his way back home. They'd soon be miles from any landmark he would recognize.

They rode for two hours, following the dirt road for a while, then smooth highway. The car made many turns. Ssam had no idea where he was going or where he'd been, especially riding in the dark. Eddie and his mother talked about the lovely weather; about the things they'd seen; about what to have for dinner; but they didn't speak of reptiles, particularly one zipped into a raincoat in the back seat. Eddie seemed to be saving this bit of news as a surprise.

At length the car slowed, turned sharply, and the woman cut its engine. Doors opened. Ssam felt the raincoat being lifted and carried through more opening doors, then set down. A door closed. Time passed.

'He's home,' thought Ssam. *'What's he doing?'* Ssam heard moving, bumping sounds, shuffling, scraping sounds. Hands lifted the coat again and unrolled it. *'Now's my chance,'* Ssam thought. As the zipper opened, he flung himself from the pocket to try to get away. He dropped in a thrashing heap on sand, smooth sand at the bottom of an empty aquarium. He darted a look around—glass walls on every side. He looked up. Eddie was covering the open top with a screen.

"Welcome to my house, George," Eddie said. "This is your place now. I hope you like it."

Ssam gritted his tiny, inward-curving teeth. Complications had piled on complications. He'd need another strategy now. He had to settle down, think, make a plan, but all that came to mind just then was, *'Don't call me George.'*

So we, too, pause to review the situation. Ssam is safe but held captive. He doesn't know where he is and couldn't find his way back if he did. It's late in the afternoon. Clearly, Ssam won't be "back soon" as his note to Needlenose promised.

Eddie, who is eight years old, thinks he has a nifty new pet. He hasn't told his mother yet so he will have some explaining to do. Surprises may be in store for Eddie, but not just from his mother. There is much he doesn't know about Ssam.

We don't yet know much about Eddie's mother, whose name is Gloria, but she'll surely soon ask, at a minimum, "Eddie, where did you get this?"

"Eddie, (ah, there she is now) where did you get this?" It was an hour later and she'd come to fetch the boy for dinner. Ssam tried to burrow into the sand.

"Get what?" said Eddie, ever the innocent little boy.

"The garter snake in your aquarium, that's what."

"Oh, that."

"Yes, that. It wasn't here this morning."

"I found him in the woods. I wanted to give him a good home."

"How do you know it didn't have one?"

'Good point,' thought Ssam.

"Out there in the woods?" said Eddie.

"Uh huh," said Gloria. "That's where animals live, you know. What if one of them took you to the woods to give you a good home, in a tree or cave or someplace? How would you like that?"

'Excellent point!' thought Ssam. *'Eddie, pay attention.'*

"I needed something for show-and-tell at school."

"It's August, Eddie. You have another month till school."

"I'll have time to learn more about him this way."

"What you should learn," Gloria replied in a patient, motherly way, "is that it's dangerous to pick up animals in the woods, especially snakes. Some can hurt you and make you sick. Don't you remember me telling you that?"

"George is just a garter snake," said Eddie. "He won't hurt me."

'I'm not GEORGE!' Ssam said to himself, his eyes starting to bulge and his ears starting to ring. Ssam can even think in a loud voice, you see.

"You're not answering my questions very well, Eddie."

"But I want to keep it, Mom. Can I?"

'Absolutely not,' thought Ssam, *'no, no, no.'*

"Why didn't you ask when you found it instead of bringing it home without telling me?"

"I thought you'd say no."

"I probably would have," Gloria replied. She looked closely at Ssam through the glass.

"Though it is a pretty thing," she said.

'Thank you,' thought Ssam. *'Now, please take me home.'*

"So, can I keep him?" Eddie asked.

"What will you feed it?"

"He's not an it. His name is George."

'My name is SSAM—SSAM, SSAM, SSAM,' Ssam wanted

to shout.

"What will you feed him?" Gloria repeated.

"He eats mice, doesn't he?" Eddie said. "He can probably find his own if I let him loose."

"Not in this house, you won't. He stays in that tank until we can take him back to where you found him. Where was that. Do you remember?"

"Near an old road, I guess."

"Which one? We were on several today."

"Where you were sleeping."

"I don't remember where that was. It might be hard to find again but then, I suppose anywhere will do. Come to dinner now." She left the room.

"You hear that, George?" Eddie said with a smile. "You can stay. We're going to be friends."

'So, this is how little boys do things,' thought Ssam. *'He sneaks me into the house and pretends I'm a project for school. He ignores everything his mother says, and when she distinctly tells him I'm to go back home what he hears is that I can stay. When it's time to take me back, he'll probably say,* "But Mom, you said I could keeeeep him."*'*

Ssam moped around the confining tank beset with disappointment. The lady hadn't mentioned when they'd take him home. Tomorrow? Next week? When? And what if they couldn't find the right place? Anywhere certainly wouldn't do! Ssam probed the tank's corners with his nose and pushed against the screen. He discovered what he'd expected; there was no easy way out.

'I wonder if Needlenose has missed me,' he thought. *'Will my friends be worried? But then, what good would it do? They would never find me. They won't know where to look.'*

He coiled up on the sand in the center of the tank and his head drooped sadly over his tail. And while Eddie ate dinner in a room down the hall, Ssam thought, and thought, and thought.

'Strategy: What do I have to work with?

'Well, for one thing, no one has shrieked, "Eeeek, a snake, kill it." That's a plus. They're even trying to be nice.

'What else? Hmmm. . .they don't know I can understand them or that I can talk, and that I can do so very loudly. They'd keep me for sure if they knew. I'll keep that a secret, at least for now.

'What else? Aha, one more thing, I have Manford's phone number. If I can get out of this tank and find a phone when no one's looking, I can call Manford and tell him where I am.

'Except. . .I don't know where I am. And I can't get out of this tank. And what's Manford going to do about it? A few details remain to be worked out, I can see.'

Thus Ssam gathered his resources—the first thing to do when you're in a jam—and made the beginnings of a plan. Eddie returned from dinner then, lifted him from the tank, and carried him around the house.

"This is the kitchen," the boy said, pointing Ssam at different parts of the room. "And here's the living room where we watch TV." They watched two minutes of the program playing then moved on. "That hallway goes to a guest room." Eddie showed everything to Ssam as if expecting him to be interested. Ssam was. He noted what he saw, particularly the location of the phones.

"This is Mom's office," his tour guide continued, going into another room, "and here's our computer. Want to play a game, George?"

'I WANT YOU TO STOP CALLING ME GEORGE!' Ssam thought loudly. Had word balloons appeared above his head, they would have held angry, black capital letters.

Eddie turned on the computer and showed Ssam what he knew, explaining things as if planning to give a quiz. Ssam would have passed. He remembered what he saw, including the instructions on the screen. After a long evening of games Ssam found to be a lot of fun, Eddie finally went to bed. He returned

Ssam to the aquarium and, alas, firmly replaced the screen.

Five days went by. Eddie paid him much attention at first, taking him outdoors, watching TV, playing computer games, but he was losing interest. Ssam spent more and more of his time alone in the tank while Eddie was who knows where.

Gloria's good intentions also seemed to fade. She'd talked once of taking Ssam back to the woods but had said no more about it. She'd been making plans for the coming weekend and those that followed, but her agendas never included Ssam.

Ssam wanted to go home. He wanted to call Manford to let him know he was okay. His MorningGlory Forest friends must surely miss him now.

Finally, the opportunity came. Eddie was tossing his pillow around his room one afternoon when it bounced off the aquarium. Eddie picked up the pillow but didn't notice it had bumped the screen aside and left an opening.

Ssam waited for evening, for them to turn out the lights and go to sleep. They dawdled about it forever, of course, watching TV, making snacks in the kitchen, talking on the phone. Eddie finally went to bed hours after dark.

"Read me a story," he said, and his mother did, some interminable tale about a long sea voyage, fierce storms, and great riches never quite realized. Eddie went to sleep. Ssam almost went to sleep. Long past midnight, Gloria retired and the house at last grew quiet.

Ssam raised his head to the top of the tank, pulled himself through the opening, and dropped quietly to the table outside. He hung from the table's edge, then wound easily around a leg and spiraled down it to the floor. He zigzagged out Eddie's bedroom door and down the hall. In the darkened living room, he climbed another table leg and reached the phone next to the couch. Magazines were strewn there. In dim moonlight coming through the front windows, he read the delivery address.

Ssam pushed the phone off the hook. It toppled backward, falling on the magazines and making little noise. He punched out Manford's number with his nose, then listened at the receiver for an answer. He heard clicking and switching sounds, then ringing: one. . .two. . .three. . .four. . .

"Hel-lo." It was Manford, sounding very sleepy.

"Manford, it's Ssam," said Ssam in a whispery voice.

"Who?" said Manford. "I can't hear you."

"Ssam."

"Sam," Manford said, not realizing what he'd heard. "Sam. . . wait. . .our Ssam? Ssam, is that you?"

"Yes," said Ssam, darting his head between the speaking and listening ends of the receiver, "but I can't talk long."

"Where are you?" Manford asked. "We've been looking for you for days. We've been terribly worried. Are you okay?"

"I'm not hurt. A little boy picked me up near the road beyond Beaver Brothers and took me home with him."

"We thought it was something like that," said Manford. "We found your tracks."

"Mine?"

"Yes, and the footprints and tire tracks, too."

"You must have really been looking to find all that," said Ssam, suddenly pleased that his friends had been so concerned.

"Does this boy keep you in his room?" Manford went on.

"Uh huh."

"In a glass tank with sand in it?"

"Yes," said Ssam, surprised. "How did you know that?"

"We used the necklace. I saw a room with clothes and toys, and something like an aquarium with you inside, but couldn't tell anything more."

"Here's the rest of it, then," said Ssam. "The address is 173 Blackwood Terrace in Rockport, Washington, though I don't know where that is. The people's name is Parkhurst." He read

Manford the number off the phone as well.

"I'm writing it down," said Manford and, after a pause, read everything back.

"Right," said Ssam. "Now please come get me. They said they'd take me back but I think they've forgotten about it. Good thing; they don't remember where to go. They might dump me anywhere."

"I'll tell the others right away," said Manford. "We'll find you, don't worry."

"Thanks," said Ssam, "see you soon." He coiled his tail around the receiver, lifted it, and hung it up.

'Good,' he thought. *'They know I'm okay and they know where I am. We'll see what happens next.'* Ssam moved silently about the house. He had no intention of returning to the tank; he'd had quite enough of that. *'Hmmm...I was exploring when they found me, wasn't I? Maybe I'll pick up where I left off.'*

Nobody noticed Ssam missing at all the first day. Eddie went to and from his room, took playthings outside and brought them back (some of them, anyway), woke up and went to sleep ten feet from the aquarium, but never once noticed it was empty. Now you can guess why there was nothing in it to begin with. If he'd ever had fish, he'd probably lost interest in those, too.

Gloria rose early and worked a full day and part of the evening in her office. She operated a travel service from her home. Eddie's dad drove eighteen-wheel trucks. He was gone much of the time but would often call in the evenings. Gloria was sound asleep by ten o'clock. There was no great to-do about Ssam's disappearance, no search for him high and low, no notice of him, or the lack of him, at all. Color the day "uneventful."

Oh, there was one small thing. Gloria was writing "bananas" on the grocery list when she noticed it.

"Eddie, did you write this?" she asked when he happened by.

"What?"

"This," and she showed him where it was written, in small block letters, *"MY NAME IS SSAM!"*

"Not me," said Eddie.

"You're sure."

"Uh huh, I wrote this one," and he pointed to where it said "cookies."

"That does look more like your writing. Hmmm, how strange." Then her mind passed on to other things and the incident was forgotten.

The second day wasn't so quiet. Gloria went to her office early that morning and found the computer running.

"I thought I turned that off," she said aloud. She passed by it to sit at her desk then looked back at the screen.

"And I certainly didn't write that!" she said.

In the screen's very center were the words, *"MY NAME IS SSAM!"*

"Eddie!" she called. He didn't answer.

"Where are you, Eddie?" She looked outside. He wasn't there. She went to his room and found him standing in front of the empty aquarium.

"George is gone," he said, sounding a trifle sad. "Have you seen him?"

"George who?"

"My garter snake; he's not here."

"You mean he's loose in the house? Wonderful! Was he in there this morning?"

"I don't know."

"You don't know?" Gloria said. "Didn't you notice?"

"Huh uh."

"Was he there yesterday?"

"I don't know."

"When did you last see him?"

"A few days ago, I think," said Eddie.

"You don't look after your pets very well, young man. Did you ever feed him?"

"No."

"Why not?"

"I couldn't catch any mice," Eddie answered. "He didn't look hungry anyway."

"How would you know whether he looked hungry or not? You'd better start hunting for him, Eddie. He'd better be back in that tank by bedtime."

"Will you help me?"

"I will if you don't find him right away, but I have some business to finish first. Which reminds me, come with me a minute." He followed to her office.

"I found this on the computer this morning," she said, pointing at the screen. "Did you do that?"

"No," said Eddie, eyes wide and innocent, "it wasn't me."

"You'd better be telling the truth because I sure didn't write it. If you didn't, either, I wonder who did."

"That's what was on the grocery list," Eddie said.

"Yes, it is. Something odd is going on around here. You'd better start looking for George."

Eddie went to his room. He looked under his bed and in his closet. He looked in all his dresser drawers and behind the desk and chair. He looked and looked for at least half an hour, then his attention wandered and he went outside.

"Have you found him?" his mother asked at noon when she made lunch.

"Not yet," Eddie answered.

"Looks like I'd better help you," she said. They began in the living room doing one piece of furniture at a time. They'd move a chair to look under it, pull out cushions if there were any, then tip it over to look at the underside. Finding nothing, they'd move on to something else. Unlike Eddie, Gloria was thorough and methodical and kept to her work.

When they'd checked the furniture, she dumped the magazine rack and looked there. She took flower arrangements out of pots and looked inside. She even took the back off the TV set in case Ssam had wiggled in there. Finding nothing in the living room, they moved on to the next room, then the next.

Ssam, meanwhile, had found a foolproof place to hide. Water pipes led into the wall under the kitchen sink and the opening was wide enough for him to crawl inside the wall. A small bonus came with this. As Eddie had predicted, there were mice. . .

Reaching the kitchen, the searchers started with the bottom cupboards. Eddie's attention was seriously flagging by now but his mother kept him to the task. They took everything out of each cupboard, then put it back. The bottom row finished, they moved appliances—stove, refrigerator, dishwasher—and looked and swept under each. There was no sign of Ssam.

Daylight was fading when they began searching the top row of cupboards.

"I'm hungry," said Eddie.

"Keep looking," his mother said. "You got us into this." They found nothing in the top cupboards, either.

It was when she looked on the very top of the top cupboards that Gloria screamed.

"Did you find him?" asked Eddie.

She said nothing, but stood pointing, her face a mask of disbelief. Eddie climbed onto the counter and stretched to see where she was looking.

There, written large in the dust was, *"MY NAME IS SSAM!"* A telltale serpentine track led through the dust to the far end of the cupboard where Ssam had found his way down.

"It's your friend, George," Gloria said. "He wrote this and probably those other messages, too! How can this be?"

"Um. . .I guess his name isn't George," said Eddie.

But this time, his mother wasn't listening.

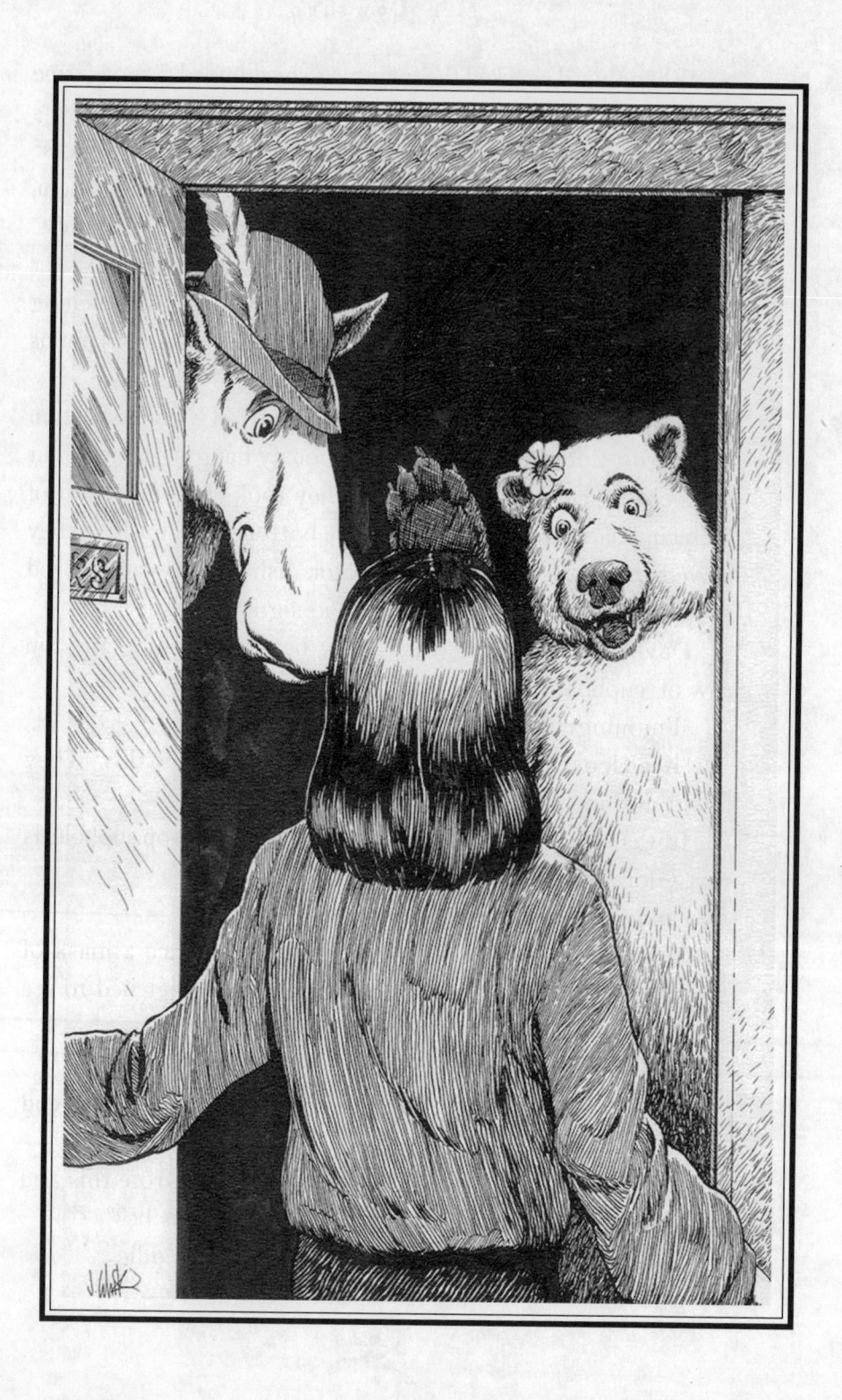

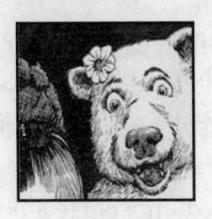

15

Rescue at Eight, Black Tie Optional

In which a visitor returns, and brings magic

[NOTE: Let's go back two days to Page 234—at the top, where Ssam hangs up the phone after telling Manford where he is—and tell that part of the story again, this time from another point of view. . .]

Manford hung up the phone. Ssam was okay! What super news! The others would want to know; he had to tell them right away. He rushed to call Flossie. She took a long time to answer.

"Hello, have you any idea what time it is?"

"I just heard from Ssam and he's okay," Manford said.

"It's two o'clock in the morning, Manford," Flossie fussed. "Didn't you notice that before. . .wait, did you say something about Ssam?"

"He just called. He said he was okay."

"Thank goodness for that. Where is he?"

"In a town some ways from here. A boy picked him up and took him home. Ssam gave me the address."

"Then we were right."

"Yes," Manford said, "we guessed pretty close. Now we have

to get everyone together. You find Golly and Needlenose and—"

"Slow down, slow down," Flossie said. "There's nothing we can do now. Go back to sleep. If Ssam found a way to call you, he'll be safe for a while."

"We should tell Needlenose. He's been really sad."

"Just go to sleep, Manford. Wake everyone up at first light and we'll get started then."

"I suppose," Manford said. "Goodbye."

"But thanks for telling me," Flossie said. "It's nice to know."

The light came on in the hall and Manford's mother entered his room.

"I heard the phone ring," she said. "Is something happening?"

"It was Ssam. He called to say he's okay."

"That's wonderful news!"

"He's in a town somewhere and we have to go rescue him. I called Flossie to get everyone together."

"At this hour? What did she say?"

"To wait till morning."

"That's probably best," Mary said.

"But I should tell Needlenose and Veronica and Golly. They'll want to know."

"Do that if you wish, but sleeping till morning first won't hurt."

"Okay, Mom."

But Manford couldn't sleep. There was so much to do! He tossed and rolled on his bed. Minutes passed by like hours. Morning would never come at this rate. He got up and left the house.

Manford walked through quiet, shadowy woods. The moon was low in the sky and gave enough light to see the pathway ahead. He moved quickly along and soon came out of the trees into

WhiteFlower Meadow. He looked up. The night sky was clear and bright with stars. The moon hovered just behind the meadow's big tree, lighting its branches in black silhouette.

"Hey," Manford said, "the moon was over there..." He looked toward MorningGlory Mountain where he'd thought he'd seen it before. Sure enough, the moon was there, too.

"Wha..." He looked back to the tree. The light behind it was moving toward him. It passed through the tree and settled to the ground near him. *It wasn't the moon.*

"Hello, Manford," it said.

"Mountain Spirit," said Manford, "hello..."

"You have news from your missing friend."

"Yes, he's okay. I'm on my way to tell the others."

"Good," said the voice, "but be careful."

"Of what?" Manford asked.

"People in cities don't always understand that you can talk, read and write, and comprehend what they say."

"Mr. Johnny does, and Mr. Turner, too."

"They came to you. They saw you in your home, the forest, and it made sense to them there. It will be different when you go to town."

"What should we do?"

"Do what attracts the least attention."

"We'll have to be clever, is that what you mean?"

"Yes."

"Can you help us?"

"I will give you this." The spirit extended a wispy arm of light. A small rock at Manford's feet began to glow. "Keep it with you. It will help you when you are in need."

"How do I use it?"

"When the time comes, you will know. Goodbye, Manford. Come visit my mountain again."

"Goodbye..." Manford said.

The light moved away from him then, through the trees

and off toward MorningGlory Mountain. The rock at Manford's feet continued to glow. He set it near the tree where he'd find it later, then galloped up Lookout Hill, down the path, and around the pond to Haystack Hollow.

"Needlenose," he called at the entrance, out of breath. "Needlenose, wake up, it's Manford."

"Just a minute," came a sleepy voice from deep within the burrow. Needlenose emerged moments later.

"What is it?" he said. Manford told him of the call from Ssam.

"What a relief!"

"I was happy, too," said Manford, "but we have lots to do. We have to rescue Ssam, and the Mountain Spirit said we'd have to be careful."

"You saw the spirit again? Where?"

"In the meadow. At first I thought it was the moon."

"I wish I'd get to see it sometime."

"We should start right away," Manford went on. "It'll be light in two hours. I'll get Golly and Veronica and meet you in the meadow then."

"Okay," said Needlenose, "I'll bring Flossie and Columbine." Manford was already running down the path on his way to Misty Falls.

The animals had not been idle in the time since Ssam had disappeared. Needlenose had seen Ssam's note in mid-afternoon and had begun to wonder when he wasn't back by dark. After checking on and off through the night, Needlenose told the others next morning there might be something wrong.

They'd started searching at once. Needlenose looked in Ssam's favorite spots, where he would lay in the sun on nice days, but found no sign of him. Manford followed the trail toward MorningGlory Crossing thinking that for some reason Ssam might have gone there. He hadn't, as far as Manford could tell.

Flossie had checked the paths around the pond and found S-marks in the sand. Veronica put her nose to work then and followed Ssam's trail to Beaver Brothers. The marks continued down the trail for a while, then disappeared. Columbine found them again a mile farther on and they traced them to a set of small footprints. There the trail ended.

From the automobile tire tracks found at the road, with the same small footprints nearby, they were able to guess what had happened. Golly followed the tire marks to the highway, noting that the car had turned north. He couldn't tell where it had gone from there.

They'd used the necklace then. Manford gathered everyone in a circle as they'd done in The Place With No Trees. In his mind, he'd seen Ssam in a boy's room, in an aquarium. As it turned out, that was where he had been; but until Ssam called with the details, they didn't know the exact location.

Dawn lit the sky slowly, turning it from starlit black to dim, pearly gray, then gradually lighter and lighter to shades of orange and pink. Flossie, Golly, Needlenose, Veronica, Princess Columbine, Mary, and Manford gathered in the meadow. Manford recounted details of Ssam's phone call, of his pre-dawn visits to everyone, and his talk with the Mountain Spirit.

"The spirit said to be careful," he told them. "People in town might think we're strange. We have to be clever."

"Was there anything more specific?" Mary asked.

"It gave me a rock." Manford found it at the base of the tree and held it up. "It said this would help us."

"What does it do?" asked Veronica.

"It glowed when the spirit touched it."

"Doesn't sound exactly useful," said Needlenose. "Anything else?"

"I don't know. The spirit said we'd know what to do when

the time came."

"Sounds like your spirit friend, all right," said Flossie.

"Carry it in your pack with your other things," said Columbine. "The necklace helped us after the spirit touched it. This might, too."

"What happens now?" asked Veronica.

Golly unfolded a map on the ground. "Here's where Ssam is," he said, pointing to a small town northwest of MorningGlory Forest. "It's about fifty road miles from here. We have to go there, find Ssam, bring him back and, as the spirit said, not attract too much attention."

"That's a long way," said Needlenose. "It would take me days to walk it."

"Golly and Flossie can fly," said Veronica. "They'd only take an hour or so."

"I could fly there, too," said Princess Columbine.

"Hold on, team," said Flossie. "Knocking on these people's door and saying, 'Hi, we're from the forest and we'd like our friend back' probably isn't the best idea. We don't know anything about them, whether they're good or bad or crazy or what. With half a dozen talking animals at their door, who knows what they might do."

"Flossie's right," said Golly.

"Let's find out something about them," said Mary.

"How do we do that?" asked Needlenose.

"You have their phone number, don't you, Manford?"

"Uh huh, Ssam gave it to me."

"I get it," Flossie said, "we'll call and ask questions like we're doing a survey."

"Good idea," said Veronica.

"Maybe something like that," Mary continued. "What time is it?"

"It's still only seven in the morning," said Manford.

"Too early for phone calls, but it is time we decided what to do. Why don't you all come to Moostery Manor for breakfast? Afterward, we'll make this call and work out our plan." Everyone thought this was a wonderful idea and followed Mary down the path.

Flossie and Manford helped her serve breakfast. The group ate at the dining room table, either in thoughtful silence or, in no particular direction, thinking out loud. It was nearly nine by the time they'd cleared everything away.

"Okay," Mary said, "let's get started."

They gathered round the phone as she punched in the numbers. She was nervous, not knowing what she would say. When a voice answered, "Parkhurst Travel Service, this is Gloria," she nearly dropped the phone.

"Hello," Mary said, trying to think quickly, "I've. . .um. . . been thinking about a trip to. . .Australia, and I wonder if you can help me."

"Sure," said the voice on the phone. "There are airline tours visiting major cities, bus tours to any part of the country, bed and breakfast tours you drive yourself, or you could rent a motor home and go where you like. Did you have something in mind?"

"I want to see scenery and animals."

"Good choice; that's my favorite, too. A private bus tour might be best. Will you be traveling by yourself?"

"No, I have a youngster to take along. He'll enjoy this kind of thing."

"How wonderful," Gloria said. "My boy, Eddie, goes with me on trips sometimes. He's crazy about animals. If you give me your address, I'll send you some brochures."

"Oh, don't go to any trouble," said Mary. "I'll just stop by and look at them. Are you at 173 Blackwood Terrace?"

"That's right."

"Will I have trouble locating you?"

"The office is in my home but it's not hard to find." She gave directions.

"Thank you," Mary said, writing the directions down. "I'll stop by sometime next week. Goodbye." She hung up the phone.

"That sounded interesting," said Flossie.

"It was," Mary said. "The lady's name is Gloria Parkhurst, she has a son named Eddie whom she takes on trips because they both like animals, and she operates a travel service from her home. Here are directions for getting there."

"Whoa, great sleuthing," said Needlenose.

"Why Australia?" asked Manford.

"It was the first place I thought of."

"Okay," said Golly, "now we need a plan to rescue Ssam. What are we going to do? Who's going to do it? Ideas, anyone?"

"We all want to go, don't we?" Manford said.

"Sure," said Veronica.

"But that may not be best," said Mary.

"Maybe Golly and Flossie should fly there now," said Needlenose. "They could look the place over and come back to tell us what it's like."

"I could do that," Golly said.

"You could, but not me," said Flossie.

"Why not?"

"A pink flamingo in western Washington? I'd be pretty conspicuous, don't you think? I'd be on the Audubon Hot Line in half an hour. The neighborhood would fill up with birders with binoculars."

"Pretend you're a lawn ornament," said Needlenose. "Stand very still."

"Great," said Flossie.

"I could go with Golly," said Columbine. "I'm very small and can stay out of sight."

"Good idea," Mary said. "You two should go when we're finished here."

"Is that the start of our plan?" Manford asked.

"That's right," his mother replied, "but we're going to need much more than that. Keep thinking, everybody."

The animals thought and thought. They offered ideas, talked them over, then fell silent to think some more.

They talked about how to get themselves into the house.

They talked about how to get the people out of the house.

They talked about disguises, about going to the house delivering telegrams or flowers, or pretending they were repairmen of some kind. They talked about creating diversions and confusions. Ideas ran hot and ran cold and often sounded like a lot of movies they'd seen.

They talked and plotted the rest of the morning, and out of all the talk eventually came a plan; a plan, they agreed, that just might work. They left the house and went outside. "Time to be going, Princess," said Golly. "Are you flying or riding?"

"I'll ride, thank you," Her Butterfly Loveliness replied, and she fluttered to Golly's back.

"We'll return by dark," Golly said, and he took off. Soon, he was just a dot in the sky far to the northwest.

"Time for the rest of you to get busy, too," said Mary.

"Okay," Manford said and he, Veronica, Flossie, and Needlenose departed to work the next part of the plan.

Which was: Figure out how to use the rock the Mountain Spirit had given Manford. If it was going to help them, Flossie had said, it would be nice to know how. They sat in a circle in the meadow trying to decide how to start. "Let's try what works with the necklace," said Needlenose. They joined wings and hoofs and paws, closed their eyes and thought about…and that was just the problem, there was nothing specific to think about like "Where is Columbine?" or "Where is Ssam?"

Manford balanced the rock on his nose and they tried again, all thinking, *'What does it do?'*

"Nothing happens," he said. "It doesn't get hot or cold, or

anything. It just sits there."

"Let's try one at a time," said Veronica.

So they each took the rock in turn and did what seemed right, pressing it to their heart, holding it in their eye, tossing it into the air. Veronica even danced around the tree with it. They thought profound thoughts and chanted mysterious verses. None of it revealed the rock's secret. Hours passed as they each tried several times.

"Are you sure you have the right rock?" said Flossie.

"I think so," Manford said. "I found it right where I left it. It was still glowing a little."

"Why did you leave it there, anyway?"

"I wasn't wearing my pack. Moose don't have pockets, y'know."

"Gee, none of us do," said Veronica. "I never thought about that."

"I would have thought you'd find a better place to hide it," Flossie said. The rock grew suddenly warm in Needlenose's paw and gave off a great cloud of fog that enveloped the four of them and the tree as well.

"What happened?" they said all at once.

"Where are you?"

"Who has it?"

"I do," said Needlenose. "It got warm all of a sudden then fogged us in."

"Okay, I see you," said Manford as the cloud thinned a bit. "What were you thinking when it did that?"

"That this was a strange way to spend the afternoon."

"That's probably not it," said Veronica. "Maybe it was what Flossie said."

"What did I say?" asked Flossie.

"Something about a place to hide it," said Manford. Another cloud burst from the rock, making their cover even thicker.

"It's a secret word rock," said Needlenose. "I'll bet it does that every time you say hide." More fog came and they saw nothing but solid white cloud.

"Let's get out of this," Manford said. They walked this way and that, bumping into each other and into the tree. They couldn't find the cloud's edge. They couldn't even see the ground.

"It's either a very big cloud or it's following us," said Veronica.

"Maybe there's also a word to make it go away," said Needlenose.

"Be careful," said Flossie, "we might make it rain or snow or freeze."

Nothing happened at any of these words so they tried others. The most obvious, "clear," dissolved the fog and they stood in sunny meadow again.

"Pardon me for being dense," said Flossie, "but what good is a rock that makes it impossible to see where you're going?"

"Maybe if you say the word softly you only get a little cloud," said Veronica.

This was the case, they discovered. They could make the cloud as thick or as thin, as large or as small as they wished, and it did follow when they moved.

"This is just what we needed," said Manford. "It's perfect. Let's go tell Mom."

Golly returned a while later. Columbine did not.

"Where is she?" Mary asked.

"She's in the house," Golly answered.

"Oh, dear," Flossie said, "is she a prisoner now, too?"

"No," Golly said. "She flew in an open door and perched on a vase of flowers. With her wings folded flat, they'll never see her. I watched through the windows and didn't see anything unusual happening inside. Either Ssam crawled back into the tank after he phoned you or they haven't noticed he's missing."

"What's Columbine going to do?"

"When everyone's sleeping, she'll find Ssam and tell him the plan."

"Good idea," said Mary.

"We figured out the rock," Manford said, and he went on to tell of their successful experiment in the meadow.

It was soon evening. The next step was for Manford, Veronica, and Golly to go to town. Manford wore his backpack; Golly rode on Veronica's shoulder. They made their way to Beaver Brothers, went on down the trail to the road, then took it in the direction the tire tracks had gone. Golly knew the way and guided them easily. They walked quickly, trotting almost, through brightly moonlit forest. They said little as they went and covered thirty miles of dirt road by an hour past midnight.

They turned into the woods at the highway, choosing to cover the next twenty miles out of sight. They reached Rockport in the dark hours of early morning and found a sheltered place in the woods to sleep. Other parts of the plan would now unfold. There was nothing for them to do until it was dark once again.

Other players in this drama were sleeping as well. Flossie, Needlenose, and Mary were sleeping. Gloria was asleep, and so was Eddie. As Golly had observed, they hadn't yet noticed Ssam missing. Columbine had found Ssam and told him the plan. Now she was sleeping, too, hidden in plain sight on a vase of brilliant tiger lilies.

Only Ssam was awake. He'd turned on the computer and was at the keyboard, pressing the keys with his nose. Large capital letters now lit up the center of the screen, *MY NAME IS SSAM!* He smiled.

Veronica and Manford slept till late in the afternoon. Golly roosted on a branch just above them.

When they woke and lay waiting for darkness, Manford

suddenly said, "There's a problem with our plan."

"What's that?" said Veronica.

"We're going to the people's house tonight, right?"

"Right."

"We're going to pretend we're people dressed up like a bear and a moose, right?"

"Uh huh."

"But we're dirty. We have dust all over us from walking fifty miles, and we're covered with dirt and leaves from sleeping here. We're a mess."

"We could brush each other off," said Veronica.

"Yes," answered Manford, "but we're still going to smell like a bear and a moose."

"So? That's what we are."

"That's the problem. They'll never believe we're people dressed in costume if we smell like a bear and a moose."

"Hmmm. . .maybe you're right."

"We need a bath."

"We can jump in a pond," said Veronica. "That's what we do at home."

"I don't remember any near here," Manford said. "Besides, then we'd smell like a wet bear and moose. We're going to need soap."

"I don't suppose you brought any."

"No, I didn't."

"Buying some at a store probably isn't such a hot idea, either," Veronica observed.

"Not really."

"There's a car wash just outside of town," Golly said.

"How does that work?" Manford asked.

"Well, I'd guess you put quarters in and get soap and water out of a hose. People clean their cars that way."

"Got any quarters, Manford?" said Veronica.

"I brought some in case we had to use a phone."

"You think of everything."

At dusk, after Gloria had spent hours searching for Ssam, and about the time she found his message atop the kitchen cupboards and screamed, the rest of the rescue plan clicked into place. From Florida-by-the-Pond, Flossie dialed the number Ssam had given them.

"Hello," Gloria said, confused and shaken by what she'd just discovered.

"Oh, hi," Flossie said. "I'm coming to your costume party tonight but I forgot what time it starts."

"Costume party?" Gloria said. "Here? There's no party here."

"There isn't?" Flossie said. "Oh, I must have the wrong number. Sorry to bother you." Flossie hung up.

"That's odd," Gloria said. "In fact, everything is odd. I don't understand what's going on."

"We'd better keep looking for George," Eddie said, "or maybe it's supposed to be Ssam."

"Don't remind me," Gloria replied.

Manford and Veronica left their hiding place a while later and found their way to the car wash. They formed a low-lying cloud around themselves and one end of the building and spent half an hour happily scrubbing and hosing each other off. Dark brown water ran down the drain the first four times they soaped each other up, but the rinse water eventually ran clear.

"I should put bows in my hair after all this fuss," said Veronica.

"Maybe I should wear a tie," said Manford.

Hidden by their cloud, they crossed town through the darkest streets and yards. Golly steered, telling them where to turn to reach Blackwood Terrace. They were three blocks away when, back at Moostery Manor, Needlenose picked up the phone and dialed.

"Hello," Gloria said, extremely wary this time.

"Hello," said Needlenose, "I'm just leaving for your eight

o'clock party. Could you give me directions?"

"I don't know what's going on, sir," Gloria said, still being polite, "but there's no party here. You must have the wrong number."

"Are you at 173 Blackwood Terrace?" Needlenose said.

"Yes."

"That's what this invitation says. Your name is Parkhurst, right?"

"Yes, but I don't recognize your voice," Gloria said. "Do I know you?"

"I don't think so."

"Why would you come to a party if you don't even know me?"

"It just sounded like fun."

"Sorry to disappoint you, but I'm not giving a party."

"What a shame," Needlenose said, "and I have this great costume, too. I look for all the world like a porcupine. Well, sorry to trouble you. Goodbye."

"I think I'm going crazy," said Gloria as she hung up the phone.

About a block away, a mysterious cloud drifted slowly up Blackwood Terrace. Few people noticed it. Those who did gave it little thought.

"The house we want is on the left where that small red car is parked in the driveway," Golly said.

The cloud floated down the street, then up to the house at 173. An arm reached out and pushed the doorbell.

"What now?" Gloria said. She went to the door and looked through the peephole. She saw nothing. Nothing, that is, but a thin white cloud with streetlights shining through it. The bell rang again. She opened the door.

There was a cloud on her doorstep. She thought that's what it was, anyway, but then it began to clear. It dissolved slowly, slowly, until standing before her were a moose and a bear. She raised her hands to her face as if to scream.

"Hi," Manford said, "is this where the party is? It's eight o'clock. We didn't see any cars parked around."

"Those are costumes, right?" Gloria said. Eddie stood just behind her, eyes wide, mouth hanging open.

"Yeah," said Veronica. "Great, aren't they? Neat special effects, too, don't you think?"

"Sure. . .neat," the lady said, sounding somewhat relieved. "You look like the real thing. But I'm not having a party. There's been some big mistake."

"Really?" Manford said. "Gee, and our ride just left. Could we possibly use your phone? We must have the wrong address."

"I suppose," Gloria said. "It's been such a crazy day anyway, why not? Use the one in the kitchen." She pointed across the living room to the kitchen doorway. She and Eddie sat down to wait, turning on the TV. Out of sight behind them, Columbine flew from the tiger lilies to the brim of Manford's hat. Manford took off his pack and dug inside it.

"The number's in here somewhere," he said. Finding a scrap of paper, he set the pack down.

"Ssam's under the sink," Columbine said softly.

Manford dialed the phone. Veronica opened the door below the sink. Ssam, waiting inside, crawled out and into the open pack.

Manford talked briefly (to his mother, actually), then hung up the phone, put on his pack, and went out through the living room toward the front door.

"Can you believe it," he said to Gloria and Eddie, "we have the wrong town. Our ride's going to meet us a few blocks from here. Thank you for your help. Sorry we've been so much trouble."

"It has been a rough day," Gloria said. "I hope you find your party." She closed the door behind them.

Outside the house, a small white cloud drifted through yards and streets and headed for the woods.

"Thanks for the rescue," Ssam said. "Boy, you really do things in style."

Inside the house, Gloria went to the kitchen to get something, anything, to drink.

"Whew, smells like soap in here," she said. She saw a scrap of paper under the phone. "What's that? Oh, they must have left it."

As she picked it up to throw it away, she noticed the writing:

Dear Gloria and Eddie,

We've taken Ssam with us. He is our friend. Thank you for keeping him safe. If you visit MorningGlory Forest again, come see us. You could be our friend, too.
Manford and Veronica

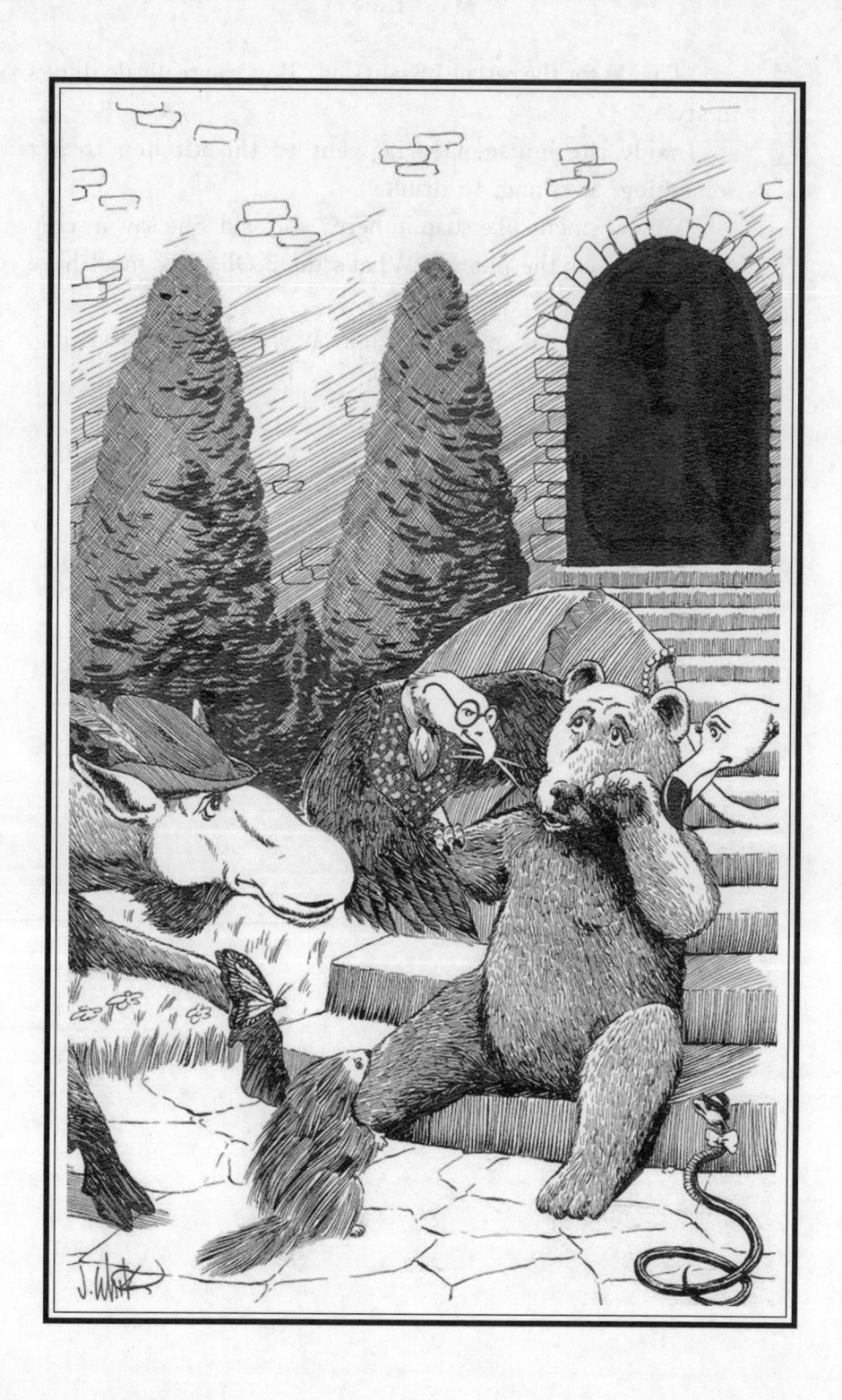

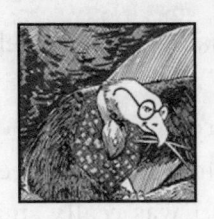

16

Journey to Long Ago
In which the animals have a holiday and stage a pageant

The hot days of August settled on MorningGlory Forest. The sun beat steadily down from a clear blue sky and the grass and flowers faded and drooped in the heat. Sometimes it would rain, cooling things off in mid-afternoon, but the clouds never lasted long. Soon it would be clear and hot again, too hot to do much of anything.

The animals rose early to enjoy the cool mornings and stayed up late for the cool evening hours. They found shady spots to rest in the middle of the day. Often, they would sleep through a hot afternoon or have long conversations about whatever might be on their minds. One day, Veronica and Needlenose lay resting under the tree in WhiteFlower Meadow, waiting for others in the neighborhood to join them.

"It's hot," said Needlenose.

"Uh huh," said Veronica, "just like last summer, and the one before that."

"Were you here then?"

"I was born here, in the cave where I live."

"I didn't get here until late last year. Then I was moving

into my burrow and having it remodeled and didn't take time to have friends."

"Too bad," said Veronica.

"What did you do here?" asked Needlenose.

"The first summer I was really small and I spent my time with Mom. She taught me to find things to eat and to be careful in the woods. That part was easy, bears eat nearly anything and almost everything is afraid of us."

"I'm not afraid of you," said Needlenose.

"Of course not," said Veronica. "We're friends, and you've got sharp quills. Even bears don't like a nose full of porcupine quills."

Manford came across the meadow and joined them then, and they saw Flossie and Princess Columbine flying up from the pond.

"Veronica's telling about what she did here the last couple of summers," said Needlenose.

"Oh, good," said Manford, "none of us were here then."

"I don't remember being anywhere last summer," said Columbine.

"I think this was before your time, Princess," said Veronica.

"So tell us more about what it was like," said Needlenose. "You were just getting started."

"What I remember most is learning things from Mom, like how to tell directions from the sun, and how to find my way to someplace and back again."

"We all learned that," said Manford.

"I didn't," said Flossie. "One direction is like another to me. Remember when I got here? I was sure this was Florida."

"We could teach you about directions," said Veronica. "Then you could fly back to Florida for a visit sometime."

"That would be kind of you, though with my beautiful new house, I don't think I'll be going anywhere soon."

"I learned about smelling things, too," Veronica went on.

"Mom taught me to recognize the scents of people and different animals along with the regular smells in the woods. It seemed an awful lot to learn after a while. Every time I thought I was figuring something out, she would come along with more."

"Mothers are like that," said Flossie.

"I never even met my mother," said Columbine.

"You didn't?" said Manford. "Why not?"

"I don't know. I just never did."

"That's strange. I guess we're lucky to have someone to learn from."

"Uh huh," said Veronica. "My mom spent most of her time teaching me to be a proper bear. It was interesting and we had great fun until she started teaching me to dance."

"What happened then?" asked Needlenose.

"She got lonely for the circus. She would show me something and we'd practice for an hour or so, then she'd get to telling stories about life on the road. After a while she'd be sad because she missed it so. I wondered if learning to dance was such a good idea."

"What did you do?"

"I told her she should go back there if that was what she wanted. That made her happy. First thing this spring, that's what she did."

"Didn't you want to go with her?" asked Flossie.

"Yes, but I was almost two then and she thought I should stay here and be on my own. I missed her when she first went away, but I kind of like it now. I've met lots of friends and we have fun."

"What else do you remember?" asked Columbine.

"Mom taught me to be careful of hunters. We would see them now and then in the woods far from here."

"What did you do?" asked Manford.

"We'd hide in the brush sometimes and hold very still. They would usually walk by and never see us. Their dogs would smell us, though, so we'd run and lead them through the woods and creeks and over mountains until they got lost and gave up chasing us. We really enjoyed doing that."

"Did anyone ever shoot at you?" asked Flossie.

"Not at us. We were too fast for them."

"Shooting doesn't sound friendly," said Needlenose.

"It isn't," said Veronica, "but it's not allowed in Morning-Glory Forest. Stay here and no one will shoot at you."

Manford suddenly started singing:

"Oh, the forest is a friendly place, a friendly place,
No one ever shoots at you, it's such a friendly place."

"Where did you hear that?" asked Flossie.

"Nowhere," said Manford, "I made it up."

Golly passed over the meadow just then and circled down for a landing.

"Hello, everyone," he said.

"Hello," said Veronica. "It looks like all of us except Ssam are here."

"I'm here," said Ssam, who was riding on Golly's back. "Golly took me soaring so I could look at things from the air."

"What did you see?" asked Princess Columbine.

"Wow, trees and creeks and valleys and mountains everywhere! We flew over our garden with the picture in it, too. It looks great from above, though some of the flowers are starting to fade."

"What are you folks doing this hot day?" asked Golly.

"Manford was singing," said Needlenose.

"What about?"

"Something about the forest being friendly," said Flossie. "Sing it again."

Manford sang once more:

"Oh, the forest is a friendly place, a friendly place,
No one ever shoots at you, it's such a friendly place."

"Is there more to it?"

"No, that's all I've thought of so far."

"Let's make up some more," said Ssam.

"Wait a minute, that reminds me of something," said Veronica. "I remember Mom telling me about a special holiday around this time of year, a holiday just for animals. People don't even know about it."

"What's it called?" asked Needlenose.

"Um, let me think..."

"Forest Friendship Day," said Golly. "It's a day animals take to have fun and be friends and be happy about living in this wonderful place."

"Why did Manford's song remind you of that?" asked Flossie.

"Because sometimes, Mom said, the animals get together and put on a play."

"I don't follow you. Any special play, like *Goldilocks and the Three Bears*?"

"No, not like that," said Veronica. "You see, it's not a play you find written down at all. You make it up as you go along, like Manford was doing."

"That sounds different," said Columbine.

"It's the Forest Friendship Pageant," said Golly. "I saw one once and it looked like fun."

"There are lots of us," said Manford. "Do you suppose we could put on a play?"

"Sure," said Veronica.

"Sounds fine to me," said Flossie. "We'll each have to think of a part we want to play."

"I'll be a princess," said Princess Columbine.

"I'll be a famous explorer," said Manford.

"That was easy," said Flossie. "Anybody else?"

"I'm thinking," said Needlenose.

"I'll be a serpent..." began Ssam.

"We're with you so far," said Flossie.

"...who is, let's see, guarding a secret place...in a gloomy castle."

"Okay, we have a castle, a princess, a serpent, and an explorer now," said Flossie, "and a deep, dark secret. This is starting to take shape."

"When is Forest Friendship Day?" asked Columbine.

"Tomorrow, the fifteenth of August," said Golly. "We should give our play tomorrow."

"Well, friends," Flossie said, "let's pull this idea together. Broadway, here we come!"

They sat under the tree the rest of the afternoon making their plans. Each eventually chose a character he or she wanted to be and they worked out the play's general theme. There was no rehearsal and no one practiced any lines. There weren't any. They planned to make the story up as they went along.

Everyone gathered in the meadow again early next morning. Golly and Flossie made trips to the store to provide snacks and refreshments for the day. Manford and Veronica brought items from their parents' show business trunks to use for costumes.

Manford's mother, most of Beaver Brothers' crew, and many curious creatures of the nearby woods joined them for the holiday celebration. There wasn't time to send out invitations but word traveled fast. The guests talked and played games through the morning; lunched and snoozed through mid day. In late afternoon, everyone gathered quietly on one side of the big tree. The seven friends donned their costumes and took their places for the play that follows.

The Castle on the Cliff

Characters:
Sir Manford, a famous explorer
Princess Columbine, a royal princess
Squire Needlenose, a simple forest creature
Golly, the Wise, venerable counselor and advisor

Veronica, the Horrible, a ferocious monster
Princess Flossie, Columbine's older sister
Sserpent Ssam, protector of the secret room

The story takes place in MorningGlory Forest a very long time ago.

Act I

Scene 1: A trail deep in the forest. It is summer. The day is hot but trees filter the sunlight and give shade. Dense brush crowds the pathway and sounds of birds and small animals can be heard. A creek flows nearby. Sir Manford makes his way along the trail. He wears an expedition hat and pack and is in good spirits. Princess Columbine, sad and downhearted, rides atop his hat, staring intently into the distance.

Sir Manford (singing):
Oh, the forest is a friendly place, a friendly place,
Exploring it is good for you, it's such a friendly place.
We've been following this trail for a week now, Princess. We should reach the castle soon.

Princess Columbine: I hope so, but I keep worrying that we've gone the wrong way.

Manford: No, I remember seeing it once before when I came this way. It looked dark and mysterious. I didn't want to go near it.

Columbine (sobbing): Oh, that sounds so terrible. If my sister is really there, we might never get her back.

Manford: Don't fret, Princess. We'll find her.

Columbine: If we get past the monster.

Manford (puzzled): Monster?

Columbine: There's something horrible that guards the trail to the castle. We have to find a way around it.

Manford: You never mentioned that. Here, let's rest a moment and go through this once again. [He stops in a clearing and sits down. Columbine flutters to the grass beside him.]

Manford: First, your sister disappeared, is that right?

Columbine: Yes, she was to be married the next day but she changed her mind. Instead of waiting and explaining things, she flew away in the night. Oh, it was so foolish of her, especially when the groom didn't show up. I guess he changed his mind, too.

Manford: Next, you heard from her.

Columbine: It was weeks later. A messenger brought a note. Flossie wrote that she was going to the castle.

Manford: Why would she go there?

Columbine: The castle was our ancestors' home for hundreds of years. Maybe Flossie thought she could live there. Maybe she thought she could find the secret room. I don't know what she might have been thinking. She gets lost so easily, I don't know how she'll even find the place. Maybe she didn't find it.

Manford: Secret room?

Columbine: There is legend of a passage to a hidden room somewhere in the castle. I don't know what's in it, if anything, or if it's even true.

Manford: Did Flossie know about the monster?

Columbine: Of course.

Manford: How would she get past it?

Columbine: She can fly, just like me. [She flies to the top of Manford's hat.]

Manford: This could get interesting. [He exits, singing.]
Oh, the forest is a friendly place, a friendly place,
Fighting monsters is the thing to do in such a friendly place.

Scene 2: Farther along the trail the same day. Sir Manford and Princess Columbine approach Squire Needlenose, a local resident.

Columbine: There's someone on the trail ahead.

Manford: Good, he'll know how far we are from the castle.

Squire Needlenose: Sir Manford, I presume.

Manford: You know of me, friend?

Needlenose: Your travels are spoken of far and wide, good sir, but who is your passenger?

Manford: Princess Columbine. We seek her lost sister.

Needlenose (bowing): Pleased to meet you, m'lady. Squire Needlenose, at your service.

Columbine: Thank you.

Manford: We're bound for the Castle on the Cliff. Do you know of it?

Needlenose: Aye, I feared as much. Leave it to a famous adventurer to pick the worst place to go. I'd turn back if I were you.

Columbine (insistent): But we must go on. My sister may be there.

Needlenose: She may, indeed. She passed this way more than a week ago. I tried to turn her back but she went on despite my warnings.

Manford: We've heard a monster guards the castle.

Needlenose: A monster it is, and if you got by 'twould be a wonder. But there's something even worse inside.

Columbine: Worse?

Needlenose: An evil serpent, m'lady. If the monster doesn't get you, the serpent surely will.

Columbine (sobbing uncontrollably): Oh, Flossie, will I ever see you again?

Manford: Have courage, sweet princess. We'll find her. Tell us, Squire, how far lays the castle from here?

Needlenose: Many days' walk even to get to the cliff. Then you must climb the steep trail and get by her to reach the castle.

Columbine: Her?

Needlenose: Veronica, the Horrible. She'll be waiting for you, 'tis certain.

Manford: Might you accompany us?

Needlenose: Me? Go up there? Not a chance of it, sir. I value my life, just as you should value yours. But if you are determined to press on, seek counsel of Golly, the Wise. He is two days' walk from here where the trail forks to the left. He lives in a big tree near a creek.

Manford: You have been most helpful, Squire.

Needlenose: Good fortune to you both.

Scene 3: Along the left fork of the trail two days later. It is near dark and raining steadily. Sir Manford searches anxiously for Golly, the Wise. Princess Columbine has taken shelter inside Manford's pack.

Manford (singing bravely):
Oh, the forest is a soggy place, a soggy place,
The trails will all turn muddy soon, it's such a soggy place.
Columbine (voice muffled): Are we nearing the spot yet?
Manford: I don't know. I don't hear a creek, and I don't know which tree might be big enough for Golly, the Wise. The Squire's directions were rather vague, if you ask me. We'd better find something soon.
Columbine: It's still raining, I gather.
Manford: Buckets, m'lady. [He hears something overhead and stops to look. A great brown bird lands on a branch overhanging the trail. He wears a white ascot, a brown vest, and wire-rimmed glasses.]
Golly, the Wise: It's not a fit night out for man or beast. Hurry, my tree is just ahead. It's dry underneath. [Sir Manford follows Golly to the tree.]
Manford: You are Golly, the Wise?
Golly: The very one, and you are Sir Manford, intended rescuer of the damsel who passed this way a week ago.
Manford: Yes, how did you know?
Golly: I'm wise, remember? Fair damsels bring rescuers. It's the way of the world.
Columbine: So you saw Flossie, too. Do you know if she made it to the castle?
Golly: I expect she did. The beast up the road has been uncommonly grumpy of late. It upsets her terribly when something gets by her.
Manford: Maybe Flossie is safe!
Columbine (hopeful): Oh, I hope so.
Golly: Getting to the castle doesn't mean she's safe, fair princess.
Manford: Can you help us, great wise bird?
Golly: You didn't come for warnings—no doubt you got those in the last scene—so, I will tell you this. Veronica,

the Horrible, lives halfway up the steep trail to the Castle on the Cliff. She awaits travelers there, but often sleeps during the hot part of the day. You may have a chance to get past her then.

Columbine: But it has been cold and rainy.

Golly (gently): Tomorrow is another day, young lady. It may be sunny.

Manford: What about the serpent?

Golly: Ssam? He'll be in the secret room, if there is one. Somewhat of a scholar, story has it. You'll have to take your chances with him, if he even exists. You two had better get some sleep now. With luck, you'll make it back to the trail and to the base of the cliff tomorrow. The day after that...

Columbine (fearful): The monster! Oh, no!

Act II

Scene 1: Ascending the cliff trail two days later. The rain has passed but the day is cool. Sir Manford and Princess Columbine climb the rocky slope slowly, looking around them at every moment.

Columbine: I don't like this at all.

Manford: Try to think of it as an adventure, Princess.

Columbine: Thanks, that helps a lot.

Manford: We've come a little more than halfway. I haven't seen any monster, have you?

Columbine (hopeful): No, maybe she'll be sleeping. [They hear a dreadful roar.]

Veronica, the Horrible (growling, then singing):
Oh, the forest is a scary place, a scary place,
I see it will be lunchtime soon in such a scary place.

Manford (frowning): She's singing my song!

Columbine (terrified): Oh, we're doomed!

Veronica: Right you are, my pretty. [She appears above them, huge and black and blocking their path] Your sister escaped me but you won't. Just come this way and we'll get it over quickly.

Columbine: Flossie's safe!

Veronica: It's merely temporary. She has to come out again, y'know, and I'll be waiting. A tasty dessert. I'm looking forward to it.

Manford: We mean you no harm, ma'am. We only seek to rescue Princess Flossie. Please let us pass.

Veronica: Mean me no harm! That's a good one. Who's your writer, anyway? [She rolls on the ground, laughing. Manford leaves the trail and scrambles along the rocky sidehill toward a large tree]

Veronica: Trying to escape, are you. Biiig moostake! I'll put an end to that. [She bounds forward toward the tree, lunging at Manford. As she passes under a low branch, however, a bushy quill tail flashes down and whacks her soundly on the nose. She falls back with a cry of pain then runs wailing down the slope.]

Manford: Squire Needlenose!

Needlenose: Aye, I thought you might need a hand, or in this case, a tail.

Columbine: Oh, thank you, Squire, but you said you wouldn't help us.

Needlenose: I say a lot of things, m'lady. Shall we go on to the castle now?

Scene 2: On the castle grounds later that day. Sir Manford, Princess Columbine, and Squire Needlenose have searched inside the castle for hours. They've found no trace of Princess Flossie. They now look outside for clues they may have missed.

Columbine: We must find her and be away before the monster recovers.

Needlenose: Veronica will be out of action for several days, m'lady. In any case, we'll be spending the night here. It's too late in the day to head back.

Manford: But where's Flossie? We've called and called, and looked in room after room on the main floor and up all the stairs. Nothing! [They look up at the castle's many peaked roofs, windows, and turrets.]

Columbine (singing):
Oh, this castle is a gloomy place, a gloomy place,
Where could Flossie have gotten to in such a gloomy place.

Manford (shouting): FLOSSIE! FLOSSIE, WHERE ARE YOU?

Needlenose (listening): No answer, good sir. All afternoon you've been calling and there's been no answer. [They round a corner toward the side of the castle set upon the plunging cliff.]

Columbine: Look! [She points to a tower window above them.]

Manford: It's her! FLOSSIE, CAN YOU HEAR ME!

Princess Flossie: Loud and clear. I was hoping you'd get around to this side pretty soon. It's almost dark.

Manford: What are you doing up there?

Flossie: Nothing much. I locked myself in, or out. I'm not sure which. You'll have to come let me out, or in, or whatever.

Manford: How do we get up there?

Flossie: Well, I can't let down my hair, that's for sure.

Needlenose: I remember a stair to the back towers, sir. I'll find it and set her free. [He exits.]

Columbine: How did you get past the monster?

Flossie: I flew over it.

Manford: Then why don't you fly down from there?

Flossie: Look, I'm supposed to be in distress. A damsel in distress can't escape so easily.

Manford: Have you looked for the secret room?

Flossie: Are you kidding? I've turned this place inside out. I'd still be looking but today I got locked in here, or out here, or something. Stupid door!

Columbine: Oh, we're so glad you're safe.

Manford: We were beginning to think you weren't here.

Flossie: I've been rooting around this place for a week. To think somebody once lived here. Say, I thought that Squire fellow was coming to help me. What do you suppose happened?

Columbine: Haven't you heard him at the door?

Manford of MorningGlory Mountain

Flossie: Not a whisper.

Manford: Hang on, we're coming up to get you.

Flossie: Maybe you do need a new writer, kiddo. What else am I going to do?

Scene 3: On the tower stairs moments later. Sir Manford has released Princess Flossie. She wears a gray traveling cape and a long string of pearls. Squire Needlenose is nowhere in sight.

Manford: I don't think the Squire was ever here. I don't see his footprints in the dust.

Columbine: But he said he was coming up these stairs.

Flossie: Let's go back down and see where he did go. [They descend the stairs inside the tower until they reach a landing.]

Columbine (pointing to footprints): That must be his trail there!

Manford: I see it. It looks like he shuffled up the stairs to this landing. . .stopped here to rest. . .and disappeared. He didn't go back down; there's only one set of footprints and they all go the same direction.

Flossie (looking around): Then something happened to him here. Maybe he leaned against a wall and it moved.

Manford: They look like rock to me. [He butts them with his head]. Uh huh, rock. Now where could that fellow be hiding? [As he sits down, a great cloud of fog erupts from his pack and envelops them. The stair landing begins moving slowly downward.]

Manford: Hey, what's happening?

Columbine: Where are you, Flossie? I can't see!

Flossie: Right here, Princess. I'm not going anywhere, not until this fog clears, anyway. [She feels the wall moving behind her.] Whoa, maybe I am! We're moving. We're sinking into the stairs! [Downward movement soon slows and stops. The fog thins.]

Manford: Look, there's an opening down here, a kind of hallway.

Flossie: The secret room! I never would have found this.

[They follow a curving hallway to a large, open room. It is a library. Shelves of books cover all four walls floor to ceiling. Squire Needlenose is seated at a table, reading.]

Manford: There you are, Squire.

Needlenose: Oh, hello. I got so interested in reading I lost track of time.

Flossie: We wondered where you'd gone.

Needlenose: Curious contraption, that stairway. [They hear a loud voice.]

Sserpent Ssam: QUIET IN THE LIBRARY, PLEASE.

Needlenose: Oh, meet the librarian, Ssam. [Ssam is coiled on a large pillow to their right. He wears a patch over his left eye and black fedora with a white band.]

Manford: Are you the evil serpent we were warned about?

Ssam (in a friendly tone): That's me. Don't I look the part?

Flossie: Oh, yes, evil.

Columbine: What do you do here?

Ssam: I'm the protector of this room, or more to the point, these books. Castles have mice, you see. Mice ruin books. I eat mice.

Flossie: A simple job description, that's for sure.

Columbine: Your reputation makes you out to be much more dangerous.

Ssam: So much the better. That way, Veronica and I keep everyone away. She let you by, I see.

Needlenose: Not exactly. I had to whack her on the nose with my tail.

Ssam: Oh, the poor thing! You probably hurt her.

Columbine: But she was going to eat us!

Ssam: No, she was just trying to scare you away. She wouldn't really have hurt you. You see, the owner of this library wants the books protected. That's what Veronica and I do. We're the security team.

Manford: What kind of books are these?

Ssam: I don't think you'd believe me if I told you.

Manford: I might.

Needlenose: Go ahead, Ssam. I think I've already figured it out.

Ssam: Very well. These books...all of these hundreds of volumes you see around you...are from the future. They are going to be written someday when the authors get around to it. Perhaps you see why it wouldn't do to have too many visitors, particularly the authors.

Manford: That is hard to believe.

Flossie: Where did they come from if they haven't been written yet?

Ssam: I don't ask questions. I just eat mice.

Needlenose: I was reading one about you, Sir Manford.

Manford: Me? Someone will write a book about me?

Needlenose: Several of them, actually. They're called Manford of MorningGlory Mountain.

Manford: May I see one?

Ssam: Just for a moment. You can't be meddling with the future, you know.

Manford (paging through the book): Wow, look at all these neat adventures! Wait...we're all in here; how can that be if this happens a long time from now?

Ssam: Sorry, no questions. Time's up now; follow me upstairs and I'll show you a place to spend the night.

Finale

Scene: In the great hall the next morning. The adventurers are preparing to depart when they hear a sad whimpering outside. They open the main castle doors and find Veronica, the Horrible, on the front steps. Golly, the Wise, is extracting quills one at a time from her damaged nose. The entire cast gathers round them as he finishes.

Needlenose: My apologies, noble beast, for thrashing your nose like that.

Veronica: Thank you, but I suspect I had it coming. In any case, I shall recover soon.

Golly: Well, Sir Manford, you rescued the runaway princess and found the hidden room and its secret. Not bad work for a day.

Manford: It has been an interesting adventure, and it's a strange secret, that's for sure.

Ssam: One that is safe with you, I'm sure. No one will believe you if you do tell. Meanwhile, you and the Squire and the fair princesses are welcome to visit any time.

Flossie (looking around at everyone): And now, before we go, shall we?

Columbine (nodding): Definitely!

All (facing the audience and singing):
Oh, the forest is a busy place, a busy place,
There are so many things to do, it's such a busy place.
Oh, the forest is a mystery place, a mystery place,
But you can learn the secrets, too, in this mystery place.
Oh, the forest is a friendly place, a friendly place,
The creatures will be nice to you, it's such a friendly place.

The meadow audience, now grown quite large, began to cheer and applaud. The cast bowed, bowed again to the continuing applause, and attempted to depart but the clapping went on. Mary, pleased with the afternoon's entertainment, led calls for an encore. The characters looked at each other, smiled, regrouped, and again sang their song, all nine verses.

"That was wonderful," Mary told them when all was done. "And to think you made it up as you went. That's amazing."

"Actually," Flossie said, "the whole play was in that book in the castle library. We each just took our own part."

"But that hasn't been written yet," Mary said, ". . .or has it?"

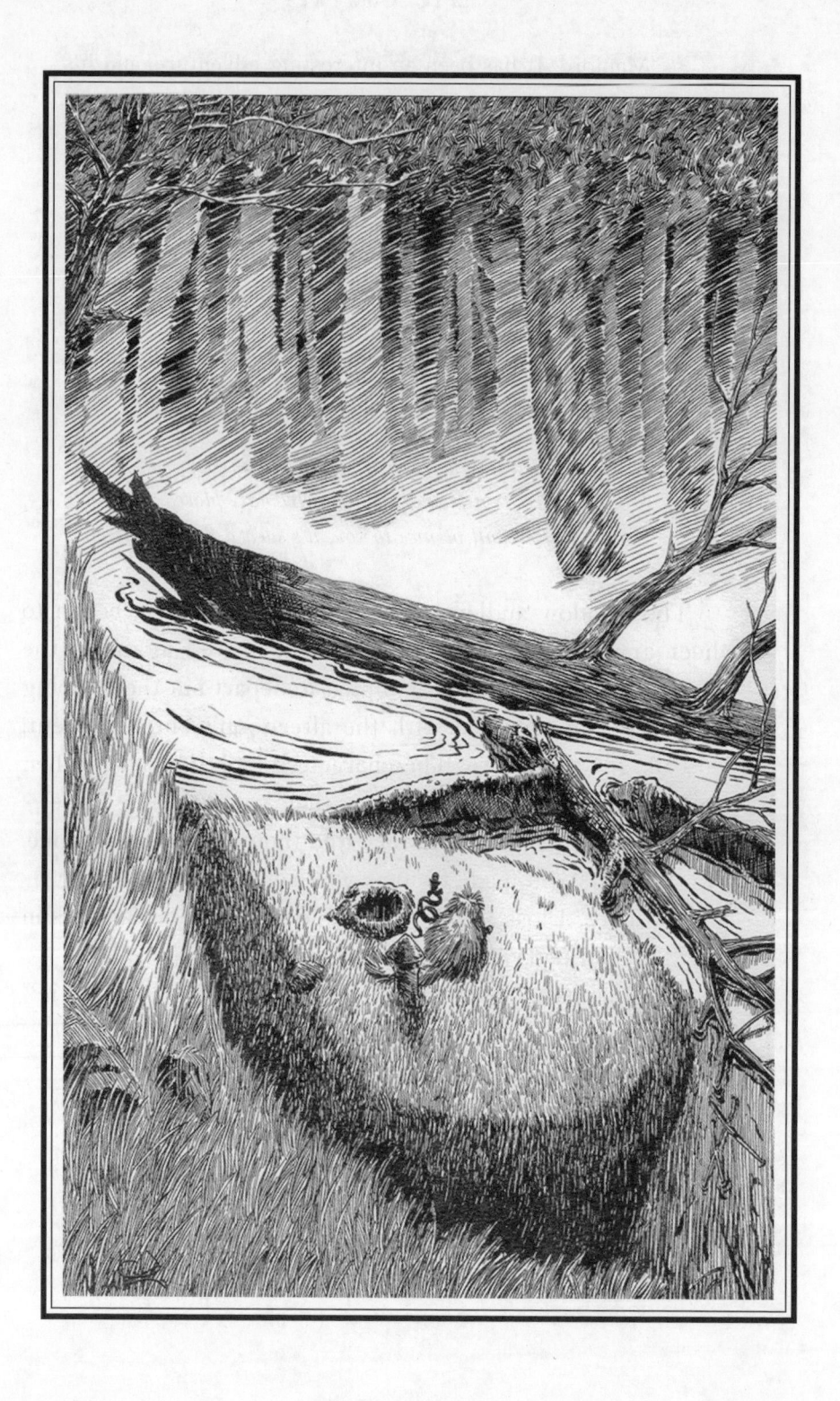

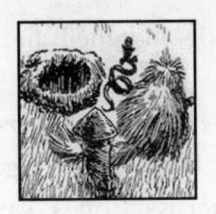

17

Of Rain and Flood and Darkness
In which Veronica brings aid and comfort

Dark clouds gathered to the north of MorningGlory Forest. Wind pushed them and they grew bigger and bigger until they blocked out the sun and made miles-long shadows on the ground. Wind blew through the forest, bending trees and driving dead leaves and dust before it. Then it began to rain.

The rain came lightly at first, making dainty circles in ponds and streams. Then it rained harder. Soon, water ran steadily from tree branches and leaves and the dust on the ground no longer stirred.

More clouds gathered then and the storm moved south. It grew to be many miles long and wide and rain began to pound the forests. Wet ground became mud, then puddles, then moving water that flowed down the trails and gullies and into the streams.

Wind shook the forest, setting trees creaking and swaying, sending showers spraying from the leaves. Sheets of water swept before the wind. Water splashed and puddled and splattered everywhere.

Lightning streaked the sky, flashing, flickering, sizzling

through the air. Thunder boomed and rumbled and the rain came down in torrents.

And the streams grew full. They rose higher and ran faster and spread beyond their banks. Crossings that were once a small step or a simple hop across stones, grew wide and deep and swift. More water came with each hour. MorningGlory Creek became a river. Instead of flowing quietly off the cliff above Veronica's cave and falling as a fine mist, it thundered and roared.

Veronica was asleep in her room. She had shut the front door tight and hadn't seen the huge cloud or heard the wind and rain; nor had she awakened in the night as the sound of falling water grew louder.

It was when water began to drip on her nose that she finally woke up and wondered what was wrong. Water drips from the ceiling in most caves, of course, and her furniture was arranged around the usual spots so it wouldn't get wet. A drip on her nose was something new. She got up to look. She went to the living room and opened the front door.

Water poured from above in a solid sheet, churning the pool at the base of the cliff into foam. Veronica stood in the doorway and listened to the roar. It was early morning. There was little light. It looked like she had suddenly awakened at the bottom of Yosemite Falls.

She wondered how the others were doing. Maybe Flossie was worried about her house. What about Manford and Needlenose and Golly up in a tree? Maybe they were wondering about her. Veronica decided to go out in the storm and check on her friends.

She moved the furniture in her bedroom so it wouldn't get wet and closed the front door. The pool under the falls had risen, but not much. Water was flowing out from the stream on the other side about as fast as it came over the falls. Veronica built a dike of dirt around the doorway just in case. Then she walked around the pool and a short way down the creek. There she took the path that led to the top of the canyon wall and on to Golly's house at GloryView.

Golly was worried. He'd been through storms at GloryView before but this was different. Clouds hung angrily above him and rain drummed against the windows and roof. Wind swayed the tree and set branches and house walls to creaking.

The house had been built to move. It was another of Beaver Brothers' creations (the one in their catalog, in fact) and was designed to bend with the tree. Just the same, it worried Golly. Not the moving about, no, birds who built nests in trees were used to that. It was lightning that concerned him. Lightning could set the house on fire. Lightning could split and topple the tree in an instant. Lightning could turn him to roasted golden eagle, and that's what was on Golly's mind.

But lightning strikes high points. With this in mind, Beaver Brothers had chosen for Golly's house a tree surrounded by many other trees, not one standing alone and in the open, and they'd made sure it wasn't the tallest. They'd also installed a lightning rod. The metal pole at the tree top would quickly direct any bolt that did strike harmlessly into the ground. Finally, they'd built Golly's lookout perch in a taller tree some distance away; thus, he had a high place to sit and survey the countryside, but it wasn't connected to his house.

So why would Golly be worried, you might ask?

Science was grand, he would say, but one just never knew, especially in a storm as fierce as this one. He paced back and forth. He sat in his study and tried to read. He roosted in his lookout but with the heavy clouds, there was nothing to see. He tried to eat. He tried to take a nap. But nothing could take his attention from the storm. The wind howled, the rain pounded down, the tree swayed back and forth. Lightning crackled in the distance; then thunder crashed and echoed through the forest again.

He wondered if he should visit the others and see how they were doing. Was Flossie okay, and Needlenose? Would water flood Veronica's cave? Maybe he should go find out. It would give him something to do.

"Hello," came a voice from below. "Are you there, Golly? Are you okay?"

He went to the porch and looked down. It was Veronica, sitting in the pouring rain and looking up at him.

"Yes, I'm fine," Golly answered. "What brings you out on such a day?"

"I've been wondering about you and the others."

"I've been wondering, too."

"Is your treehouse okay?" Veronica asked.

"Yes, yes, the wonders of science are holding steady here. No problems to report, though I think I should call it SoggyView today."

"I'm headed to Manford's," said Veronica. "Want to come along?"

"I think so," said Golly, "but instead of flying, I'll ride along with you, if you don't mind." So the two set off through the wind and the rain, heading back down the path to the creek.

Manford watched from the window of his room. The storm was exciting! The rain, the wind, the clouds, the lightning and thunder—it was fabulous and thrilling and wonderful! He'd wanted to go outside and see what it was like but his mother had said he should stay in. Not today, Manford, she'd told him. Today, he was better off inside.

Manford's house was in a dense grove of trees. It was large and white with gray shingles and shutters. There were big windows on every side. Just looking at it, you might have thought the house had dozens of rooms upstairs and down. But there was no upstairs. It was just one floor with large rooms and tall ceilings. Moose needed space and wide doorways, you see.

The house was solidly built with thick walls and huge wooden roof beams. Neither rain nor wind would harm it. Lightning wouldn't come near. Even a tree falling on it would likely bounce off or at most, break a window. It had once been a wilderness lodge, wide open, with lots of space to move around.

Looking for a new place to live, Mary Moose had seen its possibilities. She'd had the place remodeled inside and out before they'd moved in. There was plenty of room for their belongings, for Manford's friends and visitors like Mr. Johnny, and even for Manford's dad to practice dancing on his visits home.

There was no need to fear a storm. They were perfectly safe inside, which was why Manford's mother wanted him to stay home. So he watched out the window of his room, wishing he could go out, eyes alight with wonder as water ran down the glass and wind blew trees against the eaves.

He saw Veronica coming up the path. Veronica, her fur wet and dripping, with Golly riding on her shoulder, came to the front door and knocked. Manford went to open it.

"Is everything okay with you?" Veronica asked.

"In this fortress?" said Manford. "Nothing could get us here. Why don't you come in?"

"We're a bit damp," said Golly.

"That's okay," Mary said, coming to the door. "We'll have you sit near the fire for a while and you'll soon dry."

Manford led his wet friends to the fireplace in the living room where they found a warm spot to sit. Golly told about the wind and rain at GloryView and about the lightning and thunder nearby. Veronica told about Misty Falls turning to a torrent and the water foaming in the pool. Manford hung on every word, wanting to know how everything looked and sounded and smelled. He was disappointed that he had nothing to add.

At Moostery Manor, he'd felt little effect from the storm except what he'd seen from his bedroom window.

"I wonder how Flossie's doing," said Veronica. "I'll bet she's nervous about her house."

"Beaver Brothers promised she'd have no problems," said Golly. "They're true to their word. The house they built for me has been wonderful."

A look of horror suddenly spread across Veronica's face. "Oh, no," she said, "oh, no..."

"What's wrong?" said Manford.

"Princess Columbine. She sleeps on tree branches and flowers. This rain has probably smashed her flat."

"Maybe we should look for her," said Golly.

"I think so," said Manford, getting up to go.

"Nothing to worry about," said Mary, popping her head in the door. "I talked to Flossie on the phone just a while ago. Columbine is with her and they're both doing fine. They've had a great view of the storm from Flossie's windows."

"Did Flossie say if the pond was rising?" Veronica asked.

"No, she didn't mention it."

"Maybe she hasn't noticed. I'll bet the water's up three feet. Well, that was my next stop anyway," Veronica said, heading out the door. "See you folks later."

"Good-bye," Manford said. He shut the door and headed for the dining room.

"What have you been writing in your journal?" Golly asked.

"I'll show you," Manford said, and he began paging through the book. "Here's where I wrote about climbing MorningGlory Mountain."

Golly looked it over. "Only one page?" he said.

"That's all I wanted to say. I wrote about Mom and her roses here," Manford went on, pointing to pages as he turned them. "And this is about meeting Aurora. This one is about building Flossie's house, and here's where I told about rescuing Ssam."

"Would you read some of those to me?"

"Sure," said Manford, and he did. Golly nodded with approval after each one.

"Now you should write about the storm," Golly said.

"Okay, tell me again about the rain and thunder and lightning at GloryView, and the things Veronica said, too. Oh, this will be good to write about. . ."

At Florida-by-the-Pond, Flossie wasn't worried about the weather. Oh, maybe the storm had bothered her a little at first—rain beating on 270 degrees of windows; wind churning the pond to whitecaps; a sky dark hour after hour with threatening clouds—these things had given her pause. But she'd soon realized that half the world could blow away before her house would move, so she and Columbine put on some music, gathered some snacks, and settled down to talk and watch the storm from the windows.

You might think this was out of character for a bird that once shrieked and took flight at every sudden noise. But Flossie had changed since her arrival in MorningGlory Forest. She'd grown used to her neighbors and their curious ways and nothing much surprised or bothered her anymore. She'd become a sort of experienced, eccentric aunt to them all.

Princess Columbine had come calling in the early hours of the storm. She'd sensed danger in the dark clouds moving in and had flown to the safety of Flossie's porch. Flossie had welcomed her inside when she awoke and they'd been chatting non-stop ever since. Now, their conversation was interrupted by a knock at the side door.

"In this weather?" Flossie said. "Who could that be?"

"Surely not a salesman," said Columbine. News of Flossie's house had drawn peddlers tramping through the woods to offer insurance, cosmetics, vacuum cleaners, magazine subscriptions, and a dozen other things. None of their persuasive routines had made the slightest headway with steely-eyed Flossie, proprietor of Florida-by-the-Pond. She opened the door to find Veronica.

"Hello, Ms. Bear," Flossie said, "you look like you've been swimming."

"I was," Veronica replied, "and the pond's choppy today, I can tell you that. Did you know it was rising?"

"Hmmm," Flossie said, glancing out the windows. "Now that you mention it, the beach to the east has disappeared and the stream to the west is roaring along like the dam broke. How much has the water come up?"

"It's two feet from the bottom of your house."

"Oh, dear," Flossie said, looking suddenly less casual about the matter. "What should I do?"

"I'd keep the front trap door closed if I were you."

"Well, yes, I could have told you that. Does it look like the water will rise higher?"

"I don't think so. It's overflowing the bank in several places and flooding the woods. You're probably safe unless it rains for another week."

"Which part of the woods?" Columbine asked from atop Flossie's head.

"Off that way," Veronica said, pointing east beyond the flooded beach.

"That's where Needlenose lives," said Flossie. "Water will flood his burrow if it gets too high. He could lose everything. And Ssam probably doesn't swim!"

"I'm going there next," said Veronica.

"Should we come along?"

"No, you two stay here. I'll bring them back if they need warming up and drying out."

Needlenose had been digging for hours. He'd seen the pond rising and had started building a dike around Haystack Hollow at once. He'd sent Ssam to the top room of the burrow while he stayed outside to dig, pile up dirt, and make a wall. But he was losing in his struggle against the forces of nature. He'd completed the dike only three-quarters of the way around, and but a foot high at that, when the first seeping water came in sight.

Needlenose worked harder and faster but couldn't stop either the water or the unhappy feelings coming upon him. His home would be flooded. His furniture and keepsakes and treasures—his potato chips!—all would be ruined. It was hard to keep back the sadness, but he kept digging. The water kept coming; he could do nothing more.

"Need some help?" said Veronica, arriving at a run.

"Sure do," said Needlenose. "I'll be swamped before long."

"I'll dig, you build," Veronica said, and she began moving dirt with great strokes of her powerful front paws. Needlenose followed behind her, packing and shaping the earth into a protective wall. They finished the dike Needlenose had started, and then went round again.

By evening, a U-shaped wall three feet high surrounded Haystack Hollow, extending outward from where the burrow joined the hill. None too soon, either. Water overflowing the pond was soon lapping gently at the dike and slowly rising. Needlenose prowled the pathway inside, checking for seepage and leaks.

"Maybe you and Ssam should go to Flossie's house," Veronica said. "I'm sure she'd have you in."

"No doubt she would, but we'll stay here till morning. If it keeps getting worse, we'll go then."

"I'll come back tomorrow to see how you're doing."

"Thanks for your help," said Needlenose. "Everything would be ruined now if you hadn't come along."

He went back inside. He knew rooms at the top of his burrow would stay dry, even if water did come in. He was tired, but he began dragging furniture upstairs—his chair, his couch, his trunk of mementos, and, of course, his potato chip supply. Everything of value found its way to upper rooms as Needlenose worked into the night. Ssam stayed awake to tell stories and offer encouragement.

Still, the storm raged on. Water kept rising but did so slowly now as it spread more widely into the woods. The dike around Haystack Hollow held back a foot of water, eventually a foot and a half. Water soaked into the ground. The walls and bottom floor of the burrow began to feel damp. Ssam and Needlenose sat on the bed in an upstairs room, listening for sounds in the dark.

"Isn't this a NeedleNuisance," said the tired porcupine, "marooned in our own house?"

"We should get some sleep," said Ssam. "Maybe things will seem better in the morning."

"I don't feel much like sleeping, especially knowing any minute the dike could give way and fill this place with water."

"Have some potato chips."

"Wow," said Needlenose, "why didn't I think of that!" He opened a bag from the dozens he'd carried upstairs. Half of it was empty in just a few minutes.

"I feel better already," he said. "There's nothing like potato chips to take your mind off your problems." Rain continued in the darkness outside as the two talked.

"I've been thinking," Needlenose said.

"About what?" said Ssam.

"With Flossie living here for a while, and now with you moved in, I wonder if I shouldn't remodel this burrow again and make it bigger."

"Why would you do that?"

"Oh, I don't know. Flossie has lots of space in her house.

Maybe I should have more space, too."

"Just what would you do?"

"Nothing much, really. We could make a couple new rooms just by digging back farther into the hillside and hauling out the dirt. We'd get some furniture, stick up a few candles, and it would be done."

"What would the rooms be for?"

"Maybe we'd make more space for guests. I like having company. Or how about some kind of study room?"

"That would be nice."

"If the dike does break and the water does come in, maybe that's what we'll do."

"We could have a library room," said Ssam. "A place to read and study, kind of like the project room you have here upstairs. It's noisy in the living room sometimes."

"This is sounding better all the time," said Needlenose. "We could use it when we needed someplace quiet."

"We could get a computer," said Ssam.

"You think so?"

"Sure, that would be good for me. I don't have fingers but I could punch the keys with my nose. I could use it for lots of things."

"Like what?" asked Needlenose.

"It would have been helpful designing Flossie's house."

"I'll bet you're right."

"We could keep records of our adventures and draw pictures for your projects, like Manford's necklace. There are lots of things we could use it for."

"Manford could use one for his writing," said Needlenose. "Computers are good for writing, aren't they?"

"Yes," said Ssam, "but his mother wants him to learn the regular way first. Manford can use a computer when he's filled up his journal."

"Well, that makes sense. But I like the library idea. Maybe

we should think more about it."

The rain eased off for a time in the early morning hours, then began to pound once more. The waters around Haystack Hollow splashed and bubbled as great drops splattered down. The dike held, but was turning soft as it soaked up water. Thunder crashed overhead. The forest flashed white as lightning streaked through the sky and struck a huge old tree forty feet from the burrow. The tree exploded midway up the trunk.

"That was close," said Ssam, hearing the sound. "I wonder what it hit."

The tree twisted about slowly, wavered a moment, then fell through the air and landed with a tremendous splash very near the burrow.

"Must have been the old, hollow tree," said Needlenose. "I'm glad it didn't fall on us."

The tree had missed Haystack Hollow, but one of its extending branches fell on the dike and broke through it. Water pushed through the opening and gurgled into the burrow in a rush.

"Here it comes," said Ssam.

"Man the lifeboats," said Needlenose.

The water rose swiftly to the level of the water outside, stranding Ssam and Needlenose in the upstairs room. The belongings Needlenose had hauled upstairs were spared. Those he'd left behind bobbed about in the flood.

"We'll have to get out of here now," he said.

"How?" asked Ssam. "By diving down through the water in the dark to find the entrance? I don't think so; I'm not much of a swimmer."

"I'm not, either," said Needlenose. "We're going up, not down."

"How?"

"I'll dig through the roof. There's a ventilation hole here somewhere. I'll widen it and we'll crawl out."

"That will make a mess," said Ssam.

"As if we don't have one already."

Needlenose covered his furniture, then located the hole and began to dig. As dawn slowly brightened the sky, he and Ssam crawled out through the hole to the top of Haystack Hollow. The rain had stopped. The sky had cleared. When Veronica arrived as she'd promised, she found the burrow-dwellers basking in the day's first sunlight.

"Looks like you had problems," she said, seeing the broken dike and the huge, fallen tree.

"You could say that," replied Needlenose. "I wonder if I could interest Beaver Brothers in this place. It would make a fine lodge for them at the edge of this lake."

"Is everything ruined inside?"

"No, I lugged all of the things I cared about upstairs."

"What are you going to do now?" asked Veronica.

"I believe we'll accept that lift to Flossie's house," said Needlenose. "We'll come back to clean up when the water goes down."

Days later, when the forest had drained and dried, a cleaning and construction crew of Flossie, Manford, Veronica, Golly, Princess Columbine, Needlenose, Ssam, and five Beaver Brothers workers returned to Haystack Hollow to clean and rebuild.

Needlenose and Flossie carried furniture into the sunshine to air out and dry. The beavers enlarged the burrow, digging back into the hill to add the new library and another small room for guests. They removed candleholders from all the burrow walls and installed electric lights. Ssam's computer would need electricity, they said so why not do the rest of the place, too? Finally, to meet fire code requirements, they turned the escape hole Needlenose had dug into a hatch for emergency exit.

Columbine directed the cleaning efforts, restoring each room upstairs and down to Needlenose's high standard of tidiness. Golly and Ssam covered the floors with soft moss throughout. Outside, Veronica and Manford used the excavated dirt to build a permanent dike around the burrow to protect it against future floods. By the end of the second day, Ssam and Needlenose were ready to move into their new home. They were happy to be back, happy to have their home reclaimed from the flood.

Flossie had brought catalogs and she and Needlenose looked through them. They found replacements for things and furniture for the two new rooms. Ssam picked out everything he'd need for his new computer.

"Thanks for your help, everyone," Ssam said. "Work sure goes faster with so many of us pitching in. It's more fun, too."

"Yes, it's wonderful to have such good friends," said Needlenose. "Thank you all."

"You're welcome," Flossie said. "You help us, we help you. That's how it works. And we'll be counting on a burrow party soon."

"Absolutely," Needlenose said chuckling. "Ssam will send computerized invitations."

Later, in the meadow, Veronica sat quietly while Manford wrote in his journal. Manford seemed to be thinking about what to say. He wrote and stopped, wrote and stopped, sometimes looking around him or at the sky, sometimes closing his eyes. Finally, he finished.

"Is it about the storm?" Veronica asked.

"Uh huh."

"Will you read it to me?"

"Okay," Manford said, and this is what he read:

One day big clouds came and it started to rain. It rained and rained. Veronica woke up when the ceiling dripped on her nose. Wind blew Golly's tree house and he worried about lightning. Flossie and Columbine weren't worried at all. They just watched out the windows. So did I. I thought it was fun.

The rain filled up the creeks and the creeks filled up the pond and the pond filled up Needlenose's burrow. That was too bad. He and Ssam would have been okay except lightning hit a tree, but we cleaned everything up. That made them happy.

The rain is over and the sky is blue again now. The storm was interesting. Next time we have one, I want to go out in it. You can't have adventures and learn about the world just by watching.

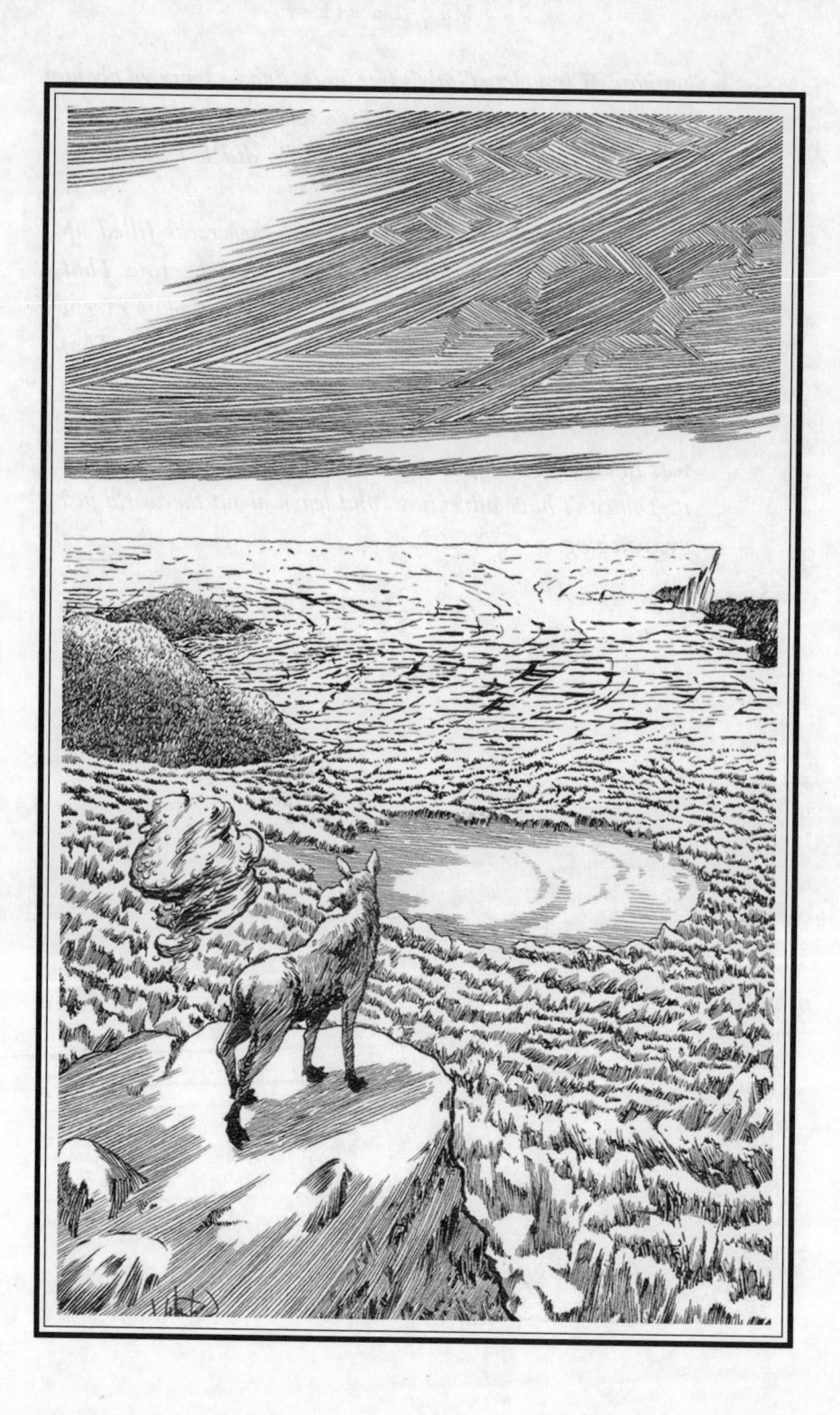

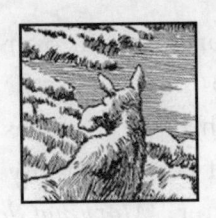

18

Ahead of His Time
In which Manford visits new worlds

[NOTE: Manford is sleeping in his room. He stayed up late reading stories last night, stories about traveling in space and time. Scenes from his reading and scenes from his adventures in MorningGlory Forest are merging in his dreams. To Manford, they don't seem like dreams at all...]

Moostery Manor was gone. The rosebushes, the yard, the long front walk, the big, front door on the gray-shuttered white house, gone. Manford lay in a stand of tall grass wondering what had happened. He'd expected to wake up in his room and go to the kitchen in time for breakfast when his mother called, but his room wasn't there. The house wasn't there. There was probably no breakfast, either.

What was there, a stately group of trees that looked like they'd been growing for hundreds of years, he didn't remember at all. *'Where am I?'* he thought. *'Where's Mom?'* He got up and looked around, pacing about the area, hoping to find something familiar. Soon he stopped and shook his head. *'There's never been a house built here. This is weird.'*

He walked into the woods. The trail was gone. The path

through the woods worn smooth over seventeen chapters of animal to-ing and fro-ing wasn't there. *'Did I miss it?'* he wondered. He looked through the trees and brush. There was no trail, no evidence of passage of any kind.

Manford heard water. *'MorningGlory Creek!'* he thought with relief. *'That's still there.'* He walked till he came to its edge. It was the creek, but it was different—deeper, wider, more set on going where it was going than on making happy sounds as it went. He turned to follow it upstream as he had months before on the first day he'd explored in the forest.

The land rose up beside the creek and he was led into a canyon. *'This looks right,'* he thought. He soon heard the waterfall, then turned the bend in the creek and saw it. It was huge and thundering. Not misty. Not friendly enough to walk under and have water splash lightly on your back. *'If I walk under that,'* Manford thought, *'I'll be washed out to sea or wherever it is creeks go.'*

He went closer and tried to get behind the falls to see the cave. There was no cave. No door, no mailbox, no sign; only rocks and a pounding torrent of water. *'What's wrong here?'* Manford wondered. *'This looks like the right place but it isn't. How can Misty Falls not be misty? How could a cave disappear overnight? Why is everything different?'* Manford didn't understand.

'The meadow, I'll check the meadow.' He backtracked along the creek, then made his way north through the woods. Soon the trees thinned. *'There it is,'* he thought, *'WhiteFlower Meadow.'* He walked around in it, looking things over just to be sure. *'Hmmm, the tree is different. It's smaller and faces a different way. And something's missing. . .the white daisies; they're gone. Now it's No-White-Flower Meadow.'*

Manford climbed Lookout Hill, stepping through the brush in the absence of the familiar, worn trail. Atop it, he looked toward MorningGlory Mountain. It was there, rising through the clouds as always. *'Whew!'* Manford thought, *'at least something's still the same. Or is it?'*

He continued on to Flossie's Pond. Yes, it was there and it seemed to be the right shape. There were trees around it. There was water in it. But Florida-by-the-Pond was gone. The house they'd labored a month to build for Flossie wasn't there. Manford was no longer surprised.

He looked for Haystack Hollow. Not there. He walked to the library and post office and store. Nothing. He went back to look for GloryView atop the ridge near Misty Falls. That was gone, too.

He made his way back to the meadow at the end of the day and sat under the tree. He'd found nothing. MorningGlory Forest was sort of the same, yet all of it was different. Worse yet, he'd seen no one. He'd found none of his friends in all his searching.

'Are they hiding? Are they somewhere else today? Am I in some strange place?' Manford didn't know. He went to sleep in the meadow, legs tucked under him, head drawn up to his side, feeling very confused. *'No point in going home,'* he thought, *'it's not there. But maybe it will be tomorrow. Maybe I'm dreaming and everything will be better when I wake up.'*

But it wasn't. The next day followed the same pattern and so did the day after that. Manford wandered all over the forest, looking for something. . .someone. He went back to nearly every place he'd ever been. Each left him with the same sort of feeling; things seemed to be the same as they'd been, yet they weren't.

"Veronica! Princess Columbine! Ssam!" he shouted. "Flossie! Golly! Needlenose!" No one replied.

He wrote notes in the dirt. No one answered. He was alone.

'I don't like this,' he said to himself. *'I'm used to seeing Mom every day. I'm used to finding my friends—maybe one, maybe all of them—and playing or going on adventures. Sure, I like walking by*

myself, but this is different. There's no one here to be with at all.'

Manford felt lonely. He felt trapped. He felt captured in a cage as big as all outdoors.

'Maybe my friends are on the outside watching me. Maybe if I look in the right place, I'll see them. Maybe they're calling to me and I can't hear them. If I shout loud enough, maybe they'll hear me.'

He settled down for another night under the tree in the meadow. He wished he had his journal. He would write about what was happening so he'd have a record. He started making sentences in his head. The words came freely and in a rush:

I have been two years in this place. Two years since I woke up not knowing where I was or how I got here. Two years of wandering, wondering, seeking. I know little more now than I did in those first moments. I am alone; that much I know. I have walked the length and breadth of this place, many thousands of miles, and have seen no one. The only signs of passage are my own. There is forest. There is water. There are mountains. There is day and night and wind and weather and sky. And there is time: day after day of endless, quiet, solitary time...

Manford stopped. *'Who's writing this?'* he thought. *'That doesn't sound like me. I would write happy things telling how much fun everything is. This sounds gloomy and depressed. Am I still Manford? Am I changed, too—sort of the same, yet different?'* He was puzzled. He hoped there was an answer somewhere.

Manford soon spent all his days in the meadow, leaving it only to drink from the creek and find leaves to eat that didn't taste too terribly bad. He wanted to be exploring but he knew what he would find—everything would look sort of the same as it had before, but not quite, and no one would be there. He began to feel sad. Two weeks had passed since he'd been caught in this puzzle. He would have to find an answer soon. He settled down under the tree to sleep as the sky grew dark yet again.

He awoke an hour after midnight. Stars were bright in the sky and the moon hung on the horizon. Manford remembered something that seemed important. *'The Mountain Spirit told it to me. . .what was it?'* The words came suddenly to Manford's mind: "I have always been here."

'That's it. That's what the spirit said. So, if the spirit has always been here, maybe it's here now. And if I can find it, maybe I can find the answer to this puzzle.' He lay in moonlit darkness and considered this idea.

'Yes, I'll go there. I'll climb MorningGlory Mountain to The Place With No Trees and find the Mountain Spirit. Then things will make sense again.' He settled back to sleep feeling better. He was going to do something. He was going to do something first thing tomorrow.

But there was no trail. That was the first thought that struck him when he awoke next morning. There were no trails in whatever world this was. Manford wished he had his backpack. He wished he had his scarf. He wished he had his hiker hat. Most of all, he wished he had his friends to come with him.

'Enough of this whimpering,' he finally told himself. *'I can go as fast as I want by myself, and I don't have to wait until anyone else is ready.'* With that, he walked out the east end of the meadow at a brisk pace, picking his way through the forest.

He worked his way uphill all morning. The forest was thick at low elevations so he couldn't see where he was going or where he had been. But he knew he should be going up, and that's where he went.

Progress through the brush and trees was slower with no trail to follow. He rested a time or two and, in places where the forest thinned, he stopped to look out over the valley retreating below. As he climbed higher and higher, he became more and more certain this was the right thing to do.

Manford reached MorningGlory Crossing atop the first mountain by early afternoon. That's what they used to call it, anyway, but here the spot wasn't marked. He crossed the second mountain several hours later, rested a while, and then started down toward the gap where the climb of MorningGlory Mountain would begin. He remembered the barren, wind-bent tree that stood marking a fork in the trail. Maybe it was still there. It would be a good place to stop for the night so he could climb the great mountain the next day.

In fading daylight, Manford saw the tree in the distance as he neared the open ridge where it stood. The tree wasn't standing anymore. The top of it lay broken and smashed on the ground. What remained of the trunk stood jagged and split as if struck by lightning. But something else caught Manford's attention. There was a sign nailed to the part of the tree that was still upright. It pointed up MorningGlory Mountain. It read:

THE ANSWER 15 min →

"A sign!" Manford said out loud. It was first thing of intelligence he'd seen.

'The Answer,' he read. *'That means I'm doing the right thing and going the right way. Good. Maybe things are getting better. But it says fifteen miles. The Place With No Trees isn't nearly that far.'* Manford was puzzled. He looked at the sign again.

'Wait, it says fifteen minutes. *That's odd. It takes much longer to climb to the top than that.'* He was still puzzled. The sky was fast growing dark so he settled down to sleep.

'What does it mean?' he wondered. *'Fifteen miles, fifteen minutes; neither makes sense. Hmmm, maybe I won't worry about it.*

The sign says the answer is that way, up the mountain. I want an answer. In the morning I'll go up there and find it.'

Manford slept soundly after a day of forging his way through brush and over the tops of two mountains. No sounds disturbed him. No creatures roamed in the night. Had he been awake, he'd have heard wind in the trees and the sound of water flowing in the distance; otherwise, there was nothing. The moon and stars shown but they made no sound.

The bright light drifting slowly down MorningGlory Mountain made no sound, either. It had started at The Place With No Trees about the time Manford fell asleep. It came up from that odd, circular room bounded by rocks and floated among the boulders strewn across the top of the mountain. Then it drifted slowly downward, taking its time. Night was well advanced by the time it reached the broken tree with the sign. The light hovered over Manford as he slept soundly. It passed on then, ranging far into the distance along the route Manford had traveled as he came up the mountain. In an hour it returned. It pulsed and glowed and grew large until the area around the tree was as bright as sunrise.

Manford opened his eyes. *'It can't be morning already.'* The light was so bright he shut his eyes again.

"Manford."

He heard someone speak his name, the first voice he'd heard since this strange adventure began. It was a familiar voice. He opened one eye, shading it with his front leg.

"Mountain Spirit?" he asked.

"Yes."

"I was coming to find you. I thought you might still be here, even if no one else is."

"I am here," the spirit said, reducing its brightness to a soft glow.

"I'm terribly confused," Manford went on. "Everyone is gone except me. The places we live in are gone. Everything looks sort of the same, yet it's different. It's like one morning I woke up in a different world. I've been looking for something I recognize for weeks."

"You *are* in a different world."

"I am? Where?"

"You're in a world fifteen minutes ahead in time from where you were," said the spirit.

"I don't understand," Manford said.

"Where you and your friends live is only one of many worlds. There are hundreds of thousands of others. They all share the same space but are separated from each other by time. Where you are now is the same place as where you were, but it's fifteen minutes ahead in time."

"That's what it said on the sign: 15 min →," said Manford. "That must be The Answer."

"Correct."

"Does that mean I've traveled in time?"

"It does."

"I don't think I'm getting it. In stories I've read, people go ahead in time a few days or years and find out what will happen to their world then. Sometimes they meet themselves there, which gets very confusing. Or they go back in time, to their world days or years earlier, to try to change something to make it come out different. That doesn't always work the way they think it should. If I'm fifteen minutes ahead, why isn't this world the same, only fifteen minutes later?"

"If you go ahead in time," the spirit said, "you don't go to the same world that much later. It isn't there yet. It's still where you left it. If you go back in time, you don't go to the same world that much earlier. It's already been there and gone."

"Then where am I?" said Manford, thinking it was awfully early in the morning for a science lesson.

"You're in the same place you were, on the same planet, and that's why things look sort of the same. But you're in a world that exists in a different time, one that has its own history. That's why it's different."

"How did I do this?"

"You dreamed yourself here."

"On purpose?"

"No, it just happens sometimes."

"Can I dream myself back?"

"That's not as easy. You might end up in the world you left or in any one of the others. Or you could go nowhere at all, which is what most often happens."

"Are the other worlds quiet and lonely like this one?" Manford asked.

"Some are, but many are very different. I can show you some if you'd like."

"Can you take me back to my mom and Veronica and all my friends and MorningGlory Forest as it's supposed to be?"

"Yes, if you'd like to go there instead."

Manford thought about it. He wanted to go home after being alone so long. But he didn't often get a chance to see other worlds. Maybe being gone a little longer wouldn't hurt.

"Show me a few of these places," he said. "Then I'd like to go home."

"Close your eyes," said the spirit.

Manford did, and when he opened them again, he was on top of what would have been Lookout Hill. The scene about him had changed completely. MorningGlory Mountain was a volcano. Smoke rose from it and flows of lava oozed down the side. The huge mountain was hundreds of feet shorter than Manford remembered, as if its top had blown away.

MorningGlory Forest was gone. Manford saw a plain of parched, lava-encrusted ground instead, its surface dried and cracked. A few trees with spiky leaves grew wide distances apart.

Swamp covered the meadow and the pond and extended south beyond where Beaver Brothers would have been. Plants with rubbery leaves as big as elephant ears grew along the edges and in places where the water was shallow. Gasses belched from the murky brown water and hung in the air as a greasy yellow mist. The air smelled foul, full of things rotting and dead.

It was daybreak. The sun streaked through a sky that was violet, orange, and, in places, a sort of blotchy greenish-rose. The colors shifted and changed, faded and brightened, and made Manford think the entire world was not feeling well.

"Where is this?" he asked the spirit, who still pulsed with a warm glow by his side.

"This world is two weeks back in time," the spirit said.

A shriek pierced the air and the ground began to shake. Below, near the edge of the swamp, two giant beasts came running across the broken ground. They were not playing, not going for a swim in the pond; one intended to catch and eat the other. The sounds of their struggle filled the air with pain.

"I'm glad I didn't wake up here," Manford said. "This is an awful place." Manford heard something behind him and looked around. A beast even bigger than the others was thumping toward him thinking, no doubt, that Manford would be good for breakfast.

"This would be an excellent time to leave," the spirit said. "Close your eyes."

"Gladly," Manford said, and the dreadful smells and sounds of that prehistoric world faded away.

A new sound came to him, a distant humming, a sort of busyness about things. Manford opened his eyes and looked around him in shock. He was standing at what would have been MorningGlory Crossing. Everywhere he looked he saw city. Houses filled every square foot of the forest, covered the meadow, and pushed up against the edges of the pond. Houses rose up and over Lookout Hill and the mountain on which Manford stood. Houses covered the next mountain and MorningGlory Mountain, too, almost to the top. The houses were small and tightly packed together. The only spots of green were occasional trees and tiny tended yards.

"Where is this?" he asked.

"You mean, 'When is this?'" the spirit replied. "We're in a world eleven hours ahead of yours. I thought you might find it interesting."

"There is city everywhere you look, house after house after house, like people packed up in boxes. I see children playing in yards, and so many boats on the pond there's not room for anyone to move."

"It's a crowded world."

"I don't see any cars or roads," said Manford.

"People here move about by thinking themselves from one place to another. It's called teleportation, though they have little need to go anywhere. They work at home, have all their entertainment at home, and shop from home, too. They only go out to special places."

"Do they travel to see other parts of their world?"

"Not often. The rest of it looks just like this, houses built over everything, even in places where it's very hot or very cold."

"The houses go nearly up to The Place With No Trees," Manford said. "Is there something up there?"

"Yes, a restaurant. It's built over what you remember as the sunken room. It has an outstanding view."

"A view? All they can see is houses."

"That's what people here like to look at."

"This is so amazing," Manford said, "worlds side by side just a few minutes or hours apart, all going on day to day in this spot that always looks the same, yet it's different. Have you been to many of them?"

"Thousands."

"Wow, you must really keep busy."

"I've had plenty of time," the spirit said. "There's another one I want to show you if you'll close your eyes again."

Manford did so. The hum of busyness faded and suddenly he was cold. A freezing wind made him shiver even through his thick hairy coat. He opened his eyes. He was standing atop MorningGlory Mountain this time, looking west to where Lookout Hill would be except it wasn't there. The pond wasn't there and the meadow wasn't there. As in the other worlds he'd visited, the forest wasn't there, either. A glacier covered everything but the mountain on which they stood and those next to it. It had come grinding its way down from the north, scouring out trees and rocks and pushing them away, burying everything under five hundred feet of ice. It had parted to flow around the mountains but nothing else could stand in its path.

Manford looked down upon the ice. The top of the glacier was ridged and broken. You could not walk upon it, even if you had four feet. The way would constantly be blocked by towering ice pinnacles or deep crevasses that changed as the glacier moved. Ridges sheared off as Manford watched, sending tons of ice crashing down. Deep cracks opened and closed making sounds like sudden explosions or deep, rumbling sighs. The sun glinted off a lake atop the glacier, a lake carried along like a pool on a cruise ship's deck. It would be much too cold for swimming, even if you could get to it.

"This world is four days ahead of yours," said the spirit, anticipating Manford's question. "The glacier moves slowly, maybe two feet a week. It slowly wears down everything along its route. As you can see, Lookout Hill has been ground down and carried away. These mountains are being carved away, too."

"Where does the glacier go?"

"The front of it has moved twenty miles or more to the southeast where it flows into a lake. Great blocks of ice continually break off and crash into the water there as the glacier moves."

"I don't want to live here," Manford said. "It's too cold and unfriendly."

"It's all of that," said the spirit.

"What other kinds of worlds are there?"

"There's one to match anything you can imagine. In one, this area is covered by water; only the top of MorningGlory Mountain sticks above it. In another, this is desert with sand dunes, cactus, and hardly any water at all. In still another, a bomb was dropped here and there's only a huge, radioactive hole."

"These places seem to have such problems," Manford said. "The creatures are nasty or the land is swampy, icy, or blowing up. They're too hot or too cold or too crowded. Are all the worlds like that?"

"Some are more successful than others," the spirit said. "Some are at war; some live in peace. Some are busy; some are deserted. In some, this area is industrial with factories making automobiles, computers or airplanes. In some it's farmland, growing wheat or corn or even dandelions."

"Dandelions?"

"Yes, yellow-faced flowers as far as you can see."

"But are there worlds that are happy and pleasant like ours? Where creatures can be friends and have a good time and where things almost always work out? Are there any other happy ending places like ours?"

"Not many," the spirit answered. "Yours is one of very, very few. That's why I like to live there."

"I think it's time to go back there now."

"I think so, too," said the spirit. "Goodbye, Manford. I've enjoyed visiting with you again. Close your eyes."

"Goodbye," Manford said. "Thank you for rescuing me, and for showing me around, and for answering my questions, and..."

Manford opened his eyes. It was morning. He was in his room at Moostery Manor. It was time to get up.

"Time for breakfast, Manford." That was his mother calling. "Wake up, sleepyhead," she went on. "I've been calling you and calling you."

'What a pleasant sound,' Manford thought, *'my mom calling. I dreamed she was gone; no, I dreamed I was gone, and I couldn't find her or any of my friends. I dreamed a lot of things, about a lot of strange places. I'll have to write them down after breakfast.'*

Another pleasant thought: breakfast. That had seemed worlds away in his dreams. He'd been eating only leaves that didn't taste very good.

"Breakfast, Manford," his mother said again. "Come on, young moose-about-town, you'll be late."

'Late,' thought Manford with a smile. *'No, I won't be late, not for breakfast, not for anything. I'm on time. . .in the right time. . .exactly where I'm supposed to be.'*

Chapter Notes

Chapter 2

The Great Bucknikov first appeared in the speech, "Bucky Plays the Palace," winner of the Yukon-Alaska Toastmasters Tall Tales contest in 1987.

Chapter 3

Directions for hopscotch are as played in northern Minnesota in the late 1940s.

Bubble-blowing research conducted on wilderness trails in Alaska, Arizona, California, Minnesota, North Carolina, New Hampshire, and Maine as something interesting to do on lunch breaks atop mountains. No, snowflakes don't pop bubbles, either.

Chapter 4

Upon completion in summer 1993, the Pacific Crest Trail was 2,638 miles long, extending between the Canadian and Mexican borders.

Chapter 5

Millie, the Dancing Bear, first appeared in the speech, "An Evening With Millie," winner of the Yukon-Alaska Toastmasters Tall Tales contest in 1985.

The "barren, wind bent tree" mentioned here and in later chapters can be found in Bly Gap where the Appalachian Trail crosses the Georgia-North Carolina border. This is the first state crossing for the northbound hiker and the scene sticks in one's memory.

Chapter 7

The hybrid tea rose is a cross between the original tea rose and a hybrid perpetual rose.

Royal Highness was an All-American Rose selection in 1963, Miss All-American Beauty in 1968, Angel Face in 1969, and First Prize in 1970. Lady X is a bit of a mystery, which seems fitting.

Browne, Roland A. *The Rose-Lover's Guide*. New York: Atheneum, 1983.

Crockett, James Underwood. *Roses*. New York: Time-Life Books, 1971.

Chapter 8

My daughter Kyra provided the Italian translation for the dragonfly's name.

Chapter 10

Finley, Bill. *Yellowstone Aflame*. California: Finley-Holiday Film Corp, 1989.

Chapter 11

Color relationships and plant preparation techniques based on "Navajo Dye Chart," an artwork by Ella Myers, Shiprock, New Mexico.

Chapter 12

Dr. Maynard Falconer of the Alaska Eye Care Center provided details for this visit to the optometrist.

Chapter 18

This story combines remembrances from a fever dream, thoughts about a hard disk crash in which Manford was held captive for a time with no backup or printout, and the lead paragraph of a novel I planned to write thirty years ago but never did. Everything has its uses.

About the Author

Mic Lowther

Mic Lowther grew up in Minnesota and worked as a computer systems analyst for thirty-three years in New York, Arizona, and Alaska. He has backpacked more than 4,000 miles in various parts of the US, half of which is the subject of his book *Walking North*, written about his family's through-hike of the Appalachian Trail in 1973. Mic spends his time working with his brothers in Minnesota (LowtherBrothers LLC), building cabins with friends in Colorado (Rocking Moose Mountain Ranch), and writing both fiction and non-fiction adventure stories in Alaska.

About the Illustrator

Jeff White

Jeff White has illustrated several books as well as comics, cartoons and spot illustrations for various publications. He has lived in New York and Tokyo, Japan and currently resides north of Boston with his wife and two hounds.

For more information about Manford and his friends
and to order books, go to:
www.manford.com